MIXED BLESSINGS

Intensive Care for Newborns

Jeanne Harley Guillemin

Lynda Lytle Holmstrom

New York   *Oxford*
OXFORD UNIVERSITY PRESS

Oxford University Press

Oxford   New York   Toronto
Delhi   Bombay   Calcutta   Madras   Karachi
Petaling Jaya   Singapore   Hong Kong   Tokyo
Nairobi   Dar es Salaam   Cape Town
Melbourne   Auckland

and associated companies in
Berlin   Ibadan

Copyright © 1986 by Oxford University Press, Inc.

First published in 1986 by Oxford University Press, Inc.,
200 Madison Avenue, New York, New York 10016

First issued as an Oxford University Press paperback, 1990

Oxford is a registered trademark of Oxford University Press

Library of Congress Cataloging-in-Publication Data
Guillemin, Jeanne Harley, 1943–
   Mixed blessings.
   Bibliography: p.
   Includes index.
   1. Neonatal intensive care.
I. Holmstrom, Lynda Lytle. II. Title.
RJ253.5.G85   1986   618.92'01   85-28968
ISBN 0-19-504032-5
ISBN 0-19-506659-6 PBK

Printing (last digit): 2 4 6 8 10 9 7 5 3 1

Printed in the United States of America

To
Eileen D. Garrigan
and
Dorothy Thomas Lytle

What measure shall I give these generations
That breathe on the void and are void
And exist and do not exist?

SOPHOCLES, Oedipus Rex

Preface

Anyone entering a maximum care unit for newborns cannot help but be struck by the complexity of hospital organization and the sophistication of hospital technology. These modern forms, however, should not blind us to the universal drama surrounding human reproduction. Such institutions and technologies are, in fact, only contemporary expressions of the fundamental need to control regeneration, to insure personal and social continuity by protecting our young against the threat of death.

Our good fortune is that in our time and society so many newborns survive to become adults. But survival in itself is an insufficient answer to the larger question posed by every birth. How will the future fulfill the promise of this new life? Intensive medical care for newborns is an intervention intended to secure the healthiest future for an infant. Yet the obstacles posed by severely premature birth and serious birth defects cannot be easily overcome. A good part of the problem lies in the care not taken to prevent these threats to infant life. Instead of a preventive approach, the overwhelming choice in the last two decades has been to address serious newborn pathologies after they happen, by developing centralized hospital services and new technologies. Despite this heavy investment, some medical procedures only partially or temporarily remedy the problems of the critically ill or damaged newborn. The result is the "mixed blessing" referred to by our title; that is, a high level of uncertainty about the benefits of this sustained treatment for the infant patient.

Our book is based on the hope that the well-being of infants who survive and of infants who cannot will have priority over the allure of organizational efficiency and medical progress. To prevent these facets of hospital organization from becoming ends in themselves requires, first, a dispassionate assessment of how the current system works. This, we think, *Mixed Blessings* provides. The second requirement is much more difficult and remains to be hammered out among hospital professionals, legislators, and the public—a working consensus about the appropriate use of newborn intensive care. When it comes to critically ill newborns, we are all parents because their fate is a matter of public as well as private decisions. Either existing hospital services help them or they do not. Either reasonable calculation is made of viability or it is not. Either responsibility is taken for survivors with long-term needs or it is not. Such choices are made daily, but not always with feeling for their enormous consequences for individuals, families, and society.

We are indebted to many people and organizations that helped us with our research and the completion of this book. Above all we wish to thank the many physicians, nurses, social workers, and administrators who allowed us to observe their work under what were often trying circumstances. The substantial service and research commitment of the staff at the main hospital where we did fieldwork, as well as at the other American and overseas nurseries where we interviewed staff, must account for the great tolerance granted our intrusions. We are therefore most grateful for the help of these professionals. As much as we would like to thank each one by name, we made the decision at the inception of our research to safeguard individual and institutional anonymity. This decision applies especially to the parents of infants in intensive care, whose presence in this hospital context was often fleeting but always marked by intense feelings most deserving of privacy. Consequently all the names used to identify the people and hospitals described in *Mixed Blessings* are fictitious.

We thank the many people with whom we discussed the research project. Among those who were especially helpful in its initial formulation were Kevin McIntyre, M.D., John Potts, M.D., Thomas Moloney, Irving Louis Horowitz, and Everett Cherrington Hughes. As we began our field research, our colleagues at Boston College, Stephen J. Pfohl, David A. Karp, and Paul S. Gray, provided methodological advice. As he has done for many others, William Silverman, M.D. provided consistent encouragement for this venture which, because of its inherent complexity, took much longer to complete than we anticipated. In 1979 as we began our research, Margaret Mahoney, then at the Robert Wood Johnson Foundation and now President of the Commonwealth Fund, advised that we should reckon on seven years from start to finish. She proved correct.

In 1980–1981 Daniel Callahan and the staff at the Hastings Center offered an ample forum for the discussion of ethical issues, along with generous office and research support underwritten by the National Endowment for the Humanities. The health policy staff of the office of U.S. Senator Dave Durenberger (Republican–Minnesota), as well as the Washington office of the American Academy of Pediatrics, provided invaluable information on legislative and legal developments relating to the Baby Doe rule.

Iain Chalmers, Jo Garcia, and the staff at the National Perinatal Epidemiology Center in England gave generously of their expertise to enlighten us on the social and political context of special care for infants in the United Kingdom. In the Netherlands J.M.L. Phaff, M.D. and G.J. Kloosterman, M.D., were particularly helpful in informing us about the Dutch system of maternal and newborn care.

We are grateful to the many people who helped us with introductions for our international site visits and regarding Brazil we thank María da Consolação Aguiar Franceschini, M.D., Frederick L. Ahearn, David Wood, Marilia Travessa Baker, and Néia Schor.

We owe special thanks to those people who read and commented upon selected portions of the manuscript: I. David Todres, M.D. (the aggressive intervention chapter and the glossary); John B. Guillemin (Introduction); Michael Grodin, M.D. (physicians); Peter Auld, M.D. (Darlene Bourne case history); Catherine P. Murphy, R.N. (nursing) and Martha Nencioli, R.N. (referrals); Graeme Fincke, M.D. (death and survival); Alan Sager and Matthew Meselson (policy); Mark G. Field and Alexander Schuller (international comparisons); Dick Batten and Jetty Westerkamp (the Netherlands); and James J. Horn (Brazil). Robert Weir, Samuel Bloom, Suzanne Potts, Raymond Duff, M.D., Irving Louis Horowitz, and James Brian Garrigan read earlier drafts of the entire manuscript and we are grateful for their comments. Of course we remain wholly responsible for the interpretations and conclusions presented, including any shortcomings.

We appreciate the efforts of James Brian Garrigan who did the major work of preparing the glossary, Robert D. Guillemin who did the necessary graphic work for our charts, F. Ross Holmstrom who provided technical assistance with computer and word processing systems, Marilyn A. Grant who designed the computer search utilizing the data base of the National Library of Medicine, Larry Snyder who provided bibliographic assistance, and Estelle Stanley who assisted in preparing the index.

Many thanks are due to Shirley S. Urban for supervising the typing of the manuscript and its revisions, assisted by Alice L. Close, Barbara Lloyd, Kathleen M. Crowell, Martha A. Roth, and Barbara Fanning. Special moral and technical support came from Lorraine B. Bone.

We wish to thank Susan Rabiner, our editor at Oxford, for her support, and Susan Meigs for her able work in marshalling the book through production and into print.

Financial support for the completion of the manuscript came from Boston College, the Commonwealth Fund, and the Mellon Foundation. We also wish to thank Boston College for generously granting various sabbaticals and leaves of absence, without which it would have been impossible to complete our field research in such diverse locales.

Contents

MIXED BLESSINGS

Introduction

Technological progress, in whatever field, always presents a paradox. As it solves certain immediate problems, it creates others that were unforeseen. In medicine, progress in the technology for sustaining lives has resulted in the successful rescue of cases once considered hopeless. The negative repercussion has been for some patients the deterioration of the quality of their lives, so that they remain alive, in a reduced biological sense, but without the capacities this society most identifies with a meaningful life: full consciousness, responsiveness to others, reflection, physical autonomy, and the capacity for affection. Still, the great promise of modern medicine is that it will give us complete and sophisticated solutions to life-threatening conditions (Thomas, 1977), for children as well as adults.

As the trend toward medical innovation continues, the question of professional and institutional directives is paramount. Following the ground-breaking work of Fox (1959), Fox and Swazey (1974), and Crane (1977), we need to know how physicians control the technology of medicine and what degree of influence is exerted by major hospitals and health care programs. No reasonable planning for ensuring the benefits of medical discovery is possible without this knowledge. The recent development of newborn intensive care presents a challenging case for analyzing the reinvention of acute care medicine for this new population of infant patients.

The main idea behind the first efforts to treat newborn patients was to create a womb-like environment that would allow sick infants, suffering from the complications of premature birth, to grow. In 1880, French obstetrician E. S. Tarnier put a modified poultry in-

3

cubator to use for newborns at the Paris Maternity Hospital. Curiously enough, the promotion and eventual acceptance of the infant incubator was based on exhibits mounted at world fairs and expositions (Silverman, 1979). An associate at the Paris hospital, Dr. Martin Couney, began this effort at the 1896 World Exposition in Berlin, where crowds thronged to see the tiny survivors in their "hatcheries." Couney's last demonstration of the incubator and of the careful feeding and handling of premature newborns was at the 1940 New York World's Fair. By that time, popular interest in the exhibit had waned and medical professionals had recognized Dr. Couney's substantial contribution to the care of these small infants.

Following World War II, and especially in the last twenty years, medical care for newborns has taken on the aspects of adult medicine and become disease oriented. Premature birth still presents the greatest jeopardy to newborns; it is the primary cause of death in neonates (infants in the first month of life). Now, however, prematurity is perceived in terms of discrete pathologies and their treatment, not simply as a condition to be outgrown. For example, premature infants commonly suffer from a stiffness of the lungs that is appropriate in the fetus but seriously hinders breathing in the newborn. This condition is called respiratory distress syndrome (RDS) or hyaline membrane disease (HMD), and is often the primary diagnosis on the chart of a newborn admitted to an intensive care unit. An infant with RDS is immediately put on a respirator until, after a time, the lungs develop and become more flexible. Similarly, many premature infants are born with a fetal opening in the heart, called patent ductus arteriosis (PDA), that weakens circulation and breathing. This opening in the underdeveloped heart usually closes with time, but physicians increasingly opt for heart surgery or drug therapy to repair it quickly. In the same way, the brains of premature infants are particularly susceptible to bleeding. Even for small infants, surgery is used to reduce the effects of hemorrhaging.

Each of these clinical procedures, as well as others used in newborn intensive care, has been adapted from adult medicine. Neonatologists, the pediatricians who specialize in the care of newborns, are in charge of the whole body of the patient and must be familiar with many pathologies and their treatment. The recent history of medical care for newborns reflects the complexity of this responsibility. There have been numerous false starts and dead ends have plagued clinical attempts to refine respirator therapy, to counter infection, to cure infant jaundice, and to streamline the administration of anesthesia, antibiotics, and blood transfusions for the infant surgical patient. In attempting to solve some problems, physicians inadvertently harmed their patients with untested methods, such as water-misting incubators and epsom salts enemas. The drug chloramphenicol was once widely used in nurseries until it was revealed to be the cause of the fatal "gray syndrome" in newborns. At another point, some infants treated with high levels of oxygen developed permanent blindness, called retrolental fibroplasia (RLF). Such haphazard problem solving, as Silverman (1980) argues, demonstrates the lack of scientific method in pioneering new therapies for newborns.

Despite the early mistakes, justifiable claims can be made for current respirator therapy for neonates, for real progress in treating infant jaundice, and for improvements in surgical techniques for newborns. Improved neonatal survival rates are frequently reported after intensive care units for newborns are established. There have been from 23 percent to 42 percent declines in death rates after the institution of regional intensive care facilities for newborns (Hack, Fanaroff, and Merkatz, 1979; Budetti et al., 1981:28–33).

One impressive measure of progress is found in numerous studies showing improved survival rates for very premature newborns treated with intensive care. The newborn weighing less than 2,500 grams at birth is usually considered premature or, more rarely, suffering from retarded growth. The infant born at 1,500 grams or less is considered to be of very low birth weight. It is only within the last decade that this subgroup of newborns began to be treated routinely in intensive care units. The results indicate decided improvement in their chances for survival. Budetti et al. (1981) pooled the data from available reports and concluded that the death rate per thousand for newborns weighing 1,500 grams or less went from 722 in 1960 to 184 in 1976. Similarly, the death rate for infants born weighing 1,000 grams or less declined from 919 in 1960 to 475 in 1976 (1981:30–33). These data are from small samples, often twenty to thirty infants, and from studies whose scientific rigor might be questioned. Nonetheless, it is generally believed by practitioners today that very low birth weight infants should be treated as viable patients for whom prognosis is improving (see Figure 1).

The clinical emphasis on very premature infants brings with it a high mortality risk. Low birth weight infants are almost forty times as likely to die in the first twenty-eight days of life as are full-term newborns. Infants born at less than 1,500 grams run a risk of neonatal death nearly 200 times greater than that for normal birth weight infants (Shapiro et al., 1980). In the United States, low birth weight

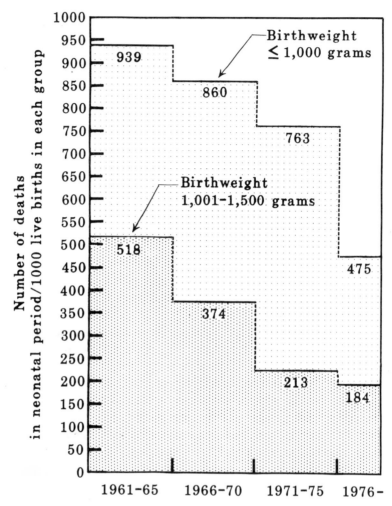

Figure 1. Pooled neonatal mortality data, 1961 to 1976. (From P. Budetti et al., 1981, p. 32)

occurs in only 7 percent of live births but accounts for two-thirds of neonatal deaths. This statistic has remained almost unchanged since 1950 (McCormick, 1985) and represents a continuing challenge to physicians. Whereas pediatricians fifty years ago had to be concerned with infectious diseases, the problem area for today's clinicians is prematurity.

Following the trend toward treating very small premature infants, the potential viability of newborns as small as 500 grams has been raised. By international standards, this birth weight is the dividing line between fetus and infant. Breaking the 500-gram barrier is a goal commonly discussed among neonatologists who, even if almost never successful, have already increased expectations that late fetal viability (for example, twenty-four to twenty-seven weeks of gestation) is equal to that of the full-term infant.

If we ascribe to vitalism, that is, the belief in the value of human life in the reduced biological sense, then all efforts to save "ultra-preemies" are justified. This position, however, ignores the growing concern about broader criteria, such as the patient's capacity to experience and enjoy life (McCormick, 1974). Survival rates for small newborns have apparently improved. Yet there is ambiguity surrounding the overall physical conditions of the survivors. Premature infants are highly susceptible to neurological disabilities and congenital anomalies, conditions from which practitioners may not be able to save them. Physical development in childhood is difficult enough to measure when medical therapy is not changing. When the hospital treatment of whole populations of premature newborns intensifies, the long-term follow-up of patients' health is even more difficult to assess because the standards of care keep changing.

One general rule still stands: the lower the birth weight, the greater is the infant's chances of having permanent, serious disability. The premature infant is five times more likely than a full-term infant to be hospitalized in the first year of life (McCormick, Shapiro, and Starfield, 1985). Several recent studies show long hospital stays and poor outcomes associated with very low birth weight (Kumar et al., 1980; Britton, Fitzhardinge, and Ashley, 1981; Guillemin and Holmstrom, 1983). Recent studies also pinpoint infants born at 900 grams and less as poor risks for survival and normal outcome, with medical and rehabilitation costs far exceeding the potential productivity of these patients as adults (Boyle et al., 1983; Walker et al., 1984; Kitchen and Murton, 1985). The neonatal care of some of these borderline cases has cost a quarter of a million dollars, not counting handicapped services, institutionalization, or the financial responsibilities assumed by parents.

In addition, a general increase in the incidence of cerebral palsy has been linked to aggressive intervention for newborns (Mac-Farlane and Mugford, 1984:186–187). Still other reports have suggested that while newborn intensive care has improved survival for infants in the first days of life, death rates have increased for newborns in the ensuing weeks and months (Hack et al., 1980; Sells et al., 1983; MacFarlane and Mugford, 1984:37–38). That is, death for some severely ill newborns is only delayed, not avoided. Finally, there is concern among some practitioners that iatrogenic consequences of treatment continue to affect newborns. These include the persistence of blindness from oxygen therapy, chronic lung disease (called bronchopulmonary dysplasia or BPD), and permanent injury from misplaced tubes and many X-ray tests (Singleton, 1981).

Practitioners are just beginning to pose these questions about the efficacy of newborn intensive care. As Dr. Mildred Stahlman, at the Vanderbilt School of Medicine, has written:

> Has newborn intensive care been a success or failure? Neither answer can be unqualified. Spectacular gains have been made in the survival of infants with increasingly low birth weights, and costs, both tangible and intangible, have been equally spectacular. (1984:36)

INSTITUTIONAL EXPANSION AND PROFESSIONAL OPPORTUNITIES

The recognition of outcome problems has come after the widespread expansion of intensive care for newborns and indicates an important new phase in evaluating the service. Yet the faith of many physicians in neonatology remains undiminished. In a 1984 poll of pediatricians in Massachusetts, the physicians almost unanimously recommended the referral and transfer of 600-gram infants. The great majority of these pediatricians also indicated that they did not consider the 700-gram infant an experimental case (Todres et al., 1986).

This strong vote of confidence for newborn intensive care is based on more than new technologies. An efficient, often regionalized system of referrals guarantees that many newborns in medical need will be efficiently transported to an intensive care nursery. Currently, between five and six hundred such units exist in the United States. Each depends on a consistent flow of newborn patients either from nurseries within the same hospital or from other hospitals. Along with a general trend toward centralizing obstetric services, the transport of newborns to regional centers is based on the idea that it is more efficient to move patients than to establish high-technology centers in local communities. This regionalization of intensive care for infants relies on efficient transportation by ambulance, helicopter, plane, or boat. It also relies on the efficient administration of interhospital services and cooperative relations among professionals.

Regional neonatal intensive care units (n.i.c.u.'s) provide the tertiary or maximum level of care and tend to be located in major medical centers. The upgrading of technology and the growth in activity of the Level III nursery have offered pediatricians a new employment niche. The Level II nursery offers a lower level of intensive care for the newborn and is often found in large community hospitals or in conjunction with the Level III nursery in the major medical center. Increasing opportunities for neonatologists are also appearing at this intermediate level. Since the numbers of American pediatricians have almost doubled in the last fifteen years (McKinlay, 1982), the development of all intensive care nurseries comes as a boon to the specialty.

Unlike the private practitioner, the neonatologist typically works for the hospital and cannot treat referred patients without its enormous backup of physical resources, personnel, and management. Board certification in neonatology became possible only in 1976, an indication of the newness of the field. The subspecialty's development is closely linked to the growth of contemporary corporate medicine and how it shapes professional behavior (see Bloom and Wilson, 1979). Its highly specialized subject, newborn pathologies, and the critical condition of the n.i.c.u. patient earn neonatologists considerable autonomy from the hospital administration. The latter is often pleased with the volume of patients and high use of hospital resources generated by the active n.i.c.u.

In turn, neonatologists have to adapt to working according to an institutional model in which teamwork becomes an integral part of decision making. As Janowitz (1960:9) has described for the modern military, consensus replaces individual initiative. In neonatology, physicians are closely involved with corporate educational goals. Level III nurseries are usually located in teaching hospitals and support physicians-in-training either as fellows in neonatology or as residents in pediatrics. Senior or attending physicians in the n.i.c.u. both teach the resident house officers and rely heavily on their services to give maximum coverage for patients.

For many physicians, the Level III nursery represents progressive medicine because its senior staff is often actively engaged in clinical or laboratory research. Unlike community-based practitioners, neonatologists concentrate on the physiological development of the fetus and newborn, crossing over into biochemistry and genetics in their research. The general activity of the high-level n.i.c.u. is linked to progressive medicine, although not necessarily to science, by its exploration of the viability of very premature infants. Without these enterprises, newborn intensive care would be simply an emergency hospital service.

Neonatologists in regional centers are also in a good position to develop administrative innovations, such as the use of computers to coordinate referrals from community hospitals. On a more ambitious level, computers are used to compare clinical records on a regional basis, with participating hospitals entering their data via a telephone interface to a central computer (Butler, 1978).

Like physicians, nurses have found new opportunities in newborn intensive care. The administrative duties that are part of the referral system are often shared by the nursing staff. The fragile condition of the infant patients demands constant surveillance, most of it provided by nurses who are capable of emergency intervention if necessary.

The challenges and stresses in newborn intensive care have the same source: the life-threatening condition of the newborn. The successful rescue of an infant from death or permanent injury gives tremendous satisfaction to the staff. At the same time, high rates of death and illness depress physicians and nurses alike. From the staff's perspective, the heaviest burden of newborn intensive care is the constant pressure to make immediate, correct decisions in the face of 15 to 30 percent mortality rates. The metaphor of warfare for high-technology medicine (Smith, 1974; Childress, 1984) is especially apt in the n.i.c.u. Boring routines alternate with clinical skirmishes, frequent exposure to death, an emphasis on body counts (survival statistics), and, for some, mixed feelings about the heavy artillery of hospital technology.

Most neonatologists in a recent poll indicated that they were satisfied with their jobs, but some 20 percent reported symptoms of anxiety (ulcers and chronic headaches) because of their work (Clarke et al., 1984). N.i.c.u. nurses often report job burnout, and physical and emotional problems (Marshall and Kasman, 1980). Yet emphasis in the tertiary nursery is so squarely on the treatment of patients that few staff members have the time to ponder these reactions. The use of therapeutic support groups has had uncertain results for intensive care staffs (Tyson et al., 1984). There is little time and few rewards for staff members themselves to assume the role of patient.

Newborn intensive care is an area of uncertain career possibilities for social workers and psychologists, not because the need for their services is lacking but because most units concentrate on emergency medical care for infants. Family problems and staff stress are not just secondary service concerns; they represent emotions and perspectives strictly compartmentalized from the clinical work of the Level III nursery.

PROTECTION OF THE INFANT PATIENT

The concentration on the medical needs of the newborn patient is a major innovation, an important elaboration of the medicalization of childbirth. The definition of childbirth as a medical crisis and of pregnant women as patients is a recent historic phenomenon (Wertz and Wertz, 1977). Now that hospitalization for childbirth is nearly universal in the United States, it is unlikely that the medical management of reproduction can be sharply reduced. In specific instances, such as the rising rates of cesarean deliveries in the 1970s, a combination of public and professional concern can curtail some unnecessary intervention. After extensive media coverage and government inquiries, the maxim "once a cesarean, always a cesarean" that unnecessarily exposed many women to surgery is no longer gospel among obstetricians (Guillemin, 1981). Still, in everything from the medical management of diabetic mothers to fetal monitoring to newborn intensive care, the technological investment in childbirth remains high.

Increasing focus on the individual newborn, rather than on the mother or family, has been characteristic of the last decade or so. In the early 1970s, pediatricians were willing to consider the newborn in the context of the family, even to the point of withholding treatment from an infant with anomalies. The classic case in the literature was a Down's syndrome newborn whose parents refused permission for a relatively routine operation to relieve intestinal blockage. Without the operation, the infant starved to death (Gustafson, 1973). Recounting an identical case and others involving defective and premature infants, Duff and Campbell (1973) described the parent–physician conference in their n.i.c.u., a process whereby difficult treatment decisions were reached largely on the basis of parental authority.

During the 1970s, a coterie of philosophers, physicians, and lawyers was quick to perceive the potential violation of newborn rights in this decision-making process (Weir, 1984:59–223). The distinction between the infant born dying and the defective newborn is central. No one involved in the ethical debates about newborn patients advocated treatment of essentially hopeless cases. Instead, attention focused on the criteria for describing "a life worth living" that medical treatment could reasonably assure or simply could not. Among the newborn patients not born dying, are there those whose lives, if prolonged, would be so full of suffering or mental or physical incapacities that treatment could not be considered beneficial? The severity of the condition of newborns with spina bifida, a spinal lesion causing gradations of neurological damage, raises this question. For some clinicians, notably Lorber (1971), there must be a clinical cutoff point past which newborns with severe defects are, by policy, not treated. For others, it is preferable to avoid conjecturing about the future quality of life and concentrate on immediate medical goals, that is, the repair of the spinal lesion and hydrocephalus.

Judgments about the future lives of very premature infants present a different order of problem solving. For example, Ramsey (1978) notes the experimental aspect of treating extremely small newborns. He suggests that categorically limiting vigorous intervention on their behalf would be more moral than treating these patients as a means of improving care for future patients, that is, as experiments.

Another important aspect of the ethical controversy surrounding newborn patients concerns who is the best guardian of an infant's interests. In a much-cited article on caretakers' legal responsibilities, Robertson and Fost (1976) warn that the letter of the law strictly protects the infant against parents and physicians who might give their own interests priority. Traditionally, parents have been given great discretion in deciding the fate of the defective or critically ill infant. An underlying assumption in the ethical debate is that unquestioning trust in either parents or physicians is not sufficient to safeguard the vulnerable newborn.

Today, a much more protective attitude toward the infant patient prevails than when Duff and Campbell described the parent–physician conference. In part, this greater sense of protection has to do with the prevalence of modern family planning and the intention of many couples to have fewer but well-cared-for children. In a larger historic sense, the role of children in the family has changed, with parents assuming more costly and long-term responsibilities for their offspring. Today's children are more invested with sentiment as they become the consumers rather than the producers of wealth (Zelitzer, 1985). That is, the infant has a new symbolic value in our times as opposed to historic episodes when children, as farm or factory workers, actively contributed to the family economy. The power of the antiabortion movement reflects this emotional valuation of the child without recognizing, however, that once born, the infant in Western society needs substantial human and material resources to survive.

An increased sense of protection of the newborn with birth defects is reflected in government efforts to enforce what is called the "Baby Doe" regulation. Ironically, despite the vastly increased medical attention being given today's newborns, recent public and governmental reactions have centered on the potential neglect of hospitalized infants. Whether to give or withhold treatment from infants with congenital anomalies has been the main issue. For example, in the 1983 Indiana Infant Doe case, treatment for a Down's syndrome infant with abnormalities of the throat was in question. In consultation with physicians, the infant's parents decided that surgery to correct problems of the trachea and esophagus should not be carried out. Like the Down's syndrome infant discussed years before, this infant could not be fed by mouth and so died in the nursery. Before the death occurred, conflicts among hospital staff members resulted in a court case to obstruct the parents' decision. Although the courts upheld the parents' position, the case of Infant Doe had widespread repercussions. The media presented it as an example of child abuse. State legislatures reacted with laws directly intended to protect such infant patients. Most important, the U.S. Department of Health and Human Services (DHHS) initiated the Baby Doe regulation to protect infants with abnormalities as handicapped persons covered by existing law. The exclusive emphasis was and remains on the undertreatment of newborns, with no reference to the risks of overtreatment.

The Baby Doe regulation has gone through several formulations and has precipitated a number of important lawsuits (Annas, 1983; Rhoden and Arras, 1985). Professional pediatric and hospital associations have disputed the style with which the federal government sought to act on its concern for the infant patient. Initially, DHHS required the posting of a federal hotline telephone number to encourage the reporting of possible infant rights violations. Squads of federal officials demanding medical records responded to such tip-offs, none of which revealed instances of abuse. Subsequently, the government retreated from these methods, but not from the position that infants with abnormalities were particularly liable to medical neglect.

In each formulation of the regulation DHHS has insisted on aggressive intervention for all newborns, except those whom nothing can save from imminent death. Little leeway is given practitioners concerned about treating infants who may die within the first year of life. No room is evident in the regulations for consideration of permanent, severe disabilities. To the contrary, so-called quality-of-life factors are specifically denied in the process of deciding whether to withhold treatment from a newborn patient. This exclusion is in part the result of the influence of antiabortion groups and advocates for the disabled, who joined with physicians, hospital administrators' lobbies, and other professionals to negotiate with DHHS concerning the final phrasing of the rule. As a result, the current Baby Doe regulation tends to preempt physician discretion by requiring maximum intervention in virtually all cases (Rhoden and Arras, 1985).

The Baby Doe rule could lead to overtreatment practices as unfair to newborn patients as medical neglect. Neonatologists who want to consider the long-range consequences of treatment may be deterred from doing so. For the obstetrician with doubts about the viability of a newborn and fears of legal action, referral and transport of the infant to an n.i.c.u. may resolve the professional dilemma without benefitting the newborn. Even before the Baby Doe regulation, newborn intensive care nurseries admitted and treated fundamentally untreatable patients. Will the regulation deepen this problem in the effort to protect certain newborns from neglect?

On another front, congressional legislation (Public Law 98-457) now authorizes state child abuse agencies to oversee the welfare of hospitalized newborns. The federal government, as part of the Baby Doe regulation, encourages hospitals to establish special committees (Infant Care Review Committees) to discuss and make decisions about difficult cases. These same committees would ideally contact state agencies to alert them to the need for protective intervention, for example, custody or adoption proceedings. In this way, committees and state agencies would become involved in decisions for the newborn along with physicians and parents.

The effort to regulate intensive care for newborns is more than a product of a general protective sentiment about children. With efficient referral systems, infants tend to get separated from their parents, either geographically or by the barriers imposed between the n.i.c.u. and the outside world. Parents have not become less trustworthy; they have become more remote from the process of medical decision making for their infants.

The newborn patient is indeed vulnerable to bureaucratic routine and impersonal service, to decisions made for professional and institutional reasons. Not only is the technology of neonatal intensive care complex but so too is its social organization. Concern that an infant could become lost in this system and be exposed to inappropriate treatment is justified.

COMPARATIVE AND POLICY ISSUES

Medical care for critically ill newborns is appreciated in every industrialized country both for its contribution to the live birth rate and for its link to progressive medicine. There is moral gratification in supporting programs that rescue infants from death. Advances in neonatal medicine, such as the improved survival rate of very low birth weight infants, are heralded even in countries, such as France, with a heavy commitment to prenatal care (Wynn and Wynn, 1976).

In the comparative cases examined in this book, newborn intensive care is revealed as a service that can be integrated into a variety of health care systems based on socialized medicine, or on a mixture of public and private insurance funds, or in a Third World context that defines the service as a luxury for the wealthy.

As with all medical services, the practical question is one of need. If the focus of intervention is only on childbirth, then the need for newborn intensive care is paramount. There is, however, another perspective that emerges clearly in the analysis of health systems in other countries. Unlike the United States, other industrialized nations have central government controls that potentially restrict costly technologies. England and the Netherlands are two examples we compare. In these countries, neonatal intensive care tends to be integrated into a larger plan for perinatal services, that is, health care for the pregnant woman and the newborn, as well as cradle-to-grave health insurance. Between these two economically advanced nations, the clinical need for newborn intensive care differs. Rates of premature birth, for example, are greater in England than in Holland (MacFarlane and Mugford, 1984:218). Within the constraints of its health care system, England is moving quickly toward the American acute care solution to this problem. In the Netherlands, there are relatively fewer infants needing intensive care, and those that do are larger and in better health than the patients ordinarily seen in high-level nurseries in either the United States or England.

The strong association between premature births, the principal cause of neonatal death, and poverty helps explain this difference. Poverty, as the experience of poor housing, malnutrition, and low income, has been more or less eliminated in the Netherlands. The same is not true of England or the United States. In both these countries, high rates of infant death tend to be localized in extremely poor communities. Developing nations present an even more vivid picture of the repercussions of poverty on newborns, with death rates six and seven times greater than those in industrialized nations. In Brazil, the third comparative case we present, the same problem of prematurity that troubles a minority of American births affects enormous numbers of newborns. However, newborn intensive care at the level of technology and personnel found in a Level III unit in the United States is not the public policy solution there. High-technology reproductive medicine is available, but primarily for the very wealthy. Otherwise, the problem of reducing infant death remains a matter of improving public health programs and resolving social class inequities.

Is newborn intensive care, which now costs approximately five billion dollars per year, a luxury service in the United States? The efficiency with which the nation has moved toward regional centers has increased the access of infants in critical condition to high-level technology, apparently without discrimination based on parental finances. Federal and state reductions in Medicaid funds could destabilize the current equity in referrals and make it a fiscal liability for hospitals to accept welfare-funded or charity patients. Inflation in hospital costs is another potential source of destabilization. The pursuit of the very low birth weight frontier carries an enormous price tag, with hospital charges for one experimental case potentially equal to the charges for ten routine cases (Guillemin and Holmstrom, 1983).

Effective as an acute care strategy, newborn intensive care is not the only way to attack the problem of premature births. A recent report by the Institute of Medicine proposes preventive measures to combat prematurity, specifically during pregnancy. This is not a new idea; the World Health Organization and countries with socialized medicine have long promoted the identification of risk factors during pregnancy as a means of preventing troubled births. The relative resistance to universal prenatal care in the United States is puzzling, since "policymakers and health professionals have enough information at present to intervene more vigorously to improve pregnancy outcome" (Institute of Medicine, 1985:1). The Institute's report also pointed out that nonwhite mothers, teenagers, and mothers with less than a high school education are most at risk for giving birth prematurely and, unfortunately, are most likely to receive no prenatal care or counseling.

At present, public and professional enthusiasm for treating newborns in intensive care units far outweighs that for guaranteeing

American women prenatal care. Protection of the infant is perceived within the dramatic framework of childbirth as a medical crisis. This is the perspective of a broad constituency—medical practitioners, antiabortion groups, the media, and parents themselves—focused on risks at birth. Yet after a decade of rapid development, newborn intensive care has reached a crucial stage of reassessment, like the second-stage evaluations characteristic of such medical innovations as therapy for childhood leukemia (Warner, 1975). The controversy around the Baby Doe regulation signals a broadening forum for discussing the clinical dilemmas in the intensive care nursery. The role of professionals in determining humane and equitable standards of medical care is fundamental. As the ethicist Paul Ramsey (1970:130) has enjoined, practitioners should envision the whole patient, not just the diseases. In the treatment of newborns, this approach requires reflection on the future life experience of the child. To do this in the emergency atmosphere of the neonatal intensive care unit is as necessary as it is difficult.

The typical high-level nursery appears to be isolated from corporate realities and national programs; in reality, it is not. As proof of the complex institutional nature of this important service, current discussion is no longer limited to cases of physicians' ethical dilemmas. Rather, complex issues of organization and research goals are now beginning to be addressed. The benefits and deficits of regionalized referral for infants, for pregnant women, and for families, for example, are unclear and need discussion and evaluation. The allocation of resources for high-risk cases, for short-term clinical care, and for long-term needs, is another vital policy issue.

There is an equally pressing need for instituting authoritative follow-up studies of the health of newborn survivors so that referral and treatment decisions are more accurately based on outcome data. This research, as Silverman (1985) and Chalmers (1983) have argued, must be scientifically rigid and on a large scale to produce credible results.

The focus of our research is on the complex organizational imperatives that have directed the growth of newborn intensive care. While an excellent assessment of the ethical dilemmas in this area has been published (Weir, 1984), the bureaucratic dynamic in newborn intensive care generally overrides the individual physician's or nurse's authority, just as it has undermined the guardianship role of parents. Pediatricians are managerially and technically in control of this important hospital service. Yet, as with other salaried professionals, their work is integrated into a hierarchical service organization, limiting their autonomy and breadth of knowledge (Mills, 1951:112). The corporate impact on this medical specialty has great repercussions for infant patients, their families, and society.

RESEARCH METHODS

A first step to the broader view of newborn intensive care is an understanding of the Level III nursery, the pivot of the referral system and the environment that produces definitive standards in neonatology. This maximum care setting should, according to professional and government guidelines, offer a full range of consulting and technical service for an indefinite period of time. The ratio of physicians to patients often reaches 1:4 or 5. The ratio of nurses to infant patients is just as often 1:2 or 3.

Newborn intensive care begins with emergency survival measures, but only by the narrowest interpretation does it remain limited to the initial rescue effort. The resources of the Level III nursery amplify survival medicine to fuller and more experimental dimensions, such as corrective surgery and even organ transplantation. The medical technologies most important to the tertiary nursery are the small pressure- and flow-adjusted respirators, intravenous feeding refined for newborns, x-ray films to monitor lung and heart development, and antibiotics. Phototherapy (sets of lights placed over incubators to cure infant jaundice) and blood transfusion equipment are also essential. Level III nurseries are increasingly involved in neonatal surgery, which requires an operating room and equipment adapted to the newborn.

In addition to neonatologists, neonatology fellows, house officers, and nurses, the Level III nursery also provides a wide range of consulting specialists: experts in nutrition, gastrointestinal disease, radiology, pharmacology, neurology, cardiology, and surgery. The supporting laboratory facilities are commensurate with acute care services for adults.

Our interest in researching medical care for newborns took us to a Level III nursery in a large pediatric hospital in the eastern United States. Northeast Pediatric Hospital (a pseudonym) is a nonprofit teaching hospital serving a densely populated city and the surrounding suburbs. It has an international reputation for basic and clinical research. The Level III nursery at Northeast Pediatric is small (about fifteen available incubators) and affiliated in a joint program with two other large hospitals, one with a Level II nursery and the other a maternity hospital with a mixed-level unit.

We entered the life of the Level III unit by going to what are called interdisciplinary rounds—weekly discussions of problem cases by nurses, social workers, physicians, and other consulting professionals. This we did for six months, while also attending seminars, conferences, and hospital-wide discussions of cases in neonatology. Then, with the permission of the physician director of the n.i.c.u., we began the daily recording of the unit's activities. Morning work rounds, the bedside discussion by staff of the patient's medical condition, gave us the best understanding of treatment norms and familiarized us with technical language. We made a point of being at the nursery for much of the working day and in the evenings, including after family visits were over, when the staff had time to relax. All admissions to the n.i.c.u. are, by definition, emergencies, so we had to learn how to fade quickly into the background or to be helpful in minor ways.

Over an eight-month period, we followed a consecutive series of 103 admissions. After this, from 1980 to 1983, we began to make site visits to other intensive care nurseries, to test our observations at Northeast Pediatric and to gain a comparative perspective on national and international variations in neonatal care. We visited and interviewed staffs at fourteen Level III newborn intensive care units in this country and at comparable nurseries in England, the Netherlands, East and West Germany, France, and Brazil.

Our comparative work informed us of how newborn intensive care was expanding in the nineteen-eighties, becoming established in a diversity of hospitals—teaching and non-teaching, for-profit and non-profit, urban and suburban. In so doing, it became exposed to pressures that the small, research-oriented nurseries where it originated seldom or never felt. The infants treated today in newborn intensive care are smaller, sicker, more likely to suffer from drug withdrawal symptoms or to be infected by the AIDS virus, and, as survivors, less likely to have their medical bills reimbursed than even ten years ago. Some nurseries, usually those in troubled inner city neighborhoods, are chronically overcrowded; others have overexpanded and struggle to keep beds full. Parents of n.i.c.u. patients now have a national organization, Parent Care, and speak openly of the need for informed consent.

Nonetheless, despite diversity and change, our comparative work also showed us that the Level III unit in the elite teaching hospital remains the respected source of neonatology's clinical standards and goals. This dominant organizational model for saving newborn lives, communicated nationally and internationally, is the primary focus of *Mixed Blessings*.

I
Professional Roles and Responsibilities

1

The N.I.C.U. Physicians

> This is the kind of place in which people assume you can be a brilliant administrator in the morning, a brilliant clinician in the afternoon, and a brilliant laboratory researcher in the evening.
>
> *Neonatology Fellow*

> The n.i.c.u. is not like other services. The risks are greater here and you have to watch what you do.   *Attending Physician to a Resident*

Physicians' confidence in the efficacy of early and maximum medical intervention gives newborn intensive care its main impetus. In the major hospital setting, neonatologists in high-level nurseries are granted great professional authority in treatment decisions. In return, the hospital demands of these employees the management of a highly efficient acute care unit, coupled with high-caliber patient surveillance. The professional prerequisites for this kind of work are considerable: firm commitment to rescuing critically ill infants, tolerance for frequent exposure to death and dying, acceptance of quick and impersonal contacts with patients and families, and exceptional technical skills under emergency-room pressures.

The professionals capable of meeting these demands are organized in hierarchical teams that reinforce the authority of senior physicians. The physicians' junior colleagues are fellows in neonatology (physicians seeking advanced experience in the field) and resident physicians training in pediatrics, along with skilled nurses.

PHYSICIANS' COMMITMENT

Senior physicians in newborn intensive care are the strongest advocates of aggressive intervention. Whether or not they are certified neonatologists by the American Academy of Pediatrics, the directors and attending physicians in many neonatal intensive care units act with a sense of mission appropriate to the proponents of an expanding field firmly linked to an acute care service. They generally

23

believe that maximum emergency intervention is the best available medical treatment for prematurity and other problems affecting newborns. In pediatrics, optimal neonatal care begins in the delivery room, with a neonatologist to provide emergency intervention. This precaution should extend to access to the n.i.c.u.

Despite its brief history, neonatology supports several generations of physicians. Most of the pioneers of the subspecialty, now in their fifties and sixties, are no longer in clinical practice. The majority have moved to administrative positions within pediatric hospitals or head pediatric departments in large general hospitals. Because the service has expanded so rapidly in the last fifteen years, many Level III nursery directors and senior physicians are relatively young pediatricians, in their forties, who have risen quickly to the top echelons because of a combination of clinical and organizational skills. As a Northeast Pediatric neonatology fellow (who later rose to the rank of attending physician) put it succinctly:

> This is the kind of place in which people assume you can be a brilliant administrator in the morning, a brilliant clinician in the afternoon, and a brilliant laboratory researcher in the evening.

Saving Lives

Despite the pressures of work, the calm, even matter-of-fact demeanor of the three senior physicians at Northeast Pediatric seldom betrayed any ambivalence or uncertainty. Sometimes, when not on duty or during a cafeteria lunch, an attending physician would admit feeling worn down or question how many years of clinical work any neonatologist could stand. In general, however, enthusiasm for the work ran high.

The simple explanation for the positive attitude of senior physicians might be the enormous gratification of rescuing infants from death. The observation that the intensive care nurse's morale is high because she is saving lives (Strauss, 1968) applies as well to n.i.c.u. physicians, especially those in an expanding service. Counting only survival rates, senior Level III physicians have much to be glad about when a regional program is put into operation. The inauguration of a new unit usually decreases recorded perinatal mortality rates right away, providing an instant boost to staff morale. This rate decrease is particularly predictable when there is no competing service in the same region. As the director of a Level III unit in a new pediatric hospital in the Midwest put it:

We've made a real difference here, not just in the mortality rates in the city, but over an entire region, even into [the adjoining state]. There are infants who wouldn't be alive now if we hadn't started this unit.

Even without this claim, the employment of neonatologists in central and research-oriented hospitals helps to explain, first, how they tolerate work in which medical crises and death are pervasive, and second, how they identify with the progressive mission of neonatology.

Order and Efficiency

The corporate structure of hospitals does much to reduce the emergency aspects of newborn intensive care. Individual cases admitted to a Level III unit may be disastrous, but the routine administration of referral, admission, and discharge normalizes the unceasing encounter with extraordinary rates of sickness and death. A bad work day for the unit is one when orders get mislabeled, plasma is unavailable, death certificates are lost, consulting physicians break appointments, and the transport ambulance is late. A good day is one when this rational system successfully imposes organizational predictability on the unpredictable incidence of patients' physiological failures.

Depending entirely on the hospital for their patients and practice, senior n.i.c.u. physicians often use corporate models of efficiency to represent how well they are utilizing the system and how well the specialists and the hospital are serving patients. Productivity records, measured by admissions and the discharge of surviving patients, are commonly displayed or circulated in units as proofs of progress. These are the kinds of records that unit directors have to present to upper-level hospital administrators, to trustees, to health systems agencies, to community organizations, and to the mass media, in order to justify the value of the service. Unit directors and senior physicians also work to establish the referral network through their contacts with obstetricians and pediatricians in other services and hospitals. The more successfully neonatologists cultivate referrals of patients, the more admissions to the unit they have. The more admissions they have, the more valid is their claim for increased hospital space, technology, and personnel. Since the Level III nursery is designed to accept potentially untreatable infants, this effort to increase referrals is not limited by narrow constraints regarding patient status.

Technological Truths

The good morale of senior n.i.c.u. physicians is also sustained by the conviction that the methods of neonatology are constantly improving. Over the last twenty years, the adaptation of many adult therapies to the treatment of full-term infants has been successful. The presumption in neonatology is that progress will continue undiminished at the same rate and prove as equal to the challenge of saving very low birth weight neonates as it has to saving more developed newborns.

N.i.c.u. physicians, in their attitudes about the procedures, machines, and medications of their trade, ascribe to what Marcuse (1982:147) called "technological truths." That is, paramount importance is ascribed to technology and to technical expertise. Technology is "an instrument of expedience," in hospital care, the sole pragmatic means to the end of curing. Advanced technology also "inspires the belief that its use fosters a progressive, rational order." Thus, entire hospital services are organized around machines. The use of the respirator in the n.i.c.u. is a prime case in point. The machine's size, pressure, and flow capacity have been finely tuned to the needs of premature infants who suffer from lung immaturity (respiratory distress syndrome). At the Northeast Pediatric unit, where most infants were premature, most of the staff's time was devoted to evaluating and managing oxygen therapy. The clinical objective was "weaning," the graduated, numerically ordered decrease in oxygen, for example, from 100 percent at transport, to 60 percent during the first day, to the withdrawal of respirator support on the second or third day. The refinements of respirator pressure and flow (as sales representatives point out) now allow great flexibility and control and offer an increased potential of giving small newborns growing time while their lungs develop.

The extensive use of the respirator organizes n.i.c.u. physicians' and nurses' behavior around the fundamental question of "dial up" or "dial down." Surveillance of patients translates into an active diagnostic search for information on respiration. Nurses at Northeast Pediatric took frequent regular blood samples for blood gas tests. Physicians depended heavily on the twice-daily review of x-ray films to evaluate the condition of infant lungs. Discussions at work rounds centered on the relationship between lung functioning, the relatively known quantity, and the far more mysterious functions of other organs and systems—brain, heart, kidney, liver, bowel, circulatory, digestive, immune, and nervous.

Resident: "We've got to wean this baby down."

Attending physician: "The respirator's your constant in all this. What you've got to do is balance the other information—on the gut and the apnea spells—against the guarantees of this machine."

Research Orientation

Consulting specialists at Northeast Pediatric sometimes joked that the neonatologists were bent on creating the artificial womb and were working backward to in vitro fertilization. The sincerity and enthusiasm of senior n.i.c.u. physicians in their mission to save babies should not, however, be underestimated. The following describes a highly committed, newly certified neonatologist.

> Her face lit up as she told me that one way to look at premature birth, the way she looked at it, was that the infant needed to get out of the uterus, that the infant needed medical help. For some reason, such as toxemia, it could no longer survive in utero. Then the baby needed the best medical help.

The nontechnological truth of newborn intensive care is that, after initial emergency intervention, larger, intact premature infants have the best survival and developmental chances and just need time to grow, under close surveillance. With the selection in the n.i.c.u. of extremely premature and damaged infants who require a great deal of medical intervention, there are fewer guarantees of good outcome inherent in the technology. As one senior resident put it, "In the back of my mind, I know that the more we do, the more we have to do, and the worse shape the baby will be in. We're all the king's horses and this is Humpty-Dumpty."

Neonatologists have responded to the challenge of saving increasingly smaller and seriously disabled infants by moving into basic laboratory and clinical research. This is partly a function of the location of most Level III nurseries at major hospitals where research is encouraged and supported. Medical journals in pediatrics and obstetrics are replete with articles on fetal development and neonatal responses to therapy. Such reported studies are often based on small samples from a single clinical setting, and publications have a fragmented and suggestive quality (not unlike other medical research) that makes direct application to clinical practice difficult. Nonetheless, there is a sophisticated research base that sets the neonatologist apart from many pediatricians and obstetricians. Scientific inquiry into the production of surfactant in unborn sheep lungs or the investigation of neonatal reactions to fluid intake legitimizes neonatologists as experts above the "hands-on" level of the ordinary local practitioner. This is an important professional claim in the context of the major medical center. In addition, the research in neonatology justifies hope in technological progress and fortifies the belief that, with enough determination, time, and money, all physical obstacles to infant survival and perhaps fetal viability will be conquered.

As neonatologists pursue the ends of progressive medicine, they have expanded the treatable newborn patient population. In general, the neonatologists' belief in medical progress expands the criteria for n.i.c.u. admission and, consequently, the numbers of treatable patients. The overlap of professional and institutional interests, at this point, is optimal insofar as the selection for more patients who are clinically interesting—even experimental cases—also means hospital beds filled and resources used to capacity.

A final reason for the good morale of senior n.i.c.u. physicians may be that, because junior colleagues do the bulk of case work, attending physicians can keep some distance from the strains of intensive care. Senior physicians are at the top of the unit hierarchy and have the power to delegate responsibilities. At the same time, these neonatologists determine the general treatment policy that staff members must follow.

THE EDUCATION OF RESIDENTS

Required and Intermittent Service

The demands that a subspecialty service like neonatal intensive care can make on pediatric residents' time are limited. Therefore, within a teaching program, an n.i.c.u. relies on residents to do a brief, required term of service but does not count on their long-term involvement. The socialization of young physicians, and the related issues of values and commitment, which can be fully dealt with in training at the specialty level (Light, 1975), are less applicable in subspecialty rotations. Instead, those who direct neonatology units must rely on the general dedication of residents to the service of patients and their prior socialization as physicians.

The demands for professional help are so heavy in newborn intensive care that residents may find themselves required to spend more of their training time in the n.i.c.u. than they would want.

Finally, the American Academy of Pediatrics (1980) felt the need to set guidelines limiting the proportion of residency time spent in this area. In some units in the United States, residents still spend as much as one-half of their clinical hours working in newborn intensive care. The deciding factor is the overall investment that a hospital and pediatrics program makes in a regional system as opposed, for example, to general pediatrics.

Many young physicians drawn to pediatrics identify with the public service values that the field represents and are willing to confront what Abbott (1981) called "publicly charismatic disorders," those mixtures of medical and human problems from which older and higher-status practitioners prefer to retreat. The current popularity of pediatrics and family medicine among young physicians implies a new interest in family and community needs. The professional mission of neonatology appeals most to a few residents interested in intensive care technology, administration, and research. Therefore, senior n.i.c.u. physicians must manage residents who represent a variety of career ambitions, letting them learn n.i.c.u. skills without doing harm to high-risk patients.

In exposing residents to a heavy volume of cases, newborn intensive care puts each resident on the front lines of clinical work, often without addressing the complexities of nonmedical problems. The rigors of residency training expose candidates to a barrage of case materials. As Bucher and Stelling noted in their account of residents in internal medicine:

> [T]heir focus was on the sheer volume of clinical experience. There was a litany which we heard over and over again from these residents which might be paraphrased: "Given the ingredients of this program, it is inevitable that you will learn and increase in competence." (1977:186)

As a subspecialty offering intensive clinical experience, neonatology is highly specific in the range of problem-solving techniques to be learned. The first priority in the n.i.c.u. is placed on narrowly defined clinical skills to meet emergency needs. It is essential that new residents during their first rotation be quickly educated or else infant patients will be in serious jeopardy. To accomplish this, staff physicians use methods that emphasize the importance of correct responses to purely medical problems.

The Importance of Supervision

In the Northeast Pediatric n.i.c.u., attending physicians consistently emphasized to the residents that they should not act independently. For example, almost the only time Dr. Cartwright, a controlled, low-keyed attending physician, ever came close to expressing anger was when she discovered that one of the new residents had not reported an evening admission to her. Using a calm but severe tone, she explained to him that the n.i.c.u. was not like other services: "Attendings are here for you to call." The precautionary approach required that the resident always have backup, especially when alone, isolated from the team, or without access to an expert. On transport duty, the new resident would be paired with a nurse experienced with community hospitals and with keeping small neonates stable in an ambulance or helicopter. As for night duty, the time of greatest autonomy for the resident, attending physicians told residents not to hesitate to inform the senior physician of problems and to call for assistance. Rather than proceeding alone, a new resident faced with an infant in failure was expected to reach immediately for the phone. Experienced residents had much more discretion and often managed multiple "crashes" or difficult procedures on their own. Said a third-year resident after one such long night's work, "You can do it. You can make the decisions, even though you feel like rats are running through your mouth."

In teaching new residents to handle (and not to create) emergencies, emphasis was put on the one-to-one relationship between the resident and attending physician, rather than between resident and the neonatology fellow. The fellow did most if not all of the technical training of residents, but the attending physician was promoted as the ultimate authority in clinical emergencies. This point was made metaphorically when a new resident naively asked why the fellow (also new to the staff) had put his name and home telephone number in large characters on the unit blackboard. Residents had already been instructed to consult the list of attending physicians' numbers on the lounge bulletin board. Another resident brightly quipped, "That's his business number." From there, the nurses and the fellow himself developed a comic scenario in which the fellow was an itinerant vender of respirators "to gypsies who stole premature infants." Thus the fellow's authority in emergency situations was underplayed.

Mastery, Confidence, and Instrumental Skills

In doing long-term field work at Northeast Pediatric, we were able to observe attitudinal changes in residents new to neonatal intensive care, as well as the more sophisticated behavior of experienced residents. The progress from hesitancy to self-confidence in these physicians seemed to take several six-week rotations. A particularly optimistic senior resident proclaimed:

> There's just a great high, a great feeling of power when you know you can handle anything that comes up. Intensive care is different that way. After five months of rotation, you feel in control.

Before that feeling of power and control is achieved, there are many moments, even days, of anxiety. Frader (1979) described the beginning of each rotation in pediatric intensive care as a "trial by fire" for house officers and a period of increased uncertainty for nurses and attending physicians. Initially, residents focus on technical concerns as they try to master the mechanical devices, monitors, and clinical procedures associated with intensive care.

For the first weeks, the new n.i.c.u. residents appeared relatively stunned by the pressures of n.i.c.u. work. Said one nurse, "I always feel sorry for the new ones. Some of the other nurses like to bully them, to bring them in line. But I always feel they need all the help they can get." In the early weeks, residents apologized for their technical incompetence, such as having to make multiple tries before achieving a successful spinal tap or intubation.

By about the fourth week, most novice residents could claim improvements in their skills and would call upon the rest of the staff team to witness a particularly good line placement or a successful spinal tap. The apologies concerning multiple failed tries also ceased, to be replaced by expressions that normalized repeated frustrations. That is, residents came to understand that these especially small and critically ill infants presented problems with which any skilled clinician would have difficulty.

New resident house officers also came to understand the high level of frustration tolerated in the unit. At first view, the senior staff appeared to be in perfect control of crises. The professional demeanor of attending physicians, the professional behavior of the nurses, even the occasional black humor of the neonatology fellows presented the image of an experienced team into which the novice resident comes as a bit of a bumbler. At second view, the residents understood work stresses shared by the entire staff as a function of the selection for difficult cases. Toward the end of the initial six weeks of rotation, even humor on that score was possible. As one resident joked to another:

"We've had twenty-five pounds of PFC [persistent fetal circulation] brought into this unit in the last month and most of it by you [as transport physician]."

THE ROLE OF THE FELLOW

As experienced pediatricians, fellows in neonatology have the authority to direct residents. However, they are structurally marginal to the team hierarchy. In the recent past, the neonatology fellowship has been a major source for the recruitment of Level III attending physicians. As places in prestigious hospitals have been filled, the fellowship has also taken on the function of educating neonatologists for other n.i.c.u. positions. These include directing new Level III or II units in underserved areas or staffing expanding units.

At Northeast Pediatric, the neonatology fellow played a crucial role as mediator between attending physicians and residents, partaking in the authority of the senior physicians and also in the learning of the residents. Three of the five fellows were already veterans of several six-month tours of service in the Level III nursery. One newcomer, Dr. Richmond, expressed some of the anxieties of managing the unit for the first time as he waited after hours for the arrival of a new admission:

> Dr. Richmond described how last week he had been in charge of the transport and admission of a baby who had been "in blooming health." He felt he had made a mistake on that and said in addition: "I felt I got treated like dog-shit for that admission." The whole event caused him stress because he thought that the baby would need a total exchange because of its bili [bilirubin] count at transport. So he went home to get some sleep and told the resident in charge to call him when the exchange [total transfusion] would have to be done and he would come in and supervise it. Theoretically the exchange should have taken place around two o'clock in the morning. Dr. Richmond said, "I woke up in a cold sweat at five o'clock, thinking I had slept through the call." It turned out the baby hadn't needed the transfusion at all. "I just don't want to go through that again. It's better if I stay here and wait."

A major part of the fellow's responsibility is described by Goffman, discussing the director of team performance: "Whether it is a funeral, a wedding, a bridge party, a one-day sale, a hanging, or a picnic, the director may tend to see the performance in terms of whether or not it went 'smoothly,' 'effectively,' and 'without a hitch,' and whether or not all possible disruptive contingencies were prepared for in advance" (1959:97–98).

The work of teaching residents was divided between attending physicians and fellows. The pedagogical approach of each allowed the residents to distance themselves from unremitting death and critical illness. Attending physicians continually drew the attention of younger physicians to the generalizations to be drawn from specific cases. At rounds, the senior physicians frequently made reference to published studies and used specific cases to instruct residents in the norms of pathology: "This is a classic case of RDS." "This ETT [endotracheal tube] complication is common in long-term cases." "Ordinarily, a PFC [persistent fetal circulation] case like this doesn't last long." Attending physicians were also in charge of formal teaching, selecting a particular clinical subject and conducting weekly seminars.

Neonatology fellows offered a more technical education. They had to school residents in quickly adjusting to the very small size and extreme fragility of n.i.c.u. patients. Some residents had already practiced intubation on cats before their rotation began, but even they needed coaching to work successfully with 600- and 700-gram newborns. Doing spinal taps and placing intravenous and arterial lines were other skills supervised by the fellow. In themselves, none of these were new techniques for the residents to master, but this seemed to add to their frustration. As for the fellow, he or she was often put in the difficult position, as trainer, of being the target of resentment:

> Trainers tend to evoke for the performer a vivid image of himself that he had repressed, a self-image of someone engaged in the clumsy and embarrassing process of becoming. The performer can make himself forget how foolish he once was, but he cannot make the trainer forget. (Goffman, 1959:158–59)

Challenging the fellow's authority was typical of the residents' behavior. In the three groups of residents we most closely observed, there was always one young physician, in each instance a man, who played the role of antagonist to the fellow. Each of these residents maintained that role regardless of which fellow was supervising. The tenor of this criticism directly related to the evaluation of therapy. Thus, Dr. Marsh, a resident on his first rotation, persistently questioned the use of antibiotics recommended by Dr. Hok, his first supervisor. Two weeks later, when Dr. Richmond took over, this resident continued to question decisions concerning antibiotics and even expanded his expression of doubt to include other areas, such as nutrition and transfusions. Although new to the supervisor role, Dr. Richmond met the challenge head on, as the following account illustrates.

> Dr. Marsh went on to point out that this is day three of ox and gent [two antibiotics, oxacillin and gentamicin]. He proceeded with a few comments on antibiotics, concluding that he doesn't mind continuing with gent but that it is toxic alone. He wants to use another drug, amacasin. Dr. Richmond brought him up short, saying: "What is our experience with it around here? Do we use it here?"
>
> *Dr. Marsh:* "No, not really. But it's practically the same as penicillin."
>
> *Dr. Richmond* (darkly): "There's probably a good reason why it's not used here."
>
> Dr. Marsh looked crushed.

This interaction between a newly arrived fellow and a resident on his first rotation represents an unusually direct confrontation, since neither had really mastered the more subtle physicians' rules of challenge and put-down. At rounds, the more experienced fellow ordinarily deflected a challenge about treatment by changing the subject, recommending discussion later, or by referring the issue immediately to the rest of the group.

An important function of the fellow was to foster team consensus about treatment. This consensus, and the discussion preceding it, provided a rationale for the course of treatment and a check against clinical uncertainty. At the end of each case discussion at work rounds, the fellow would ask for an immediate treatment plan. Usually the resident presenting the case would offer suggestions, or the primary physician who was in charge of the case would formulate a plan of tests and surveillance. Before the plan could be stated, collective agreement would have to be reached on the nature of the infant's problems. If there was hesitancy about defining those problems, then the team had to agree at least on the right diagnostic approach.

If they chose, the fellows could relieve the staff's tension with joking and teasing. A new resident who had vigorously ventilated an infant in respiratory failure would be told that the manual resuscitation using a bag device made for muscular neonatologists. Or, a resident's exasperation with spinal taps would be turned into a joke about a career in shoemaking ("tap! tap!"). Third-year residents confident enough in their work also could stage humorous scenarios, provided the right fellow was in charge. At one time, when there were five long-term, difficult cases in the unit, one of the residents, Dr. Reilly, used a spare moment at morning rounds to sit down in a rocking chair (used by nurses and parents when holding infants) and declare that he was "the oldest survivor in the unit." He talked about how he had spent many years in the n.i.c.u. The two other residents joined in with jokes about not being able to face the outside world because there was not enough oxygen.

There was great variation among fellows in their sense of accountability to patients and families. This was evidenced in seemingly small ways, but the effect on residents' and nurses' behavior was clear. The only female fellow, Dr. Hight, was at one extreme. She conducted rounds deemphasizing the ritual of moving from one isolette (infant incubator bed) to another, thus distancing the group from the patients. At the other extreme, Dr. McCord made it a rule to include a brief assessment of the parents' situation as part of each resident's daily presentation. This fellow also attended social service rounds (which was rare for physicians to do), and encouraged residents to do the same. On a return visit to the Northeast Pediatric unit, after basic research was completed, one of the researchers was in the lounge talking about Dr. McCord, who then walked in:

> *Researcher:* "Are you aware of the fact that you are unique among the fellows in the emphasis you put on the family situation?"
>
> *Dr. McCord* (smiling): "No, I'm not."
>
> *Nurse:* "Yes you are. You're kidding."
>
> *Dr. McCord:* "I don't feel that I have good contact with other people, other fellows here, enough to say that. Relative to a number of issues, we're on different planets. I'm not at a point in my career where I can go to the higher-ups and make suggestions for change, but I believe that cases should be approached broadly."

The breadth of influence that an individual fellow in neonatology can exert is limited, however, by the technical level of his or her responsibilities, the temporary nature of the position, and the overriding authority of the attending physicians.

CASE "OWNERSHIP"

One fundamental way of integrating new residents into the n.i.c.u. staff was to assign physicians the responsibility for individual cases. Theoretically, each patient had a doctor and that doctor had primary responsibility for directing treatment. Residents consistently claimed the right to have the final word on assessing their patients' needs. The descriptive expression, "This is Dr. Gould's baby," or, in confrontation, "This is *my* baby," were commonplace in the discussions of cases. Among residents on their first rotation, insecurities about skills and authority were played out competitively on the subject of case ownership. A resident assigned a particularly difficult case would be under pressure to analyze the infant's condition competently, and the greatest pressure would come from the two other residents. If an infant had problems with urine output, the primary physician had to research articles on kidney functioning in neonates, fluid maintenance, and Lasix (a diuretic), or risk having one of the other residents appear more knowledgeable about the subject. The potential threat was that another physician would both impress superiors and have a greater say in treatment.

However, the organization of work shifts and rotations made it functionally impossible for any one physician to provide continuous personal care to a patient; instead, the unit team worked at this collectively. The residents alternated night duty so that, in a team of three, each would be on duty for two nonconsecutive nights per week, and turns would be taken for Sunday evening coverage. The resident on night duty usually had the responsibility afterward of presenting cases at eight o'clock morning rounds and, after filling out report forms, would be free until the following morning. On the third day, the same resident was expected to come in for afternoon rounds and stay for night duty. Under these conditions, the responsibility for patients' treatment would shift from one primary physician, when he or she was on night duty, to a set of residents supervising patients during the day, to the next resident taking night duty, and then back to the primary physician in the morning.

The "quick cure" cases, which accounted for most admissions, would be in and out of the unit before the resident could begin to have personal input in the treatment; the tried-and-true routines of ventilator support and intravenous feeding solved most patients' problems. At the end of a rotation, the current residents' ownership of cases was passed on to the next set of house officers. The idea of case ownership, then, had no necessary connection to consistent personal advocacy for the patient.

In addition, residents at all levels were highly sensitive to what they saw as a lack of uniformity in the clinical approaches of attending physicians and fellows. Within the subspecialty, their superiors had carved out individual niches in nutrition, lung development, kidney disease, or computers. These different interests made for slightly different patterns of diagnosis and treatment. Regarding intensity of therapy, one recently certified attending physician, Dr. Simmons, was more enthusiastic in treating borderline cases than were her colleagues. When she was on service, the decision making shifted toward more aggressive support for all infants; the authority of her position was enough to override junior physicians' and nurses' opinions. The unit director, Dr. Karp, and another senior physician, Dr. Cartwright, were more open to staff input, or, perhaps more accurately, they understood the necessity of n.i.c.u. teamwork and were confident of their ultimate control of treatment decisions.

MISTAKES AND EXONERATION

The subject of medical mistakes has been well covered in the literature, often as it applies to an individual practitioner performing a single radical procedure, such as major surgery. With regard to procedures, newborn intensive care goes beyond addressing a single pathology with a single therapy. Instead, the entire age-specific condition of the newborn requires complex and general support. Even when a pathology is localized, the therapy is characteristically a fine-tuning rather than a single radical intervention. Decisions about oxygen maintenance, nutrition, and giving antibiotics have to be made daily, sometimes hourly. In addition, these decisions are continuously subject to the interpretations of many physicians and nurses reading frequently elicited diagnostic data: x-ray films, blood gas levels, blood urea nitrogen tests, and other laboratory tests.

The high level of monitoring in the n.i.c.u. does not eliminate mistakes per se, but it does make it unlikely that a mistake will go unnoticed for any length of time. In this sense, clinical peer review is an ongoing process integrated into daily work. At Northeast Pediatric, the supervision of residents was close, residents took their primary physician's role seriously and competitively, and the nursing staff was active and experienced. This system of checks is akin to the "routine surveillance" that controls the behavior of surgery residents (Bosk, 1979).

Because patients are at high risk, the distinction between skill evaluation and patient evaluation often blurs in emergency medicine. In newborn intensive care, a judgment error based on the choice of an incorrect treatment approach (Bosk, 1979:45–51) can happen first in the delivery room, for example, when an infant born dying is referred to the Level III nursery. Then n.i.c.u. physicians have to do the best they can and be prepared to fail. As the population of patients expands to include new categories of even more serious complications of prematurity and illness, the evaluation of performance and outcome becomes even more problematic: was the therapy wrong or the case hopeless? Exoneration, relief from blame, frequently comes into play when treatment is mishandled; a physician is defended as having done everything possible "under the circumstances."

As a good example of this, a resident at Northeast Pediatric, Dr. Frank, was on night duty in charge of an infant weighing less than 500 grams who had survived for a week. The previous night another resident had noticed respiratory problems and had "pinked the baby up" by increasing the oxygen flow in the respirator. On this particular evening, however, Dr. Frank interpreted the infant's trouble in breathing as a possible blocked endotracheal tube. He repeatedly attempted to insert a new tube, but failed. The infant died. At morning rounds, Dr. Frank explained what happened:

> It's gory. He looked bad, crappy. I pulled the tube about 10 p.m. Thought it might be blocked. I tried to put a tube in. Twice it looked [as if it was] in, but I couldn't hear any breath sounds. No breath sounds. Bagged. Transilluminated—right pneumothorax. We pulled out air.

At this point, the attending physician, Dr. Cartwright, cut short discussion of the case and after rounds had a private conference with Dr. Frank. Then, the resident recounted in detail what had happened:

> *Dr. Frank:* "The baby looked terrible. He had a tiny tube. All day people had said we should replace it with a bigger tube. I went to intubate it. I intubated three times. Each time it would go in, but I wouldn't hear any air move. I called [a senior physician in pediatrics]. My guess was I had gone in too far. And I probably punctured [a lung]. There was a big pneumothorax and we just couldn't do anything. For a good five to ten minutes the baby was being bagged and was stable before he crumped [deteriorated]."
>
> *Dr. Cartwright:* "Did you see it [the tube] go through the cords?"
>
> *Dr. Frank:* "Yes, I was able to."
>
> *Dr. Cartwright:* "If you go just one centimeter past the cords, that's enough."
>
> *Dr. Frank:* "The mistake was I should have put a needle in [the chest]."

For the rest of the conference, Dr. Cartwright, without admonishing Dr. Frank, went over the techniques of intubation, asked about Dr. Frank's calling in a senior physician (not on the unit), and defended the expertise of the night nurses, which Dr. Frank had questioned.

Two corrective priorities were revealed in this incident. One (impersonal) was to improve technical skills; the other was to improve relations with backup personnel. The first priority was expressed in a brief conversation between the unit director, Dr. Karp, and Dr. Cartwright at a pause during rounds:

> *Dr. Karp:* "I'm sorry about the Brock baby."
> *Dr. Cartwright:* "To last that long is an achievement."
> *Dr. Karp:* "To last that long and then to have a mechanical problem— that's not too much of an achievement. But it will tell us a little bit about how to handle the next one."

The second priority, relating to backup personnel, balances the purely technical corrections. Faced with difficult medical problems or a combination of medical and social dilemmas, the organizational reflex of the n.i.c.u. is to poll the reactions of the team immediately involved and then act. Senior physicians and the full-time nursing staff were the mainstay of this consensus process. Their framework for evaluation was normative experience—"the way we do it here"— rather than formal guidelines.

Dr. Frank's disregard of this review process resulted in his receiving more criticism than would be expected just for his lack of skill in intubation. He did not confer with the night nurses about pulling the endotracheal tube and yet expected them to give wholehearted support to his unilateral decision to re-intubate. He was also criticized by another resident and several nurses for not telephoning the fellow on call, Dr. Braun, who was known for his special skill in intubating extremely small neonates, and for not calling the n.i.c.u. attending physician. To refer again to Bosk's (1979:51) taxonomy of errors in medical decision making, Dr. Frank's real mistakes were normative, that "conduct [which] violates the working understandings on which action rests." Thus, when a normative error occurs, "the mistake renders it impossible to consider the person making it—in legal terms—a just and reasonably prudent individual." So it went for Dr. Frank, specifically in relation to the nursing staff. Less than ten days after the failed re-intubation, Dr. Frank found himself on night duty handling another emergency case. This time he claimed to have "polled" the night nurses about his decision to isolate an infant with severe infection, but the nurses who came on duty in the morning were unanimously convinced that he had acted uncooperatively and was insensitive to the nurses' input.

The interplay between correctable technical skills and the "safety catch" of group review is also evident in the routine maintenance of life support systems, and especially in the gradual withdrawal of these supports as newborns grow healthy. Attending physicians defined the unit policy for oxygen maintenance, feeding, and other routine treatments. N.i.c.u. fellows reinforced this overall policy. The work of residents and nurses in the n.i.c.u. more frequently involved fine-tuning of the support system than emergency interventions, such as Dr. Frank's.

There are, of course, gray areas in which policy does not carry. Very small neonates should not be given oral feedings, but as they get bigger, the question of withdrawing the intravenous line must be discussed. Sometimes the line is drawn too soon and, because an infant cannot tolerate oral feedings, the intravenous line has to be replaced. If made cooperatively, changes in treatment that were followed by setbacks in the infant's condition were perceived as medical problems, but they were not moral problems. Over time, the course of patient treatment might be changed, reversed, and exhibit inconsistencies as the composition of the staff and the infant's responses varied. As long as decisions were subject to daily collective review, with an individual physician or nurse taking no undiscussed unilateral action, the atmosphere surrounding patient care was relatively untroubled. The participation of junior physicians and nurses in treatment discussions satisfied the democratic ethos of the group but had little substantive impact on treatment policy.

When serious errors of judgment were made, as happened infrequently and almost always on transport and night duty, they were immediately made public within the sphere of the unit. The reaction of the other staff members was, again, to exonerate the physician or nurse, provided the error was admitted and the one who made the mistake indicated a learn-from-experience attitude. Group reaction was more favorable if individuals collectively reviewed their decisions. In Dr. Frank's case, his admission of having perhaps misjudged the need for re-intubation was made only to the attending physician. To the rest of the staff, he maintained, "In other places they wouldn't even try to treat an infant that small." Factually, he was perhaps right, but his defensive attitude did not reassure other residents or the nurses that he would not make the same mistake of unilateral action in the future.

It is questionable that n.i.c.u. physicians need to fear extreme punitive sanctions, such as expulsion from the team. Service expansion dictates an increased need for personnel, and the difficulty of the work makes senior physicians grateful to get and keep new recruits. For example, several core members of the nursing staff assumed that Dr. Frank would not be given the chance of another rotation in the n.i.c.u. Dr. Frank's superiors proved less pessimistic about his educability and accepted him back six weeks later.

Even daily collective review cannot prevent medical mistakes. Turnover in n.i.c.u. personnel makes it difficult to pinpoint who was at fault or correct mistakes except by reference to abstract standards or policy.

At one point, the Northeast Pediatric unit staff discovered that a certain test, which should have been done soon after birth, had not been given to a very premature infant. Signs of cretinism became evident and a late test for thyroid dysfunction proved positive. The problem with the error was that treatment to minimize the symptoms was begun later than it could have been. The infant, born weighing 710 grams, already had multiple anomalies and pathologies that the unit had addressed efficiently, but a major problem had been missed. For this mistake, there was no collective remedial action or exoneration, since the actual staff team responsible for the mistake had dispersed weeks before. The residents had gone on to different rotations, the fellow had changed, and there had been turnover in the nursing staff. The n.i.c.u. staff who made the discovery were stunned and embarrassed. A nurse, in retrospect, described what happened:

> *Nurse:* "For two months they [the parents] thought she was okay, just a preemie. We thought so too. Then we found out. We picked it up from PKU [phenylketonuria test]—it should have been done earlier. We missed it. So she missed getting medication. [The secretary-receptionist] went through the record and said it's missing. Oh, yeah, we'll do it now. Now we have new standards."
>
> *Consulting physician:* "Once you get burned, you change."

The breakdown that this particular mistake represented was in the area of diagnosis, where few mistakes ever occurred because the unit at Northeast Pediatric invested heavily in testing. It was not uncommon for infants to undergo x-ray tests five or six times per day and to have blood gas levels determined several times per shift. Ultrasound tests and computerized axial tomographic (CAT) scans were made less frequently but were still routine. The reaction to the error of the overlooked test—to create new standards that would make the early screening of premature infants for phenylketonuria (PKU) routine—was totally in keeping with the high value put on precautionary measures. Yet the move to tighten standards circumvented broader problems, such as responsibility for the child's long-term physical development and the parents' reactions to the condition of their child. The staff grew ambivalent toward continued n.i.c.u. treatment for this difficult infant (a living reminder of an error), but also felt obliged to continue treatment. As one nurse put it, this baby would "be here as long as the pyramids." In fact, the infant spent three months in the Level III nursery and was discharged to a Level II unit for further care. Her parents were told that she had multiple problems, which was true, but they were not informed that the most serious of them, cretinism, might have been avoided.

LEARNING ABOUT PHYSICIAN–FAMILY RELATIONS

The emergency atmosphere surrounding each admission to the n.i.c.u. makes it virtually impossible for the staff to attend simultaneously to clinical problems and family reactions. At what time, then, in the history of a case does the resident address an infant's parents? At Northeast Pediatric, the informal orientation of the new residents by the attending physician included no suggestions about how to structure relations with parents. Rather, residents followed the lead of the nurses, who took the initiative to contact parents and who felt responsible for prodding the residents in the same direction. Some residents clearly enjoyed communicating with parents; however, only one of the twelve we knew best made the blanket statement that "talking with parents is the best part of this work."

For the most part, residents could count on the nurses to handle daily communications with parents. The responsibility for maintaining relations with the family was part of nursing ideology and the majority of parents' phone calls and visits were handled by the nursing staff. The nurses shielded the residents from contact with families. On night duty, for example, the nurses would answer calls while the resident slept, so that he or she would be fresh and rested in case of an emergency.

THE CRITICAL STANCE

In his study of residents in a pediatric intensive care unit, Frader (1979) describes a two-step process whereby, having mastered mechanical devices, monitors, and technical procedures, the attention of young physicians shifts to emotional and philosophic issues. In the two sets of novice residents we observed, this shift to abstract issues never happened. The pressure to be clinically adept was on them until the last day of their service, and there had been virtually no break in their work schedules to allow formal reflection on either their feelings or ethics. The more experienced third-year residents, though, had achieved a degree of professional detachment. They became capable of the kind of medical generalizations in which the attending physicians had schooled them, not psychological or moral statements. The senior resident was often an able critic and could afford to be, since she or he was at the point of departing from specialty training.

Service in newborn intensive care, if it consistently shuts out consideration of the parents' perspective and problems of long-term outcome for patients, can curtail the resident's learning about the larger, more disorderly, and yet, perhaps to him or her, more professionally gratifying world of community practice. The dilemma for the trainee is a classic one for professionals: to acquire a high level of peer-defined expertise (being a lawyer who is "all case and no cause," "an actor's actor," or "a physician's physician") or to meet the more broadly defined needs of clients. Many pediatricians opt for community practice. One third-year resident envisioned a time in the future when he would do just that:

> Then I'll be on the other end of all this [he nodded toward the area where the sickest infants were]. I'll know all about the worst things that can happen and I'll be able to understand what a hospital like this offers. But I won't have to deal with the worst cases every day and every night. No thanks.

On the other hand, in an elite pediatric program in which senior physicians emphasize the value of clinical skills, residents might just as easily identify with a more narrow definition of professional work. For example, a second-year resident commented on how the maternity hospital affiliated with Northeast Pediatric divided labor among house officers:

> Dr. Lee said that, at Women's Hospital, the new residents do the interesting case work, while the junior and senior residents do what she called "scut work": admissions, obtaining social information about parents, and handling minor (not seriously ill) cases and a greater range of cases. The first-year residents get to concentrate, to work slowly on more difficult cases, and this Dr. Lee found enviable.

Senior residents were more confrontational about the neonatologists' clinical approach. In the following exchange, Dr. Reilly, a senior resident, questions the decision to put an infant back on antibiotics.

Dr. Reilly: "Why was she put back on the same antibiotics? I feel comfortable without antibiotics. This is just the nature of the reflex we're developing in taking care of this kid. It's just the neonatologists' view of antibiotics."

Dr. Richmond: "But you haven't seen how fast kids die—they can go in an hour."

Dr. Reilly: "This kid has never seen anything without antibiotics."

Dr. Richmond: "So what's another few days?" (The group laughed.) "You have a kid next door [in the next bed] with gent-resistant organisms."

Dr. Cartwright (attending physician): "[Dr. Richmond] is right. Ninety-nine percent of the time one or two of those things you look for [in the culture] will be suspicious."

Dr. Reilly: "My point is that this is a reflex, not a judgment."

The decision was made to maintain the infant on antibiotics, as a precaution.

More broad criticisms of neonatology and the service were rare. In the following exchange among two senior residents, a visiting medical student, and a young consultant, Dr. Crow, it is the consultant who takes the critic's role regarding heroic support of severely brain-damaged infants:

Dr. Reilly: "Yeah, we're being underwritten by [a large school for the mentally handicapped]. But [Dr. Simmons] is very optimistic about the IVH [intraventricular hemorrhage] outcome."

Dr. Crow: "They'll be gorks for the rest of their lives."

Dr. Reilly: "I suppose we should shut [the support] off."

Medical student: "How many of those kids will make it to [elite] Medical School?"

Dr. Reilly: "Actually 100 percent. That's how we supply the house staff. But [Dr. Simmons] is optimistic about them."

Dr. Crow: "They're trying new things and the guinea pigs are the parents."

Dr. Zeld: "I know the kid will have a lot of problems two or three years down the line, but we go ahead."

Dr. Crow: "I hate to be a part of it. I rush intralipids to a kid so he won't die of starvation. Each specialty pushes the frontier back but the squash men [neurosurgeons] are in the worst trouble."

The ability of members of the n.i.c.u. team to be reflective and critical about medical care was greatly restricted by the level of commitment necessary just to perform competently in that high-pressure setting. Many pediatric residents will never work in an intensive care unit again or even in a large centralized hospital. Even among fellows in neonatology, there is a new generation of private practitioners who consult for multiple hospitals and therefore escape the continuous strain of newborn intensive care.

In the next chapter, we look at the nursing staff that functions in this same demanding environment. As skilled n.i.c.u. nurses seek a professional life distinct from the physicians' model, they confront the most difficult problems of integrating the technical with the social dimensions of newborn intensive care.

2

The N.I.C.U. Nurses

It's been fascinating to take nursing from a job to a profession.
N.I.C.U. Nursing Coordinator

Nurses talk about "liking." They like a patient or a parent. Or they don't like them. That's not what physicians do. We stick to facts.
Neonatology Fellow

In the newborn intensive care nursery, two sets of professionals, the physicians and the nurses, determine the caliber of patient care. While senior physicians set the standards for n.i.c.u. treatment, nurses play a major protective role in monitoring each newborn's medical condition. Directly or indirectly, nurses can also promote a social perspective on difficult clinical decisions, in contrast to the purely analytic approach of medicine.

THE DIVISION OF HOSPITAL LABOR

Every occupation, Everett Hughes observed, has "a *mandate* to define what is proper conduct of others toward the matters concerned with their work." In the case of the physician, the mandate may "include a successful claim to supervise and determine the conditions of work of many kinds of people; in this case, nurses, technicians and the many others involved in maintaining the modern medical establishment" (Hughes, 1958:78).

The roles of physician and nurse complement each other, but often imperfectly:

> There will probably always be in this system . . . someone whose role it is to make ultimate decisions. . . . This is the role of the physician. He has and jealously guards more authority than he can, in many cases, actually assume. There will probably always be in the system, complementary to this position, another of the right-hand-man order; a position which defers to the first but which, informally, often must exceed its authority in order to protect the interests of all concerned. The nurse occupies this position. (Hughes, 1984:308)

This directly subordinate relationship to physicians was not always characteristic of the nurse's role. Prior to the development of modern nursing, women in religious nursing orders worked in hospitals and answered to an ecclesiastical superior; at times, they even flouted physicians' directives (Freidson, 1970). Ironically, Florence Nightingale's pioneering work in the Crimean War both raised the status of nursing and historically curtailed its autonomy. Initially rebuffed by the military physicians, Nightingale responded by requiring all her nurses to give service only when requested by doctors.

> Nightingale thus required that what the nurse did for the patient was a function of what the doctor felt was required . . . All nursing work flowed from the doctor's orders, and thus nursing became a formal part of the doctor's work, . . . *Nursing thus was defined as a subordinate part of the technical division of labor surrounding medicine.* (Freidson, 1970:61)

Although nursing attained dignity by associating itself with medicine, this association erected barriers to nurses' finding a position independent of medicine. Today, the relationship is especially problematic within the hospital because it is here that it is most difficult to escape the structural subordination of nursing to medicine (Glaser, 1966; Freidson, 1970; Fitzpatrick, 1977; Aiken, 1983). Leaders in nursing have correctly perceived that small clinics and community health care centers offer nurses more autonomy. Hospital work offers opportunities related to new technologies but can discourage the professionally aspiring nurse.

> [Nurses take] prestige where it is most obviously and easily gotten, namely from the technical and life-and-death tasks. . . . Thus, dependence on the medical profession threatens the policies of the aspirants for independent professional status while it serves the interests of the rank and file. (Glaser, 1966:27)

Neonatal intensive care, like intensive care in general, is affected by this dilemma and thus presents a paradox for nurses seeking recognition as professionals in their own right. On the one hand, the high technology of the specialty lets n.i.c.u. nurses take on additional technical tasks and thereby advance their status. On the other hand, the technology of intensive care is centralized in physician-dominated hospitals, thus limiting the nurses' decision-making autonomy.

The same dilemma holds for organizational skills. The administrative complexity of the newborn referral system has created new positions for nurses, for example, the n.i.c.u. nurse-manager, who coordinates relations between the professional staff and the hospital administration and also is on the lookout for internal conflict between team members (Gribbins and Marshall, 1984). These new managerial roles, however, remain subordinate to the authority of physicians. The role of the n.i.c.u. nurse reflects the heightened clinical, research, and administrative responsibilities of neonatologists without changing the conventional hierarchy.

The neonatal units we observed varied in the clinical skills and administrative responsibilities of the nurses. Northeast Pediatric was at the high end of the continuum in both regards. The nurses used complex clinical skills; for example, they resuscitated infants in emergencies (assisted their breathing manually with a bag and mask), dealt independently with doing blood gas tests and with minor changes in oxygen levels, and participated in team resuscitation efforts. Several nurses in the unit were permitted, on the basis of experience and training, to start intravenous feedings and insert other lines.

The Northeast Pediatric n.i.c.u. nurses were organizational innovators who had adopted a participatory management or team approach, combined with primary nursing, to structure their responsibilities. This eliminated the traditional nurse-supervisor role in favor of a more democratic group model. The nurses had in their favor the relatively small size of the unit (fewer than twenty beds) and consequently of the nursing staff (approximately thirty nurses) to facilitate the sharing of responsibilities. Most important, they had the steady support of the unit's physician-director, who understood the fundamental reliance of the unit on the nursing staff. Every Level III unit tries to meet the governmental and professional guidelines for a 3:1 patient-to-nurse ratio. This labor-intensive characteristic of the n.i.c.u. was acknowledged by a Northeast Pediatric attending physician:

> The nurses really do the care. I talk a lot, but the nurses give the care. If a bus ran over me, the unit would still run. But if it ran over all the nurses, we'd have to shut down.

More than did the residents, who circulated through the unit on rotation, the senior physicians relied on the stability, skills, and high morale of the nursing staff. The Northeast Pediatric n.i.c.u. nurses used their impressive skills, innovative organization, and strong camaraderie to argue for greater professional recognition. Their hope was to increase both their technical skills and their part in decision making, and they were insistent that their achievements be acknowledged. However, treatment decisions remained firmly in the hands of physicians. There were barriers to autonomy that the n.i.c.u. nurses at Northeast Pediatric could not overcome.

PARTICIPATORY MANAGEMENT

Nurses in the Northeast Pediatric n.i.c.u. instituted an innovative organizational model of "participatory management" that included, in the nurses' language, primary nursing, peer review, and staff development. The nursing coordinator who instituted this new organizational structure described its explicitly professional goals:

> The basic assumption is that nurses are professional and they do want to monitor the quality of the care. It's been fascinating to take nursing from a job to a profession. I wanted to see if those theories we learned in school could work. I took it as a challenge. . . . It took one year to get the new approach in place and then six months of polishing. [The nurses] wouldn't live now without primary nursing. They wouldn't live now without peer review.

Authority, division of labor, and professional rewards were the three key issues addressed by the new model.

Authority in the Collectivity

In collectivist organizations, the goal is to abolish the pyramid of authority and to forgo administrative hierarchy (Bernstein, 1980). There is a consensus process to formulate problems collectively and to negotiate decisions. "All major policy issues, such as hiring, firing, salaries, the division of labor, the distribution of surplus, and the shape of the final product or service, are decided by the collective as a whole" (Rothschild-Whitt, 1979:512). Decisions made by this process have the backing of the moral authority of the group.

The n.i.c.u. nurses at Northeast Pediatric defined their group as the source of nursing authority and held numerous meetings to arrive at a consensus about group problems. However, they did not meet as a group on every issue. The nursing coordinator explained:

> Participatory management, democracy, and laissez-faire: In the beginning the staff had some confusion between these three concepts. They had to realize that not every decision would be made at a meeting of everybody. And they had to realize that it did not mean everyone does their own thing à la laissez-faire.

Setting goals was important, and although the aims were defined by the members, the coordinator took an active part in orchestrating these aspirations during the organizational transformation:

> I sat and talked with each [nurse] for forty-five minutes and said, "It's your unit. Where do you see it and you going?" Then I put it all together like a patchwork. What they really needed was a plan.

Peer review, nurses' evaluation of each others' performances, was an important group activity in the new model, raising the question of whether professional groups can police themselves. The intent of peer review was to monitor quality, and the nursing coordinator explained how the nurses gained experience with the procedure:

> What happens when you start participatory management? In peer review, people start by saying the positive. They learn to use it for various reasons—termination, raises, problem solving.

Peer review included confrontation about professional shortcomings, which can be a delicate matter. The coordinator mentioned that the physician in charge of the unit had quite candidly said to her, "I'd be scared if I had to go through it."

The nursing staff thus instituted a forum for evaluation and enforced sanctions lacking in the formal and informal training of residents. Nursing peer review could lead to such sanctions as unfavorable schedule changes, work-time reductions, and shifts in responsibility to the point where the individual nurse was partially or completely expelled. For example, one nurse, Tina, raised the subject in the unit of why another nurse, Sarah, would be called before the rest of the nurses to bring her in line:

> Sarah's fooled a lot of people, but no more. She sits here and smokes cigarettes and complains about how tired she is. The real problem is that she doesn't want to take patients. She doesn't even want to teach the trainee nurse.

Three nurses sat in the middle of the nursery talking this over. The conversation continued, with one of the nurses saying:

> Sarah is not paying attention while the trainees re-intubate. She just lets them do what they feel like doing. Even if everyone tells you you're good, you've got to keep your feet on the ground and pay attention.

A peer review meeting was held within a few days regarding Sarah. Later, the outcome was explained to a nurse who had not been present:

> *Tina:* "The upshot is Sarah won't be taking trainees anymore."
> *Meredith:* "Was that her choice or the group's?"
> *Tina:* "Both."

The sanctions against Sarah were to relieve her of responsibilities and authority in work. The nurses most committed to their work did not appear to be sensitive to nurses like Sarah who complained of tiredness or burnout. They expected an "up" and even stoical attitude toward work. In short, they were committed careerists who identified with the professional attitude of senior physicians.

The idea behind peer review was not only that performance evaluation be done, but that the evaluation be done by colleagues, that is, by nurses rather than by physicians. The nursing coordinator emphasized this autonomy:

> One physician wanted to come because he wanted to say to a nurse what a good job she had done. The group said no—because now he wants to do something nice, but that opens the way for criticism in the future. The physician was told to talk to the nurse privately.

Such collegial feedback occurred in other ways too, not only at peer review. Nursing rounds were held, typically when the physicians left the unit to review x-ray films. The nurses met as a group in the nursery, discussed cases, and listened to each other's care plans. Also, at the change of shift, departing nurses were careful to brief the nurses coming on duty.

Hiring was another important group activity in the nursing collectivity. New recruits were taught the following ideology:

> When we interview we tell all this [information about how we work] to people—let me tell you what you're in for if you come here. . . . We have an orientation for new people joining.

Hiring a new nursing coordinator was a key test point for this innovative structure, and it was required about six months into our fieldwork. The coordinator who had instituted participatory management decided to leave for another job, and her replacement had to be found.

The criteria for choosing the new coordinator were well specified and the standards were high. As the departing incumbent noted:

> The nurses have clear criteria for what they want: master's preparation, maternal and child health expertise; someone with political savvy; one of the key things—participatory management; and research skills.

The collective delegated authority for part of the process to a search committee of six nurses. This committee was deliberately composed of different kinds of n.i.c.u. nurses—for example, some who had been in the unit a long time and some who had been there only a short time—to get a variety of perspectives. The position was advertised and word-of-mouth also was used to publicize the job. If the search committee was serious about a candidate, the unit director, a physician, would also interview the person; in addition, people higher in the hospital administration had to approve any appointment. This hiring protocol is significant in that the nurses were partially autonomous. They were the gatekeepers to the position, but the unit director judged candidates in whom the search committee took an interest. The job of coordinator eventually went to a nurse from within the unit (the interim coordinator) rather than to an outside candidate.

The nursing group did not resolve all the issues with which it dealt. Some topics, notably commitment and scheduling, led to recurrent tiffs on the floor:

> *Tina:* "You part-time people piss me off. You act as if you're doing us a favor. You get paid for your work."
>
> *Margot:* "I hate to raise this subject. I've worked holidays for the last five years. I can go and work where I won't be hassled."
>
> *Tina:* "What do you mean, hassled?"
>
> *Margot:* "When I raise this question of working holidays Leslie gets really worked up. She says, 'We have this policy.' "

Minimal Division of Labor

In contrast to bureaucracies with their specialized experts, collectivist organizations minimize the division of labor. Three mechanisms are often used to decrease differentiation: role rotation, task sharing, and internal education to demystify esoteric knowledge (Rothschild-Whitt, 1979:517).

The n.i.c.u. nurses at Northeast Pediatric utilized all three of these mechanisms to minimize the division of labor. Task sharing occurred at two levels. First, all staff nurses performed bedside care. (The coordinator, the exception to this rule, was seldom involved in patient care.) Second, the staff nurses participated in their own administration. A major component of participatory management was the idea that there would be a nursing coordinator—a resource person—not an "old-fashioned head nurse." When the first coordinator agreed to institute the new model, one condition she set was that the staff would have to agree to do fifty percent of its own management (for example, budgeting).

This administrative upgrading of the staff nurses' skills and de-mystification of administrative knowledge had an effect on how the nurses saw themselves. The coordinator commented:

> Without a charge nurse, people have to solve their own problems. They take it very seriously. They're harder on themselves than I ever would be.

This upgrading also led to the possibility of role rotation for some administrative tasks. An important example, that of being the representative to the hospital at large, occurred at the time the first co-ordinator was departing. A staff nurse described the situation:

> The in-unit care will work fine even without a replacement—that's what happened before when the job was open. But what we missed out on before was getting information from other meetings and groups because we no longer had a person to represent us. . . . That problem is some-what solved this time around because we have several different nurses who do go to outside things. We like having several—we're not so de-pendent on one, and also it's a way of saying to outsiders that any nurse is capable of being the representative.

Incentive Structure: Primary Nursing

Collectivist organizations rely more on ideological than on material incentives (Rothschild-Whitt, 1979). A related point is that such organizations give people much more control over their work and therefore it is more gratifying.

Primary nursing was an important expression of the nurses' ideology concerning commitment to patients. In contrast to primary care, which is associated with small health centers and allows a diversity of health professionals to initially assess a patient's condition, "primary" as a term applied to hospital nurses or physicians indicates their taking first-order responsibility for a patient (Marram et al., 1976:2). The primary nurse in the n.i.c.u., therefore, takes principal responsibility for the nursing care of a newborn. As the nursing co-ordinator explained:

> We do primary nursing here. Marie Manthey of Minnesota—she concep-tualized it. It is one nurse being responsible for the total family unit. . . . We don't assign a primary nurse. We let, in the first twelve hours [after admission] a nurse take on a baby. That way the nurse picks a baby that, for some reason, appeals to her. . . . Anyone who feels ready to be a

primary nurse makes that commitment. The primary nurse has twenty-four-hour responsibility.

This identification with and responsibility for particular cases generated a great deal of commitment to the unit's work, allowing nurses to exercise case ownership parallel to that of the residents, but with greater continuity over time and a higher investment in family issues. Staff nurses came in on their days off if their cases demanded extra attention or if there were group meetings. A primary nurse, even if not on duty, might be called at home, for example, if the condition of her patient was deteriorating. The coordinator noted another aspect of this commitment:

> When the primary nurse's name is on the isolette, her craving for knowledge goes up—the applications for library cards go up.

Primary nursing with its twenty-four-hour concern (although not physical presence) can diminish the alienating aspects of shift work. N.i.c.u. patients require twenty-four-hour coverage. Continuous coverage, by definition, means shift work (Melbin, 1978). It also means staff interchangeability, and impersonalization. "One of the most significant consequences of the impersonalization of coverage in the hospital is the obvious decrease in individual staff members' *personal* responsibility for, and commitment to, patients" (Zerubavel, 1979:44). Primary nursing can counteract this trend and increase both personal responsibility for and commitment to patients. Its advantage for the n.i.c.u. patient, in comparison to the primary physician role of the resident, is that nurses are potentially a stable source of care.

Primary nursing at Northeast Pediatric was believed to contribute to the high morale of the nurses. The nurses who remained in the unit displayed a spirited camaraderie and solidarity. When asked if this tone was typical of nursing elsewhere, one nurse replied, "I've worked at five other places, but have never found such good spirit as here."

Education as a Vehicle for Increasing Status

The collectivist and egalitarian structure of the nursing staff did not rule out nurses' educational aspirations and the acquisition of specialized skills. Although the participatory management model tended to demystify expert knowledge and minimize the division of labor within the group, it encouraged nurses to improve their status both as individuals and as a group. The collectivity, for example, encouraged specialized training. Education was perceived as a way to improve professional standing and as a way to participate more in unit decision making and to assume new responsibilities. The coordinator explained:

> The nurses found they needed more knowledge to challenge the physician. The physician will say article X says such and such. Nurses have to learn to ask, "Is that an animal study? How many were in that study?"

The implication that nurses engaged in academic debate with physicians overstates the actual situation. Nevertheless, in nurse–physician interactions, the nurses' knowledge of clinical issues enabled them to participate in case discussions. The core group of nurses pursued knowledge both formally (in school) and informally (acquiring new skills on the job). One outsider labeled them "hotshot nurses," while a sympathetic medical consultant observed that "the pressure on them is to become like a 'mini-intern.' "

THE SUPPORTIVE ROLE OF N.I.C.U. NURSES

Despite the efforts of n.i.c.u. nurses at Northeast Pediatric to expand their professional domain, the great majority of their work consisted of doing things that physicians were reluctant to do. Everett Hughes (1984:307) noted that, in medicine, responsibility for tasks shifts from physician to nurse, simultaneously upgrading nursing and downgrading the tasks. In freeing physicians to concentrate on the central clinical problems, nurses assumed a wide range of responsibilities. These include patient surveillance, routine administrative chores, social work, unit "dirty work" (especially related to dying and death), as well as diffuse emotional tasks. The first two of these responsibilities, keeping a close watch on patients and helping the unit function smoothly, earned the nurses credit as trustworthy and rational co-workers. Physicians considered the other tasks peripheral and less essential to good patient care, possibly because the nurses were effective in distancing their medical superiors from these nonmedical problems.

Surveillance

Feeding and oxygen administration decisions, both crucial to the intensive care patient's survival, are ultimately the physician's decisions. But the task of implementing n.i.c.u. feeding and oxygen surveillance is continual and tedious. Feeding a sick, premature infant is often a frustrating, tedious task, and nurses' time, not physicians', is used to accomplish it. Nurses attend repeatedly, throughout the day and night, to feeding (whether intravenous, gavage, or bottle) and to other chores related to the gastrointestinal system (cleaning up vomit and feces, measuring and recording weight gain or loss). N.i.c.u. nurses also exercise twenty-four-hour surveillance of respirators, checking their efficiency and infants' responses. Especially at night, when the resident is asleep, nurses have considerable autonomy to take diagnostic blood gas tests and alter oxygen settings in accordance with the current treatment plan. Like other nighttime hospital employees who are less closely supervised, n.i.c.u. nurses on night duty can assume decision-making prerogatives that during the day are reserved for residents. This amplified discretion extends to emergency situations when physicians are not immediately available. Unit nurses can initiate emergency respiratory support until a physician reaches bedside. Or they can make provisional clinical responses to changes in infants' blood gas levels or other tests, for example, by changing oxygen levels.

Surveillance goes beyond simple observation of the infants. More than physicians, the n.i.c.u. nurses physically handled their patients. This hands-on contact began with a nurse's responsibility to set up a newly transported infant in an isolette, with the appropriate monitors and machinery. Surveillance extended to routine chest-tapping (physical therapy to stimulate an infant's lungs) and suctioning of mucus from an infant's throat, taking blood samples, caring for lines, open wounds, lesions, or burns, and generally keeping the infant clean and comfortable.

On occasion, nurses felt compelled to defend the clinical contribution that their watchfulness represented. For example, one day a nurse was openly contemptuous of a resident who wanted an expensive test for possible infection. The group, including nurses, resisted his suggestion:

> *Resident:* "Under a kilo-[gram] I do it because if one misses an infection, it's so serious."
> *Nurse* (with great hostility): "We [the nurses] are here to watch. We're the consistent caregivers."

Both the importance and the limits of the nurses' clinical contributions were revealed in morning rounds. The nurses participated in these discussions, but the topics the nurses most often commented upon at these rounds were surveillance (feeding, oxygen therapy management, observations of the baby's condition), family issues, and discharge. Conspicuous by their absence were nurses' comments on such topics as whether surgery should be done.

At times, n.i.c.u. nurses went beyond their own limited technical responsibilities. If done competently, such initiatives might be helpful, especially to a resident. This competence was gratefully acknowledged by the resident, but often with humor or sarcasm.

> During the morning rounds the resident made a special point of telling the attending physician how helpful it was to have had a nurse put the intravenous line in the baby. One baby needed something, another baby needed something else, and it was helpful that the nurse had taken care of the intravenous line in this case. He then laughed and said something to the effect, "Don't tell her I said so."

Another morning at rounds, a resident commented on her own frustration in trying to get a line in and reported the nurse's help at doing what she, the physician, had difficulty doing. "The baby started having blue toes and a radial line was placed by one of our illustrious nurses (laugh)." The humor reveals the tension surrounding the crossing of an occupational boundary.

Routine Administration

A referral system, especially if regionalized, requires that neonatologists and nurses both pay attention to administrative details. N.i.c.u. nurses at Northeast Pediatric were accurate judges of available bed space and often assumed the responsibility of telling referring hospitals whether to proceed with a transport or not. This was not a decision involving clinical criteria, about which nurses had nothing to say, but only about bed space.

Once an infant was admitted, the nursing staff was diligent about recording daily progress notes on the patient's clinical condition (as judged by physicians), the treatment plan (again as determined by physicians), and brief notes about the infant's parents (as the nurse saw them). In contrast, residents uniformly grumbled about filling out reports and doing other paperwork—orders for medication, for plasma, and for diagnostic appointments, and death certificates—and occasionally did them wrong or not at all. What the residents saw as "scut work," the nurses perceived as an opportunity to take on managerial authority.

The smooth functioning of the unit as an organizational enterprise meant a lot to the Northeast Pediatric nurses, and bureaucratic needs at times were seen as more important than those of patients (Murphy, 1983). The nurses espoused the goal of efficiency as strongly as did the attending physicians. Perhaps more than the senior physicians, who were relatively removed from daily patient care, the nursing staff wanted the flow of patients to be consistent, fast, and with good results. They were frustrated by long-term cases and by the sudden deaths of newly transported babies; neither circumstance allowed the nurses to work well and see immediate results. They handled the details of patient discharge and were sometimes impatient to move an infant out to an intermediate-level nursery in the community; physicians were consistently more cautious regarding discharge.

Social Work Techniques

The nurses at Northeast Pediatric regarded themselves as better family specialists than physicians and were proud of it. One nurse advised us, "You shouldn't consider the doctors as the experts on the family."

The nurses were generally supportive listeners for parents, as any sympathetic lay person might be. In addition, their nursing school education made them knowledgeable about various approaches (e.g., crisis intervention, parental bonding, grieving stages) to working with distressed families. There was some competition between nurses and social workers in this regard. The nurses, although less knowledgeable and less practiced than social workers, nevertheless had mastered the vocabulary of social work. They sometimes used suggestions from social workers or psychiatrists in their approach with families, for example, in dealing with parents in crisis, encouraging family visiting, and in presenting information to parents. Physicians of all ranks were much more reluctant than nurses to interact with parents and relied on the nursing staff for information about the family.

Expressive Tasks: Nurses as Parent Surrogates

Instrumental (task-oriented) and expressive (socioemotional) roles have been a recurrent theme in sociological theory. The traditional view holds that such roles tend to be mutually exclusive, resulting in specialists for each (Parsons and Bales, 1955). Other writers have observed that some roles combine both types of tasks (Slater, 1961). Davis (1966) found the coexistence of instrumental and expressive tasks in the role of the hospital nurse to be one of the interesting paradoxes of this occupational group.

Neonatal intensive care nurses, as noted previously, perform highly technical procedures. But even technically trained, modern-day nurses are influenced by the history of nursing in which the mother-surrogate role was so important. In a Northeast Pediatric brochure on participatory management and primary nursing, this nurturant role was linked to bonding:

> [Stress for the infant], together with the partial to total absence of the parental figures to buffer the environment, necessitates the presence of a substitute maternal figure—the nurse. A recent study has suggested that primary nursing may act to reinforce the nurse/infant bond, permitting the nurse to instinctually respond to the infant's needs with precise timing.

Substitute parenting of newborns is part of n.i.c.u. work. At Northeast Pediatric, the nurses talked lovingly even to the sickest and least alert infants. They held them and walked around with them in the crook of their arm when the infants were well enough. In general, the n.i.c.u. nurses filled in for absent or disaffected parents.

Nurses' parenting behavior was highlighted in one dramatic case. The newborn did well physically in the unit but still had a modest, correctable limb deformity. The parents, especially the father, rejected the infant and they planned to put him up for adoption. The infant's plight was accentuated in the nurses' view because he was practically perfect compared with the other n.i.c.u. patients. One nurse carried the infant around, saying, "I'm going to take him home." Another nurse bought the baby clothes. She said, "You get kind of attached to the babies; all the other babies had clothes, so I bought him some." Still another nurse, who had had difficulty becoming pregnant, considered adopting the infant herself.

In contrast, it was rare to see a physician—male or female—holding or caressing an infant. Only one physician we observed, a resident, revealed pleasure in touching, holding, or interacting with the newborns as human beings. In general, the neonatologist's role is instrumental, whereas the nurse's role is both instrumental and expressive. In the view of at least some physicians, this expressive component made the nursing staff seem less rational than physicians and more liable to let subjective factors enter into their judgments. As a neonatology fellow commented:

Nurses talk about "liking." They like a patient or a parent. Or they don't like them. That's not what physicians do. We stick to the facts.

Dirty Work

Nurses also do dirty work. As Everett Hughes observed, the work of the physician closely touches the morally, ritually, and physically unclean. "Where his work leaves off, that of the undertaker begins" (1984:306). Hughes also noted that certain tasks are defined as "nuisances and impositions, or even dirty work—physically, socially or morally beneath the dignity of the profession" (1956:23).

Many such lowly tasks are delegated to the nurses. The most striking, to the outside observer, are those associated with dying and death. In keeping with Hughes' observations, where the hospital neonatologist's unsuccessful work leaves off, that of the pathologist or the undertaker begins. The nurse in the neonatal unit is the liaison between the neonatologists who work with live babies and the people who work with corpses.

At Northeast Pediatric, when a newborn's condition deteriorated and death was imminent (although it could have been hours or even days away), the nurse kept the bedside watch. When a infant was considered nonviable, to be taken off the respirator and "held" (held while he or she died), the nurse removed the tubes and prepared the infant for the parents' arms. When there was an unsuccessful resuscitation, the physicians left immediately after the code was called and rescue work halted; the nurse cleared away the equipment, cleaned the infant's body, wrapped it, and carried it away in her arms.

Physicians distanced themselves from certain emotionally draining aspects of the unit's work by the delegation of such onerous tasks. Although the ultimate responsibility, with its emotional burden, was theirs, the physician's physical association with dying patients and the aftermath was diminished by their delegating tasks to the nursing staff. Nurses sometimes expressed their feelings about this discrepancy between the physicians' situation and the nurses':

Physician (regarding the issue of dying babies): "It's hard to let anyone die—so one goes more slowly."
Nurse (with emotion): "Hard for the house officer, but harder for the nurse to sit there and watch the baby turn blue."

In the n.i.c.u., the physician gave the order that influenced the length of the dying process, but the nurse gave the more continuous care and monitored the process.

PROFESSIONAL SUCCESSES AND LIMITS

Research on participatory organizational forms has been carried out at small-group, organizational, community (e.g., kibbutz), and political levels. A poorly studied aspect, however, is the collectivist group that is a subunit within a larger hierarchical organization. The nurses at Northeast Pediatric organized in a collectivist way within the closed world of the n.i.c.u., which was itself a part of the hospital hierarchy. How effective can this type of innovation be? As Kanter advised:

> Ideas about participation need to be enlarged by conceptions of power and opportunity; . . . Participatory systems, by themselves, do not always have positive results, unless the structures of opportunity and power are also affected by the increase in shared influence over decisions. (1977:257)

At the Northeast Pediatric n.i.c.u., nurses were responsible for their own administration and for the welfare of their infant patients. Yet their influence over the most important unit policies—admission and treatment—was indirect and minimal. Interaction between physicians and nurses in the unit revealed both the successes and limits of the nurses' attempt to win recognition as professionals.

The attending physicians respected the clinical n.i.c.u. experience of the nurses and their knowledge of unit protocol, especially in comparison with that of new residents. An attending physician, during an orientation session with three new residents on their first day in the unit, gave this advice:

> If a nurse tells you to do something, the chances are that you probably should. Nine times out of ten, the nurses are right—not always, but nine times out of ten. The nurses may not know as much about diagnoses and things like that. But they are very good observers and have, many of them, been here a long time. They know that if X happens, then usually Y follows, because they have seen it before. The nurses very often are right. However, if you feel strongly about something and do not think what they say is right, then you should seek another opinion. Do not be intimidated by the nurses.

The attending physician also suggested that residents talk over issues with nurses, rather than just give orders:

> It is important to discuss things with the nurses. They react well to discussion. It is important not to dictate to them. Also, part of your job is education and so, if you have a reason for wanting to do something, then explain that reason to the nurses. And, if they think otherwise, then they will give you a reason.

Still, the superior status of even inexperienced house officers overrode serious consideration of what any n.i.c.u. nurse would venture as a clinical opinion. Newcomers to the unit (each set of new residents) and physician outsiders (consulting physicians) both challenged the nurses' claims to more than a supportive role.

Conflicts with Medical Newcomers and Outsiders

The nurses' attempts to legitimize their claims to greater professional status were most successful with the attending physicians in the unit. These physicians, the most senior and the most permanent members of the unit, accepted the nurses' self-management and primary nursing orientation. The nurses had the most difficulty with physicians who were newcomers and outsiders.

Newcomers. Nurses had recurrent difficulty establishing their claims vis-à-vis the residents and fellows, who were the more junior and transient members of the medical team. These physicians rotated through the unit and often treated the nurses as they had treated nurses previously. The unit nurses then socialized them to the new norms about the upgraded role of the n.i.c.u. nurses. The nurses' sometimes militant socialization efforts inevitably made the residents and fellows more cooperative, more members of the unit team.

Criticism and accusations went in both directions as fellows and residents came into the unit. Nurses criticized fellows and residents if they "did not listen" or seemed "rigid" in case treatment. In turn, some residents and fellows criticized nurses for trying to make too many decisions. This difference in expectations sometimes led to confrontations:

> The fellow, a resident, and the nursing coordinator were in the conference room, having a tense talk.
>
> *Fellow:* "I think that we should have these matters settled in face-to-face confrontation, say it right out. You think we do things wrong and we think you do things wrong."

> *Resident:* "It takes time to get used to this unit because it's different from the other places we've been. You [nurses] do more."

True to form, the nursing coordinator proposed the solution, a weekly airing of problems, preferably away from the unit.

The attending physicians, although they set limits on the nurses' authority, displayed confidence in the nurses and supported them. An interesting example of such support occurred when a new resident—one who was openly critical of nurses in the unit—had a baby die on his evening shift. It was an elective re-intubation, during which the baby died. (Or, as a nurse said sarcastically to us, "It was an elective re-intubation during which the child was killed.") A medical review of the death occurred the next morning. The resident attempted to divert blame away from himself and onto the nurses, but the attending physician refused to accept his definition of the situation:

> *Resident:* "The mistake was I should have put a needle in [the chest]. The social problem was worse. There was fantastic confusion between myself and the nursing staff. I didn't know who the senior nurses were and the trainees were. It was clear something was going wrong. Everyone was blaming everyone else. The kid was crumping and dying. The controversial decision was to bag with the tube in."
> *Attending physician:* "And the real social problem? The parents?"

Outsiders. Outside physicians, those in other specialties who came into the unit as consultants, constituted another problem for the nurses. These physicians sometimes did not accept the nurses' claims to authority. Perhaps in their daily work they were not dependent, as the unit physicians were, on the continued cooperation of the nurses. A dramatic confrontation occurred between a consultant anesthesiologist and a unit nurse:

> From a short distance away we saw the scene unfold. The anesthesiologist began to raise a big fuss, raising his voice and backing off from the isolette area into the center of the unit, waving his arms. Another nurse, Maureen, left her own work to go to the side of the first nurse while the anesthesiologist was still ranting. The unit director, a neonatologist, said to the anesthesiologist, "Well I'm here nearly all the time, so the situation is under control. I've been here five years and this is the way things are done." The anesthesiologist stalked to the end of the unit to look at another baby. The nurse, who was left standing at the side of the bed, looked positively stricken.

A few minutes later, over a cup of coffee in the reception area, we talked with the nurse. Her eyes were red from crying.

Researcher: "What happened?"

Nurse: "The doctor was upset with the baby's condition and [was] questioning his own use of a certain anesthesia on this infant. He asked me a question about the baby's responses post-op in the unit and I responded in a way he found arrogant. What I said was, 'We can talk about that after you look at the baby.' Then he just blew up—at the idea of talking with a nurse about a case, I guess. I had to draw on all my assertiveness training to get through it. It showed on my face that I was embarrassed. I wish he had just taken me aside to say what he wanted instead of making a scene right in the middle of the unit. Maureen came over and gave me support. She stood her ground. She told him that this was my baby and that I was in charge of her. . . ."

Such stress from outsiders reminded the nursing staff of the uniqueness of the n.i.c.u. setting within which they had negotiated an expanded professional role.

Clinical Decision Making

Despite the unit attending physicians' support of the nursing staff, a clear line was drawn between minor treatment decisions and basic diagnoses. Nurses could have some input in the first category but not in the second. For example, a nurse could question part of a resident's plan and be supported by a fellow or attending physician:

Fellow: "And the plan?"
Resident: "Hold 'dig' [medication] and up the feeds."
Nurse: (raising eyebrows in surprise) "Why increase the feeds? Is that a
  good idea?"
Fellow: "No, it isn't."

Nurses seldom ventured into the area of basic diagnosis. When they did, the physicians were less attentive. The following is an example in which the primary nurse speaks up about heart murmurs and is subtly put down:

Fellow: "Does this kid have a murmur?"
First resident: "Intermittently. . . ."
Second resident: "I don't think so."
Third resident: "Me neither."
Nurse: "I do. I've heard it."
Fellow (sarcastically): "Then yes it is!" (At this point, however, the group
  decided that the heart was not the problem; the abdomen was the
  problem. Only later did the physicians return to a focus on "the heart
  problem.")

The n.i.c.u. nurses participated in discussions on rounds about the aggressiveness of treatment. Nurses' comments that encouraged treatment merely reinforced the general aggressive stance of the unit. However, when nurses suggested less intervention than the physician wished, the nurses' position was ignored. For example, in a case of a newborn with a fatal disease, everyone agreed it would be inappropriate to put the infant on the respirator, but the physicians planned to administer antibiotics to prolong the baby's life, thus treating more than the nurses wished:

> The nurse was sitting at the head of the bed and gently stroking the back of the baby's neck.
>
> *Fellow:* "I don't think it's fair to let someone get septic and not give antibiotics. I don't expect him to be able to fight it by himself. I don't think it's correct for him to die of sepsis. He will die of his disease."
> *Nurse:* "Anything seems futile."
> *Fellow:* "It might be futile, but I don't equate that with being the wrong thing to do."

Nurses in the Northeast Pediatric n.i.c.u. argued strongly for having treatment plans set in advance, to structure their work. They wanted to have input into those plans, but they relied on the authority of physicians to set the course of medical treatment. One reason for plans is that they assure that the nurses will have guidelines to follow in an emergency. In one controversial case, for example, the nurse was insistent, saying, "Nursing needs to know what to do when she [the infant] stops breathing."

The n.i.c.u. nurses wanted direct input in decision making. However, when they could not get it, they still had a weapon that all workers have: They could "walk slow," refrain from carrying out orders, fail to cooperate. In the various units we visited, nurses were known to be reluctant to care for some difficult or hopeless cases, for example, the anencephalic newborn or the spina bifida infant judged to be too damaged for surgical correction. Although we never saw a nurse walk away from a baby in distress, the Northeast Pediatric nurse described in the following scene strategically alludes to the possibility. The reference is in the context of a discussion about what to do in the event of cessation of breathing in a controversial case:

> *Fellow to nurse:* "How do you feel about [putting the baby back on] the ventilator?"
> *Nurse:* "I wouldn't be thrilled. I wouldn't feel bad about not intubating."
>
> The resident then mentioned some reluctant nurses' comments he'd heard.

Attending physician: "If that feeling is around we need to sit down and have a conference. That can't be a unilateral decision. People should abide by the group decision, even if they do not agree."

Nurse: "You know, some women will walk away [from a baby]."

Attending physician: "Then someone else will have to do it."

In this situation, the attending physician made reference to unit conferences in which physicians and nurses discuss problem cases. Primary nursing and the generally high level of participation of nurses in this unit's activities allowed them entry to the usually closed prolongation-of-life discussions. The alternative would have been for physicians to discuss such cases among themselves and to pronounce their decisions to the nursing staff. In some larger units we visited, this was more or less what physicians did, although not without realizing that the cooperation of nurses was essential to any treatment plan. In contrast, the approach used at Northeast Pediatric was to include the primary nurse (and perhaps her alternate) in a meeting of residents, fellow, and attending physician. As at bedside, clinical judgment was the physician's domain. And, among physicians, attending physicians had the ultimate say in approving the rare "do not resuscitate" order. However, the more ambivalent physicians were about case outcome and the less confidence they had in prolonged treatment, the more latitude nurses had to introduce social issues, such as the family's problems, or nursing attitudes. These were, however, secondary aspects that could not by themselves determine any infant's course of treatment. In conference, what the n.i.c.u. nurses wanted and got was a sense that they had participated in reaching an important decision. Having had their say, they had to abide—as the attending physician quoted above indicated—by the group's decision.

Compared with other nonmedical professionals associated with the n.i.c.u., the nurses at Northeast Pediatric had considerable presence during and influence on patient treatment. In the next chapter, we look at the role of social worker and social-psychological consultants employed to handle patients' families and, on occasion, the emotional reactions of the staff.

Like the professionals who specialize in social and psychological problems, these issues tended to be compartmentalized, separated from clinical decision making or only selectively admitted as factors influencing intensive care.

3

The Social-Psychological Professionals

> I'm sorry I wasn't called. [Physicians] see social service almost as a necessary evil. They use us when they get stuck or don't want to do something.
>
> *Social Worker*

> It took me two or three months. I walked around, got to know people. A nurse said it one day, "You know, when you first came in we didn't know what to make of all your crap."
>
> *Pediatric Development Specialist*

Every newborn intensive care unit relies, to a greater or lesser degree, on the services of social workers, psychologists, or psychiatrists. These professionals are either assigned exclusively to a unit or are available as a hospital resource. The majority, social workers, attend primarily to problems troubling the infants' families, difficulties ranging from getting welfare coverage to emotional reactions. Other experts focus on parental psychology or provide counseling support for the unit staff. The nonmedical orientation of this cadre of professionals is sharply at variance with the n.i.c.u. staff's technical approach to the newborn patients. Social workers in particular represent family and community interests that most neonatologists do not want to influence medical decisions, especially as factors in limiting aggressive intervention. Nor does the emergency room atmosphere of the Level III nursery easily admit that physicians and nurses, under tremendous stress, should be themselves clients of psychotherapists.

The domination of the hospital by medical authority is the strongest influence on the work of social and psychological personnel. The physicians' mandate of "a successful claim to supervise and determine the conditions of work of many kinds of people" (Hughes, 1958:78) extends to social service workers as well. In the Level III nursery, physicians along with nurses control the conditions of the social workers' job. They do not control the particular techniques the social workers use with clients, but they do control many vital aspects of social work, such as access to families, the range of responsibilities, and whether the social workers participate in prolongation-of-life decisions.

Second, the hospital, as an institution, is dominated by narrowly defined medical concerns. The mind-set of many, although not all, n.i.c.u. physicians screens out the social aspects of a case. Some physicians are very socially minded. Historically, one thinks of Dr. Richard C. Cabot, who in 1905 pioneered the introduction of medical social service at Massachusetts General Hospital. But such physicians, both then and today, are in the minority. Analyzing the beginnings of hospital social work early in this century, Lubove observed: "Social casework in the medical setting was not an easy concept for many physicians to grasp. Trained to diagnose and treat specific organic diseases, they did not consider it their responsibility to worry about a patient's job, relations with wife and children, and similar personal circumstances" (1965:29). Lubove's comments apply to the contemporary scene as well. The acceptance of social workers by physicians and other hospital personnel is by no means complete today.

Another aspect of social support services in n.i.c.u.'s is their enormous variability from center to center. There are differences in what occupations do support work, how family referrals are made, what tasks are seen as appropriate, and whether the clients are only the patient and family or also the unit's staff. Such variability indicates that social services are given a low priority in planning. In general, social support services are secondary to medical and nursing services and do not necessarily affect a unit's rating in the medical community.

SOCIAL-PSYCHOLOGICAL SERVICES FOR FAMILIES

An Active Social Service Program

Northeast Pediatric had an active, complex, but by no means consistent, social support program. The key figure during most of our fieldwork was the social worker assigned to the Level III nursery. She had a supervisor who often participated in multidisciplinary rounds. She also had, in turn, several students of her own who received training in the unit and handled family cases. Other disciplines were represented by psychiatrists, child-development specialists, and psychology students.

Casework is the hallmark of social work as a profession, as is work with individual clients for psychiatry. But the particular styles used in these interventions vary from individual to individual. This latitude was dramatically illustrated at Northeast Pediatric. Early on in our fieldwork, a psychiatrist, by personal bent rather than institutional design, was very involved in the unit and took the lead in social service rounds. His rotation ended six months into our fieldwork, and he was replaced by another psychiatrist less inclined to intervene. Soon after, the social worker for the unit left and was replaced by a woman with a different style. The new social worker was more inclined to intervene in cases than was the person she replaced. She became very involved in the unit and took over the lead in social service rounds.

This second social worker defined her mission as doing whatever she could to help parents have and care for their baby. As she put it, "You have to support the concept of ownership—that this is their baby." On rare occasions, this mission put her on a collision course with the physicians when they thought the mother was incapable of caring for her child. The social worker pursued her mission through a combination of strategies, including meetings with community social workers and counseling therapy.

The social worker took the initiative to introduce herself to visiting parents and to indicate that she was available if they wished to see her. Often the first step she took in a case was to provide practical support (regarding transportation to the unit, financial aid, or funeral arrangements). Such concrete support both gave assistance to and established a relationship with parents. This social worker was also an advocate of crisis intervention, believing that this approach with the parents of a critically ill infant could help them overcome their emotional trauma (see Hancock, 1976).

Exclusion of Social Service

Despite the active social service program at Northeast Pediatric, at least four factors contributed to the relative exclusion of social workers from important work in the unit. Before detailing this exclusion, it should be noted that although social workers had no authority and no direct influence on medical decision making, the information about families that they handled and interpreted did reach the unit's staff and was important in assessing the behavior of parents.

Position as Outsiders. At Northeast Pediatric, the social workers spent part of their time in the neonatology division and part of their time elsewhere in the hospital. They were perceived as outsiders with a status lower than that of physician consultants and, indeed, structurally they occupied the position of outsider. The camaraderie of the unit staff, especially among the nurses, was strong enough to set up boundaries between the "in" group and the "out" group. It took time and skill for an outsider, especially a newcomer, to cross this barrier and be accepted by the unit.

Feelings that the unit was a "different world" were expressed during social service, multidisciplinary rounds one day when, because of numerous medical emergencies, no nurse or physician from the unit was able to attend. The group, unexpectedly composed exclusively of outside consultants, considered cancelling rounds. Instead, they spent much of the hour sharing with each other their feelings about being outsiders and offering strategies for overcoming the distance between themselves and the unit staff. The discussion started off with the new social worker asking the others how one makes contact:

> *Psychiatrist:* "My experience of the first four months was of not being accepted. I scheduled time for walking around [the nursery]. With thick skin and two months later, it's just 'Hi.' "
>
> *Developmental specialist* (M.D.): "There is that dynamic in the unit. They see themselves as an interlocking support network. There is a tendency to just write you off."
>
> *Psychiatrist:* "How long did it take you?"
>
> *Developmental specialist:* "It took me two or three months. I walked around, got to know people. I offered seminar sessions. I set down some of the concepts from our side. A nurse said it one day, 'You know, when you first came in we didn't know what to make of all your crap.' "
>
> *Psychiatrist:* "Personally, it felt awful. I came with contacts, credentials. Being a physician and pediatrician—that usually smooths the way, but not here."

Position as Nonmedical and Non-nursing Staff. Social workers, unlike physicians and nurses, are not responsible for the life-and-death care of patients. This difference in responsibility gives them an advantage in dealing with family issues. Staff believed that families would feel free to express certain thoughts and feelings to the social workers that they would feel uncomfortable revealing to the doctor or nurse who had control over the care of their infant. But this position also gives social workers lower status, and they are seen by staff as ancillary. This was revealed at Northeast Pediatric by differences in schedules. For example, in the n.i.c.u., medical rounds would be held even on holidays, but if social service rounds fell on a holiday they were cancelled. It was also revealed in patterns of use. For example, sometimes social workers were not consulted even in situations in which they had defined their presence as being appropriate. Following is one such case:

> The resident told the social worker about how a baby that the social worker had followed had gotten into trouble on Sunday and died.
>
> *Resident:* "I talked with [the parents] about forty-five minutes after [the baby] passed away. The mother talked about being relieved. I talked about a 'post' [autopsy]. They did not want it. My philosophy is, they need their autonomy [regarding that decision]. They picked up his toys. It was unbelievably good compared to how ugly it could have been."
>
> *Social worker:* "It may not be the end. I'm sorry I wasn't called."
>
> The resident then apologized to the social worker for not calling her. After this conversation, the social worker commented to the researcher, "I'm sorry I wasn't called. They see social service almost as a necessary evil. They use us when they get stuck or don't want to do something."

Blurring Medical and Social Issues. Social workers were excluded from many situations at Northeast Pediatric's n.i.c.u. because they were perceived as blurring the boundaries between medical and social issues. The physicians' ideal was to keep medical and social factors separate; while they did not necessarily achieve their ideal, they worked hard toward it. Social service can threaten this conceptual compartmentalization. Social service personnel, dealing with the family, are both ideologically and structurally positioned to see the economic and emotional repercussions of prolongation-of-life cases. At Northeast Pediatric, physicians and nurses tended to reject offers of social service workers to participate actively in prolongation-of-life decisions. The following is a conversation in point. The social worker asked tentatively if she should be at a meeting regarding a difficult case and was diplomatically discouraged by the nurse:

> *Social worker:* "Do people want just medicine at the meeting?"
>
> *Nurse:* "The issues are neurological. [The infant] has BPD [bronchopulmonary dysplasia]. Some people would speak less frankly. Social work does have a strong effect on our thinking."
>
> *Social worker:* "One thing that was expressed to me before [by a physician] was that 'we try to screen the social out.' . . . About another baby conference, people said for me not to be there."

Leadership Sets Tone. The physicians set the tone regarding how important, or not, social service is to the unit. At Northeast Pediatric, the physicians indicated that social service was not central to patient care. The unit director did not attend social service rounds, the attending physicians rarely went, only two of the fellows who rotated through the unit went regularly, and residents seldom went.

The physicians also demonstrated this attitude through their statements. The unit director indicated forthrightly that participation in social service rounds was not a good use of his time. An attending physician who gave the orientation to a group of new residents minimized the importance of social service rounds:

> The attending physician told the new residents what some of the rounds were that they could attend. She listed two or three. She almost forgot social service rounds, but at the end she suddenly remembered. When she did mention it, she added that she didn't know what time it met. At the mention of social service rounds, one of the new residents joked, "We'd better be sure to be off the floor then. The nurses in the unit where we were before got to know our style very well, to know we didn't go. So the nurses would start social service rounds without us knowing and then come get us and say we had to attend."

Incidentally, the scheduling of social service rounds and this orientation of new physicians coincided, making it impossible for new residents to attend both.

Unit physicians attended social service rounds under two sets of conditions. First, an enthusiastic physician could make the difference in the degree of physicians' participation. One neonatology fellow took a leadership role in emphasizing social service. During his time in the unit, he and the residents under his supervision participated regularly. Second, when a case became a problem for the entire unit, physicians attended, just for discussion of that particular case.

The nursing leadership, in contrast to medicine, promoted social service rounds. From one to five unit nurses were present at virtually every session, but they exerted little influence on physicians:

> Several physicians were sitting and talking casually in the conference room. The nursing coordinator told the group that the room was reserved for social service rounds and suggested that they stay. The three residents and the fellow left immediately. The attending physician remained. The nurse said, "I think it would be good if you stayed, but you don't have to." The attending physician left after a few minutes.

Neonatal units vary in the way they structure social service rounds and in the amount of support that physicians give to them. At one hospital we visited, the physician who was unit director was especially enthusiastic about follow-up and social aspects of care and invited us to visit social service rounds. The most striking thing about the meeting, at which many cases were discussed, was that six doctors were present and stayed for the entire session. At another hospital, the neonatal unit staff was divided into two teams, each headed by a physician. At social service rounds, each physician team-leader directed discussion of the cases assigned to that team. Physicians' attendance was reported to be good.

Selection of Cases for Social Service

N.i.c.u.'s use two different principles for selecting cases to be seen by social service. Some units, such as Northeast Pediatric, have an approach to social service that selects only difficult cases. Other units approach each admission to the n.i.c.u. as a crisis potentially needing social service support.

Case Selection. At Northeast Pediatric, nurses acted as the gatekeepers between social workers and families. Social workers did not routinely see the family of every patient admitted but instead received selected referrals. Most often it was the nurses who brought up specific cases at social service rounds and stated that something needed attention.

In certain cases, there was competition between nurses and social workers over handling the family. For example, nurses sometimes were protective of parents, acting as advocates and stating that the families were coping well and not in need of the social worker's counsel. In one instance, the social worker and a mother met by chance in the unit's lounge and this meeting led to a scene between the social worker and a very angry primary nurse. At a later meeting, the social worker brought up the general issue of access to parents:

> *Social worker:* "I wanted to raise the question. A nurse and I had a misunderstanding. It was with the recent case with twins. The nurse said the family did not need to be seen. I casually introduced myself when I was here and the mother happened to be taking, as she said, a 'cigarette break.' She went back in the nursery afterwards and said to the nurse, 'I had my session with the shrink. I wonder what she

thinks of me.' Does anyone introduce themselves to families without checking with the primary nurse? I always just introduce myself. It's really the issue of who decides who can speak to whom."

Physician: "In [another neonatal unit] every family is met by the social worker. It was useful. . . . It is my feeling you should meet everybody and we shouldn't try to put you off. In retrospect, it's probably good the mother talked to you. She's having trouble."

Several units we visited gave social workers more free access to families than did Northeast Pediatric. At one, the social worker said she had "100 percent access." At another, the social worker said, "Every case under a neonatologist is seen by a social worker at least for an initial assessment."

Type of Cases Selected.   A small number of cases dominated the social service discussions at Northeast Pediatric. We attended social service rounds for more than a year at this unit, including nineteen of the twenty-seven sessions held in the last six months. During these meetings, forty families were discussed, but five dominated the conversations. Four of these five cases involved an infant who was medically very difficult, with all the emotional strain that that implies for both staff and parents. In addition, in two of these cases, a twin had died in the n.i.c.u. All five patients had a lengthy stay, ranging from forty days to over four months. Three of the infants had no competent family care-giver yet identified. Two of these infants' mothers—one white, one black—were young, unmarried, and in conflicted relationships with their own mothers. The third was so anxious about being a good mother that she was barely able to relate to her infant. In four of the five most discussed cases, the staff believed there was a communication problem with the parents. In three cases, the staff believed that the parents did not visit enough.

Social Service Rounds

The Appropriate Forum for Family Issues.   Medical work and social work (i.e., family work) at Northeast Pediatric were to a large degree segregated. Only certain unit gatherings were appropriate for the discussion of family issues. The daily 8 a.m. medical rounds focused almost exclusively on the medical condition of the baby. These rounds were attended by physicians, primary nurses, and by nurses interested in particular cases. In some cases (a minority), there might have been a brief reference to the family. If so, it most often concerned an aspect of the family that had a direct practical bearing on the work of the unit; for example, where parents wanted the baby to be sent upon discharge, getting parental consent for a procedure, whether the parents visited, what had they been told, whether the mother's feeding plans were medically appropriate.

Discussion of social issues took place at other times. Nursing rounds, held while physicians were on radiology rounds, included discussion of both medical and family issues. There were informal conversations in the nursery about family; for example, a social worker might stop by and talk with a physician or nurse about a case. And, of course, there was the usual behind-the-scenes small talk about clients that occurs in any service setting. Family-oriented discussion was institutionalized in the form of social service rounds, as well as in special meetings called when the staff perceived a crisis.

These social service rounds—or multidisciplinary rounds—were separated from medical work in time and space. They met once a week, in contrast to medical rounds, which were held daily including weekends. Social service rounds met in a conference room in the unit, not in the nursery itself. Medical and nursing rounds were held in the nursery and, when physicians were present, at the bedsides of the individual infants.

Assessment of Risk. At social service rounds, cases usually were presented by a nurse, who acted as a link between the medical and social service worlds. The nurse usually began by recounting the newborn's history. The opening statement conveyed basic information:

> Twenty-three-year-old mother. First pregnancy. No complications until she went into labor. Delivered vaginally yesterday. Both twins have RDS [respiratory distress syndrome]—severe. 1,250 and 1,300 grams. Have not had drastic complications. Father involved, supportive of the mother, the nurses felt. The outlook I think is good. But they're going to be in here for a long time. They're going to be sick for a long time.

Introducing another baby, the nurse said:

> A twenty-seven weeker. Still being ventilated. Still a 700-gram baby. Mom very afraid of the baby. Mom in her twenties. On the telephone her questions are appropriate, but she can't relate to the baby with the tubes in. Father is the same way. Married two weeks before the baby was born.

These brief opening statements convey the infants' and the mothers' medical and social risks. The experienced listener would know that the lower the gestational age and the smaller the newborn, the greater are the medical risks. The older or younger the mother, the higher are the medical and often the social risks. The obstetrical history—number of times pregnant, type of births—reveals how many, if any, infants a particular mother has lost. The number of surviving children gives clues about whether the mother is experienced at parenting, as well as clues about possible stress due to the demands of other children. The marital status indicates possible social risk— with single parents typically facing responsibilities beyond those of parents with partners.

The complete presentation by the nurse and the ensuing multidisciplinary conversation covered various case-related issues. These fell into five categories: (1) medical (and its implications), (2) parent–infant relationship, (3) parents' social and psychological situation, (4) staff–parent relationship, and (5) staff reactions to the case (Table 3.1).

Medical issues and their social implications set the tone of the social service rounds. The infant's condition was almost always discussed. In addition, the conversation might focus on the obstetrical and delivery history of the mother, number of children in the family, age of the mother, the level of care the infant would need after discharge (and who was available and competent to provide it), the death of a newborn (especially the death of a twin whose sibling was still in the unit), how aggressive various people think the medical intervention should be, and medical mistakes made (either at the referring hospital or the admitting hospital). Nurses (or physicians) would translate the more esoteric medical expressions for social service personnel. The nurses were well-versed in medical terms and their use of such technical language helped set them apart from and above the social workers.

The parent–infant relationship was a major issue at social service rounds. This relationship was conceptualized by staff primarily within the paradigm of "bonding," the physical and emotional attachment between parent and newborn. All the disciplines focused on behavior thought to indicate the presence or absence of the bonding process. The visiting pattern of the parents was the most frequently used indicator. Parents were expected to visit soon after the infant's admission, come back often, stay long enough, and behave appropriately during the visit (for example, to indicate their involvement by approaching the isolette, touching and speaking to the infant). Lack of visiting might be seen by nurses as a reason for requesting social service involvement in a case. This parental behavior could

Table 3.1. Topics discussed in 40 cases in social
service rounds[a] (based on presentation of 40
families in 19 sessions)

Medical	
Medical condition of baby	38
Obstetrical history of mother	23
Children in family[b]	21
Age of mother[b]	16
Level of care baby will need after discharge	11
Death of a baby	9
Aggressiveness of intervention	8
Medical mistakes	7
Parent–baby relationship	
Visiting pattern of parents	31
Child at risk	5
Parents' social/psychological situation	
Parents' psychological reactions	32
Social network of parents	16
Marital status of parents	16
Practical problems facing parents	12
Marital relationship of parents	9
Unusual family structure	5
Prior psychological/social problems of parents	5
Staff–parent relationship	
What to tell (or what told) parents	21
Interaction style of parents with professionals	10
How parents use professional help	7
Staff reactions	
Staff reactions to the case	16

[a]Topics were counted only once for each case; for example, even if
the age of the mother in one particular case was discussed four times,
it still was counted only once in this table. In addition to the topics listed,
the group discussed others, such as discharge plans, suggestions on
appropriate social service intervention, and the relationship between
social service and the unit.
[b]Age of mother and number of children were discussed for both their
medical and social implications.

lead staff to conclude that the child would later be at risk for poor
treatment at home.

The parents' social and psychological state was often discussed.
Their psychological reactions to the newborn were the most frequently mentioned problems. For example, were the parents committed to the infant? Feeling guilty or angry? Denying their feelings? Or, because of the death of a twin, were they grieving? The
social structural aspect most discussed was the parent's network of
relationships with family, friends, and professionals. Staff asked how
the network provided support or caused stress for parents, posi-

tively or negatively influencing the parents' ability to relate to the newborn. The immediate family of the mother was crucial, with a married mother in a nuclear family seen as the least problematical type. Practical problems facing parents—transportation to visit the hospital, immediate financial problems, funeral arrangements, housing—were often discussed. Social workers often helped with these practical problems as a way to begin to establish rapport with the family.

Communication with families was an important subject. Most often, the topic was what to tell (or what was told) to parents. The staff and consultants discussed whether the parents had been kept well informed, whether the parents should come in to talk, and some-times, whether the parents had been told but, due to emotional trauma, could not comprehend the message. They also evaluated the manner in which parents used professional help. For example, were the parents too independent of or too dependent on the professional staff?

The staff's subjective reactions to cases were expressed at social service rounds on two levels. There was the usual behind-the-scenes gossip that indicated the positive or negative feelings that staff had about cases. More important, social service and psychiatry were in-tended to be a resource for staff as well as families. Thus, when nurses were having emotional difficulties with a case, they could air this problem at social service rounds and expect therapeutic feed-back.

Assessing risk to the child is the overarching goal that unites the five issues of social service discussion. Although "child at risk" is tabulated only five times in Table 3.1, that frequency is misleading. This theme becomes most explicit in extreme cases in which people believe the child might be grossly mistreated or neglected, but it is an implicit issue throughout social service rounds. The multidisci-plinary group looks hardest for clues to help them make judgments about parenting ability, adequacy of future parental care, and, if there are deficiencies, the need for social service intervention.

There were also some variations on this theme of risk to the in-fant. The group was often concerned about the effect of difficult cases on the staff's morale, focusing on the ability of the professional care-givers to continue their work and on the fact that the enthusiasm of staff to work on a case was influenced by the parents' reactions to the newborn. If parents were ambivalent about an infant, the staff's commitment to care-giving could be negatively affected.

Psychiatric Referrals

Discussion during social service rounds at Northeast Pediatric could lead to psychiatric referrals for parents, including those whose newborns were in very serious medical trouble. These case referrals were sometimes more difficult psychologically and socially because of strained relations between the n.i.c.u. staff and the family; therefore, the psychiatrist would be asked to intervene as a peacemaker. Professionals in the employ of organizations may serve not only (or not even primarily) the individual client but protect organizational interests as well (or instead) (Field, 1953; Daniels, 1969). Not surprisingly, social service and psychiatry personnel at Northeast Pediatric provided therapeutic intervention and also served the unit's goal of managing parents. Two examples from our early fieldwork suffice.

In the first case, the psychiatrist became involved when the infant's father insisted on continued aggressive treatment, even after the aggressively oriented unit team finally had given up hope. The psychiatrist listed the medical problems:

> The baby had multiple medical problems, each one of which would have been major: lung disease, necrotizing enterocolitis (bowel deterioration), minor heart anomaly—patent ductus arteriosus—and, most serious, major brain bleeding (intraventricular hemorrhage) by exam and by CAT [computerized axial tomographic] scan—devastating, big-league brain damage. Each illness compounded, layer upon layer. Every few days something major, some new major thing happened.

The psychiatrist described his therapeutic goal and approach with the father and mother of the infant:

> Even in the grandfather's dying year, the father thought his father was strong. Now he was likewise denying how sick his child was. The mother identified with the unit and was pulling away from her husband. The dynamics split them. My goal was to pull them together: (1) to get her to see that her future lies with him, not with the nurses; (2) to make him see he had overestimated his father's strength and similarly the baby's strength.

The psychiatrist alluded to organizational goals:

> The father refused to negotiate over the withdrawal of care. He got paranoid over two issues: (1) cost—that the hospital might not pay, and (2) experimentation—he thought some experiment was being done. He said, "Don't do it [don't withdraw treatment]. Keep the baby alive." The attending physician wanted to slow [therapy] down—as an indication that

the damage was so severe. The father couldn't bear that. That's when I stepped in.

The second, and contrasting, case is one in which the father initially insisted that the infant was too damaged to be treated, even though by n.i.c.u. standards the newborn was essentially healthy. It was reported at social service rounds that the father told the fellow, "I have decided that the baby won't live." But the fellow informed the father that the newborn could recover, and the baby made rapid progress. The nurses, upset that the parents did not want the infant, presented the case:

> He's being put up for adoption and it's causing some real strained feelings in the nursery because we've been seeing other babies with neurological difficulties. The parents only came in once. He had respiratory distress, but quickly was okay. The mother bonded right away, kissing, etc. But the father focused only on the [minor deformity]. After surgery, there will be little noticeable. But the father said to us he could not accept a child that was not perfect. We communicated with the parents for the first few days, and then they said, "Don't call."

The psychiatrist made it clear that he understood why the nurses were upset and he offered to speak to the parents:

> I want to see [the parents] alone, not as part of a nursing conference. If I get to the dirt, I'm not going to be able to talk with others around. In the long run, it may be better for the baby not to be in that situation. I won't talk to them with the idea of convincing them to take him, but it would be with the idea of exploring the issues.

In this case, rather than trying to bring the parents around to the point of view of the staff, the psychiatrist reinterpreted the situation to the staff and offered an alternative view. He pointed out that if the parents were that rigid, maybe it would be better for the baby if he went to adoptive parents. The important point, however, is that the psychiatrist's services vis-à-vis the parents were solicited when the unit staff's attempt to manage the parents failed.

THE STAFF AND STRESS

The staff's reliance on psychiatry for the members' own problems was limited and erratic. When the second psychiatrist replaced the first, he offered only a weekly session, to anyone interested. One or two nurses sought counselling, but their sessions were interrupted by other staff members' walking into the lounge. Physicians, when they felt the strain of intensive care work, avoided consultation with the psychiatrist.

The pervasive belief in the unit was that staff professionals should not switch roles and become clients themselves. The "detached concern" characteristic of physicians' demeanor (Fox, 1957) was the ideal. This was so not simply because physicians were in charge but also because the heavy pressure of acute emergency care and high patient death rates put a special onus on those who displayed emotion. Emotional outbreaks (by either staff or visiting families) could distract from and potentially undermine the high level of care demanded by fragile newborns.

As is typical in intensive care units in general, the nurses were presumed to be especially vulnerable to emotional fatigue and exhaustion. The n.i.c.u. nurses' closeness to patients was greater than that of attending physicians and more continuous than that of house officers. That the nurses were women probably contributed to the expectation that they would be more overtly troubled. Still, everyone's idea of proper professional conduct tended to the stoic. Female physicians in the n.i.c.u. were, if anything, more reserved and dispassionate than their male colleagues. Professionally minded nurses were disdainful of other nurses who let their emotions intrude into their work. The nurse described as "lazy" by the nursing leadership in the last chapter described herself as being exhausted and smoking too much out of sheer anxiety. Another nurse left the unit because she felt she could not control her anger—at the physicians, at everyone.

The antidote to burnout was twofold—a combination of security provided by those in authority and well-defined work responsibilities. This pattern follows Cherniss's (1980) analysis that structured work curtails alienation among young service professionals. Junior physicians and nurses want senior physicians to shoulder the burden of clinical decisions. Senior physicians in return are relieved of the difficulties of communication with parents. Sherman described this in the n.i.c.u. at New York Hospital–Cornell:

> The presence of a medical hierarchy and ability to delegate responsibility to superiors is an important buffer against anxiety and responsibility in both house staff and nurses. Feelings of isolation, impotence, and discomfort engendered by physicians['] having to report "bad news" to parents and staff is dealt with by allowing communications between parents and staff to occur via nurses primarily. This is one way physician[s'] anxiety is allayed on the n.i.c.u. Thus, nurses and house officers often diminish their anxiety by pushing decision-making up the chain of com-

mand, whereas those at the top tend to diminish their anxiety by push-
ing communication of "bad news" down the same chain. (1980:40)

The more experimental and difficult the cases, the more this com-
plementarity of responsibilities becomes essential to the unit.

At Northeast Pediatric, the authority of supportive attending
physicians was a safety net for residents and nurses handling crisis
cases. The clear organization of work responsibilities structured the
situation further, so that staff could lose themselves in their difficult
work. Quint's observation that the hard work of intensive care "helps
the nurses minimize their conscious involvement with the patients
and also keeps them from thinking about those who will not make
it" (1966:53) applies to physicians as well. The staff's greatest anxieties surface when directives are unclear, roles overlap, and social
and medical issues blur.

Rotation as a Teamwork Problem

Even with security and well-defined tasks, mutual professional support became a problem each time there was significant turnover in
the Northeast Pediatric n.i.c.u. team. New residents, for example,
needed to transform their individualistic and competitive attitudes
to the cooperative spirit required for teamwork. It was equally true
when a new fellow or attending physician came on board. The approach to patients, and the approach to nurses, differed enough
among these physicians to change the unit's atmosphere. In contrast, nurses had greater consensus, less authority, and much less
turnover in service, making their influence a more steady one. In
combination, the unit physicians and nurses composed and re-
composed new groups at least every six weeks. As Zerubavel observed about hospital medical teams:

> Group boundaries often constitute moral boundaries as well, and many
> teams develop their own unique ethos which distinguishes them both
> from teams who work on the same service on other rotations and from
> teams who work on other services during the same rotation. (1979:71)

The nursing staff frequently took responsibility for cheering up
the unit with small rituals—pastries for a departing foreign resident, a cake to celebrate a small infant's achieving 1,000 grams. To
foster group solidarity, they insisted that grievances between physicians and nurses be aired. If the new residents were balky or a
more senior physician (such as the new fellow described in Chapter
1) misunderstood policy, the nursing leadership became confronta-

tional. The pronouncement, "We have to talk," proceeded formal, behind-closed-doors meetings.

If status and sometimes social class differences separated physicians and nurses, work experiences united them. Getting through a difficult resuscitation, weathering a long transport, and enduring infants' "crashes" on night duty created strong ties of mutual respect. As residents became more experienced, they could contribute to the smooth functioning of the team and make work more tolerable, at least until the next rotation. One neonatology fellow went out of his way to pick teams of seasoned residents, to ensure good team spirit and a high level of expertise. This goal of maximizing camaraderie was, of course, at odds with the goal of educating new recruits.

Troubled Client Relations

Cherniss, among others, linked burnout in service professions to troubled relations with clients. This commonsense conclusion becomes an understatement with regard to newborn intensive care. The psychological state of the staff cannot be calculated independent of the medical conditions of n.i.c.u. infants. Nurses' typical reactions—fatigue, emotional breakdowns—have been well described (Marshall and Kasman, 1980; Duxbury et al, 1984). Generally, patients who left the unit quickly in an improved state helped improve the staff's morale. Conversely,

> . . . prolonged stays and poor prognoses . . . tended to make nurses see their efforts as inadequate. At that point, nurses' morale began to sag in the unit. (Cassem and Hackett, 1972:1429)

Physicians' reactions to frustrating cases are the same. The worst event for both physicians and nurses is the death of an infant. The combination of frustrating cases and death, an unpredictable but inevitable occurrence in a Level III nursery, deeply affected the mood of the unit team. Even outsiders could sense the depressed atmosphere in the unit under the strain of multiple difficult cases compounded by deaths, especially those of infants more than a week old. The collective emotional cycles characteristic of hospital life have been described for staff (Light, 1975) and patients as they react to staff changes (Coser, 1979). In the high-level n.i.c.u., the team reaction is shaped by fluctuations in patients' clinical conditions, not by social relations with patients. A profile of the unit's year, in terms of cases staying in the unit twenty-eight days and over and the deaths of patients by length of stay, is shown in Figure 3.1. Three times, in January, June, and December, an infant treated for several months in the n.i.c.u. died. Because of the accumulation of difficult cases toward the end of the year, the last of these deaths was perhaps hardest for the staff, and hardest of all for the nurses who remained after the house officers had moved on to other rotations. The personal identification of nurses with the infant patients created a constant tension between the nurses' wanting to invest emotional energy in caring for the infants and their fearing the pain of loss. In a unit crowded with difficult cases, the entire staff's emotional tolerance for medical heroics decreased.

In the same way, a series of victories—the successive quick rescues of "good babies"—would buoy spirits and make the staff optimistic about persisting in maximum support for high-risk cases. These shifts in attitude did not alter the staff's basic commitment to intensive care, but they could make a difference in the management of individual long-term cases. For example, an infant who stays in the unit but does not progress becomes a source of frustration. It is difficult for the staff to be uncertain about the treatment approach and also to maintain consistent enthusiasm. As we outline in Chapter 8, uncertainty and ambivalence about a specific case can be compounded by other difficult cases in the unit and can contribute to a shift toward curtailing care. Or, on an equally subtle level, simultaneous clinical successes will be generalized into collective optimism for a marginal case.

In addition to the especially traumatic deaths, the n.i.c.u. staff at Northeast Pediatric witnessed one or two deaths of newborns each week, most of them infants a few days old. We do not know precisely the repercussions that these had on the staff. In general, as Lifton (1979) reminds us, high exposure to death results in a personal identification with death. In the area of childbirth, in countries such as the United States that have relatively low newborn death rates, frequent exposure to neonatal death may have direct repercussions on how individuals perceive reproduction. The nurses were frank about the hesitancy with which they, as young women, approached pregnancy. One nurse, agreeing with another nurse that she did not think having children was worth the risk, stated flatly, "Here we see the worst of it." Another unit nurse became pregnant and gave birth during the time we were conducting our research. Her infant suffered from a congenital anomaly that his mother, as she told the story, discovered herself. She had to argue with the

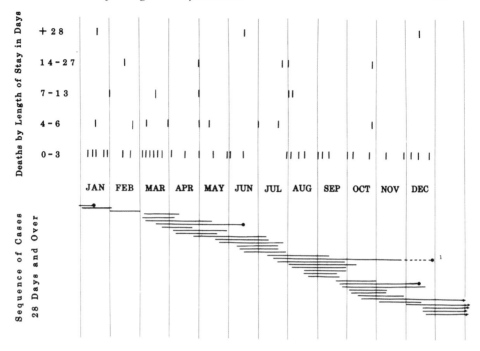

• **Deceased**

1 **Infant transferred to another unit**

Figure 3.1. Newborn deaths and long-term cases over a 12-month period in the n.i.c.u.

staff at another hospital to have it treated correctly. As feedback to the n.i.c.u. nurses, this story confirmed the risks of childbearing and the incompetence of experts—not a particularly reassuring message. Still another nurse, not pregnant herself, made this observation:

> When n.i.c.u. nurses or doctors are pregnant, when they have troubles with babies they are taking care of, that's when they themselves start bleeding or have other troubles with their own pregnancies. That's scary.

Nor are male physicians immune. One attending physician told us about his feelings when his wife was pregnant. He said that working in the n.i.c.u. made one "lose perspective" and that when his daughter was being born he was a "nervous wreck" for fear that something would go wrong.

Good relations with parents could be an antidote to burnout; some house officers and nurses were genuinely gratified to be a source of support to families, even only briefly. As professionals, the nurses were better equipped to have satisfactory relations with parents, even the parents to whom they had to bring bad news. Crisis intervention and grieving therapies are part of modern nursing curricula. Although they put the parent in the role of patient, such approaches at least admit the value of staff–family communication. Physicians, on the other hand, are not usually educated to deal either with death (except as an indication that they have failed) or with distraught parents. This lack is not likely to be addressed for residents in the Level III nursery, where priorities are clinical and dissociated from social problems. Nor were senior physicians compelled to promote client relations as a source of emotional satisfaction for the staff. To the contrary, successfully coordinated teamwork was more pertinent to the clinical care of patients. With frequent changes in group membership, the unit staff was continuously motivated to invest their emotional energy in creating a smoothly functioning professional team.

As we see in the next section of this book, the clinical challenge of treating critically ill newborns has a momentum of its own, separate from and even antagonistic to relations with families.

II

Clinical Decisions and the Patient's Career

4

Where Patients Come From: Referrals

These [babies] are the dregs—after the hurricane has come and taken all the good ones away.   *Neonatology Fellow*

The babies are butchered before we get them. And you can't do anything about it. The doctors protect each other.   *Nurse*

The strong belief of neonatologists in their field is the professional dynamic of newborn intensive care. The institutional dynamic is the referral system, a network of professional and hospital services.

This chapter begins our analysis of the path, from referral to discharge, the infant patient takes through the medical system, or, to use the sociological term, the institutional career of the client (Goffman, 1959). With the development of neonatology, the newborn was seen for the first time as an individual patient capable of an independent clinical history, apart from mother and family. The modern American hospital virtually guarantees that the sick infant's career as a patient will involve a heavy concentration of personnel and technology. In the nationwide trend toward regionalizing intensive care for newborns (Sugarman, 1981), the chances for the newborn patient to have a multiple-service or multiple-hospital career, moving from obstetric to pediatric care and from one level to another of hospital care, increase.

REGIONALIZATION OF NEWBORN INTENSIVE CARE

The greater the claim a central hospital makes to progressive childbirth technologies, the greater is its capacity to recruit referral patients, both mothers and infants. The regional service that directs high-risk patients to tertiary (i.e., maximum) care facilities exists in highly sophisticated forms in all industrialized countries. Its benefits are intended to be practical:

> The basic premise of regionalization is that a given area needs only one or two centralized intensive care facilities which provide highly technological and costly health care for serious illness, with many more primary care or general facilities which are locally based and provide less costly, less specialized services. (Sugarman, 1979:110)

Professional groups argued for the regionalization of perinatal care, citing many practical advantages (Ryan, 1975).

This rationale underlay the early development of n.i.c.u.'s in the 1960s and 1970s. The Level III unit was intended to occupy the apex of a three-tiered system serving infants of high, medium, and minimal medical need. An individual newborn might never have more than Level I care or might be referred directly to a Level II or III nursery. Having been treated in a Level III nursery, a recuperating infant might be referred back to a Level II or I nursery for prolonged surveillance.

At Northeast Pediatric, infant referrals to the Level III nursery reflected the centralization of hospital services and the simultaneous

Table 4.1. Case referrals for 1977 to 1979

	No. of cases		
Cases referred from:	1977	1978	1979
Affiliated general hospital	28	38	59
Affiliated maternity hospital	27	46	33
Community hospitals and other sources	267	246	252
Total	322	330	344

Table 4.2. Case discharges for infants admitted in 1977–1979

	No. of cases		
Cases discharged to:	1977	1978	1979
Home	73	33	22
Affiliated general hospital	24	34	45
Affiliated maternity hospital	17	24	29
Other Northeast Pediatric divisions	21	32	35
Community hospitals and others	124	159	154
Pathology department	63	48	59
Total	322	330	344

closure of low-intervention maternity services in local communities. With declining birth rates and the high expenses associated with maintaining current quality-of-care standards, many community hospitals nationally have shut down their maternity services. Simultaneously, large hospitals have been developing a full range of services, vertically integrating the levels of reproductive medicine, including neonatal units. By virtue of a joint program in neonatology, Northeast Pediatric received referral patients from two such large hospitals, one a nearby general hospital (with a Level II nursery) and the other a nearby maternity hospital (with Level II and III nurseries).

The mainstay of referrals to Northeast Pediatric was not, however, these two hospitals. Instead, a constellation of sixteen suburban hospitals within a fifty-mile radius was the routine source of referred patients. Most of the patients came from Level I and II nurseries and, if they survived, were transported back to local community hospitals (Tables 4.1 and 4.2). The Northeast Pediatric Level III nursery was almost exclusively devoted to premature infants, with a small number of other pathologies represented (Table 4.3). The path of treatment, ideally, was simple. An infant would be transported in, cured, and sent back to the local hospital. As in emergency wards (Roth, 1963), the ideal path was quickly traversed and, in reality, most surviving infants were discharged within a week.

RELIANCE ON REFERRING PHYSICIANS

From the point of view of the patient and family, the gatekeepers to the tertiary center are the local practitioners. The sick neonate's chances for high-level treatment depend on the initial physician's decision to refer.

From the point of view of personnel in the Level III nursery, the issue is recruitment of cases. Like any service organization—a church, a corporate law firm, or a university—the n.i.c.u. competes for clients. N.i.c.u.'s, like the hospitals in which they are housed, exist in a competitive "hospital market" (Russell, 1979). The viability of the n.i.c.u. and the professional mission of neonatology both require a patient population with which to work. As the number of n.i.c.u.'s in a given geographic area increases, the competition among hospitals for clients becomes a greater issue. The most significant factor in this institutional competition is professionally based, that is, the dependence on referrals from obstetricians, general practitioners, and

Table 4.3. Primary admitting diagnosis and mortality, by month, in the Northeast Pediatric n.i.c.u. for 1979, and subsequent mortality

			Diagnosis		
	RDS	Heart/brain pathologies	Asphyxia/meconium aspiration	Sepsis/ Other	MCA
January					
30 admissions	17	3	2	6	2
8 deaths	5	1	1	—	1
February					
19 admissions	7	3	5	4	
4 deaths	2		2		
March					
32 admissions	20	3	4	5	
8 deaths	6	2			
April					
32 admissions	16	6	3	5	2
6 deaths	4	1			1
May					
35 admissions	15	3	3	10	4
3 deaths		1	1		1
June					
35 admissions	17	9	3	3	3
2 deaths	1	1			
July					
34 admissions	22	2	2	8	
7 deaths	6	1			
August					
29 admissions	18	3	3	5	
4 deaths	3		1		
September					
23 admissions	11	4	4	3	1
4 deaths	4				
October					
24 admissions	17	1	2	4	
5 deaths	4		1		
November					
23 admissions	9	5	5	3	1
2 deaths			1	1	
December					
28 admissions	19	5	1	1	2
6 deaths	1	2		1	2
1979 Totals					
344 admissions	188	47	37	57	15
Percent distribution	55	14	11	17	4
59 deaths	36	9	7	2	5
Percent distribution	61	15	12	3	8

RDS, respiratory distress syndrome; MCA, multiple congenital anomalies. Almost all these infants suffered from prematurity as their basic problem.

consulting pediatricians aware and approving of newborn intensive care.

Medical specialties can be divided into those that are client dependent and those that are colleague dependent (Freidson, 1960). In other words, either they depend on clients who self-refer or they depend on referrals from other physicians. Neonatologists are colleague dependent—they get their cases not from the decisions patients make themselves but from the decisions of referring physicians, especially obstetricians. This dependence results in a strained relationship between neonatology and obstetrics and a bias in the direction of the n.i.c.u.'s receiving difficult cases.

Neonatology and Obstetrics: An Ambivalent Relationship

Merton and Barber (1963) and, more recently, Coser (1979) have encouraged the sociological study of ambivalence. The sociological focus, complementing the psychological, looks at "the processes in the social structure that affect the probability of ambivalence turning up in particular kinds of role-relations" (Merton and Barber, 1963:93). This theoretical essay continues, zeroing in on the "case study" of structured ambivalence in the relationship between the therapist's role and the patient. Using ideas from Max Weber, authors Merton, Merton, and Barber speak of "living off" the problems of clients:

> Social and professional norms dictate that professionals are not to advance their own interests at the expense of their clients. Yet the interests built into the professional situation have a dual character: removal or solution of the client's problem inevitably extinguishes the professional's source of livelihood. It is in this objective sense that professionals have an institutionalized stake in trouble, that they "live off" the troubles of their clients. Small wonder, then, that clients often suspect, at times expressly, that professionals are using their authority primarily to serve their own interests at the expense of their clients. (1983:36–37)

Much of what these authors observed can be applied to the relationship between the neonatologist and obstetrician (or in some cases, between the neonatologist and community pediatrician). In general, one can substitute the word "obstetrician" for "client" in the above, and the analysis holds. The interests of neonatologists also have a double character. Neonatologists are to solve the obstetricians' problem of what happens when the "perfect baby" does not appear, by providing maximum professional expertise and command of hospital technology. At the same time, neonatologists live off obstetricians' problems. They make their professional mark and their livelihood from the referral of problem newborns.

The two medical specialties need each other. Obstetricians need neonatologists who, with their reputation for having a solid research base, are the recognized authorities on newborn care. Neonatologists communicate to obstetricians and other community physicians the standards of newborn viability and the proper techniques for pretransport care. Obstetricians are under great pressure to diminish both the mortality and morbidity associated with childbirth. Since most obstetricians are private practitioners, the legal pressures for them to refer even marginally viable infants to an n.i.c.u. are tremendous. The recent Infant Doe regulation requiring maximum care for handicapped newborns has accentuated these pressures. Even before the regulation was proposed, obstetricians were under pressure to refer infants who might be too high-risk for the Level I nursery staff or liable to add to a hospital's neonatal mortality rate. The promise to parents that their infant will get the best possible care and the private physician's desire to shift the ultimate responsibility for a borderline case constitute the most enduring incentives for referral.

Ensconced in central hospitals, neonatologists in Level III units want patients and encourage the referral of tough cases. Obstetricians can use their act of referring as medical and legal proof that they have provided for the best possible care. The structured ambivalence in the obstetrician–neonatologist relationship becomes, as is discussed later, particularly problematic in relation to the issue of how to give corrective feedback to erring obstetricians without offending them to the point that they will no longer refer cases.

Relations between obstetricians and neonatologists are ambivalent and most strained in regional systems, especially those in which the major hospital has no maternity services and receives referrals only from other hospitals. But problems also occur when both the n.i.c.u. and the maternity service are in the same central hospital. Thus, the ambivalence seems to be related primarily to medical specialization and the patterned relationship between these two specialties, rather than to the issue of referral within or between hospitals.

At Northeast Pediatric, where the n.i.c.u. received exclusively interhospital referrals, relationships with community obstetricians were a major problem. In its referral relationship with the two nearby major hospitals, the n.i.c.u. staff experienced relatively little friction with obstetricians because known and trusted pediatricians made referral decisions. Hospital-employed pediatricians in both these nearby hospitals strongly influenced judgments about the initial delivery-room resuscitation and care of newborns and about the appropriate referral of high-risk cases to Northeast Pediatric. Difficult surgical cases, for example, were frequently channeled from these two nearby hospitals to the Level III nursery at Northeast Pediatric because neither of the other two hospitals could match the quality of its facilities and consulting surgeons. In these cases, problems of dealing directly with obstetricians were therefore eliminated for Northeast Pediatric's unit staff.

Within a major general hospital, however, the same antagonisms occurring between community obstetricians and neonatologists in regional units were characteristic of relations between obstetricians and pediatricians, even when their work was nominally integrated with a perinatal program. The two specialties compete over when the authority of the obstetrician ends and the authority of the pediatrician begins. Both specialties now emphasize the unpredictable risks surrounding childbirth. The unforeseen professional consequence of this emphasis has been the increased presence in teaching hospitals of the pediatrician in the delivery room as the arbitrator of newborn medical care.

At one general hospital with both services, the neonatologists were supposed to be called to the delivery room for all high-risk births. But the attending physician complained that it was not always done. An n.i.c.u. junior resident added:

> There's another one where we weren't called, a mother with preeclampsia. . . . I would have expected that we would have been called for such a thing.

On the other hand, there was the potential for being called too often by obstetricians:

> They get passive-aggressive. We got called at 4 a.m. for an extra digit. We went running up and said, "There's an extra digit. An extra middle finger (laugh)." The senior resident in the n.i.c.u. added "You know what you can do with your extra digit (laugh)."

Ambivalence may occur in either organizational model. However, interhospital referrals may mean greater cultural and certainly greater geographic distance between the referring and receiving organizations. This distance compounds the problem of communication and service. As the regional system expands and as neonatologists publicize their increased competence in handling extremely low birth weight and damaged infants, a major disturbance occurs in the rational order of the referral system based on a quick turnover of cases. The disturbance comes from the increase in the referral of patients of little promise, that is, more borderline cases requiring a greater investment of service (and often longer hospital stays) with less-than-optimal outcomes.

Selection for Worst Cases

Level III n.i.c.u.'s are designed to care for the most critically ill newborns. The point of referring is to send on to the specialist the cases that one's own hospital or a lower level unit is not prepared to handle. The result is that the Level III unit is a center for the worst cases, that is, the sickest, highest-risk, most difficult infants. It is here that the very low birth weight baby (less than 1,500 grams), the baby with multiple congenital anomalies, and the baby who is the result of a delivery room disaster are found. This bias is accentuated in interhospital referrals. For example, research done at a San Francisco center that accepted both in-hospital and out-of-hospital referrals compared the two groups. The transported infants had higher risk levels and their death rate was approximately three times that of the infants born in-hospital (Phibbs, Williams, and Phibbs, 1981). The concentration of difficult cases thus is greater in the referral center that receives many or exclusively interhospital referrals.

Like other major U.S. medical centers, Northeast Pediatric had a national and even international reputation for accepting nearly hopeless or particularly complex n.i.c.u. cases. Its commitment to research, clinical innovation, and physician education was reinforced by a full array of hospital resources: laboratory facilities, the most modern diagnostic equipment, the latest in oxygen and intravenous therapy, complete surgical facilities, and a heavy investment in unit personnel and consulting specialists. Like comparable units, the Northeast Pediatric n.i.c.u. also communicated to local physicians and hospitals that its staff was willing to take almost any case and try to make a successful rescue. A fellow, commenting upon the presence of difficult cases, said, "These [babies] are the dregs—after the hurricane has come and taken all the good ones away."

This kind of patient mix is both demoralizing and challenging to the staff. As deaths and damaged babies accumulate in a unit, it negatively affects the mood of the unit, especially the mood of the nurses and residents. But even the most difficult case (even a case that some call a mistake) can be regarded, especially by senior physicians, as a challenge.

Latent Experimentation

All major teaching hospitals, where most Level III nurseries are located, promote research and innovation. In newborn intensive care, the major experimental impetus is not in changing technical procedures but in the active recruitment of new, more premature, infants on which to test existing procedures. The refinements of diagnosis, oxygen therapy, intravenous nutrition, antibiotic administration, and surgery already have been worked out on infants weighing more than 1,500 grams. The clinical challenge is to apply the same therapies successfully in the smallest newborns. The n.i.c.u.'s mandate to provide emergency service combines with the subspecialty's research mission to increase recruitment of cases once considered hopeless. With no external limit on referrals or admissions, each unit has the flexibility to experiment without a scientific protocol and without rigorous inquiry into the relationship between heroic intervention and outcome. The first step in this latent experimentation is the open referral and admission policy. The second step, discussed in the next chapter, is treatment policy or how aggressively treatment is given in borderline cases.

The institutional goal of keeping beds filled and using hospital resources to capacity is rarely acknowledged within the n.i.c.u. Instead, physicians often invoke progressive medicine to justify the admission of infants weighing less than 1,000 grams or less than 800 grams or even less than 500 grams. These cases represent a chance to see if a slight movement of the respirator dial or a new combination of drugs or a different management of fluids will make the difference between death and survival.

The phrase used by n.i.c.u. staff is "being on the frontier," that is, on the edge of new knowledge. One factor that perpetuates the latent experimentation is that this frontier keeps moving; what was the frontier a short number of years ago is now known territory. And the expectation is that the frontier will keep on moving and that by taking marginal cases one will maximize outcome in the long run.

The receptivity of Northeast Pediatric to marginal cases was communicated both by word and deed. For example, in an orientation session for new residents, one resident asked about limits:

Resident: "Are there lower limits [like age and weight] when we get a transport call?"

Attending physician: "No—if you get a call, you just go. There aren't limits unless it's something like 300 grams. You can't make the decision over the telephone. You have to see the baby."

The unit in fact admitted very low birth weight newborns. Perhaps most striking was the admission of a 480-gram infant referred to the unit thirty-six hours after birth. The baby died after nine days in the n.i.c.u. One attending physician commented to the unit director that it was an accomplishment just to keep the baby alive that long.

TRANSPORT

The phrase "technology and medicine" brings to mind medical equipment per se. Yet n.i.c.u. regionalization, in its sophisticated form, depends on other kinds of technology as well: high-speed transportation, medically equipped vehicles, rapid communication, and, in the more advanced networks, computerized programs for matching the infant with an available transport team and hospital bed.

Northeast Pediatric was linked to a backup network of several other n.i.c.u.'s. These units competed for patients but also cooperated at some minimal level; namely, if one unit was full, procedures existed for finding a bed in another unit. The Northeast Pediatric transport team consisted of an n.i.c.u. nurse and a physician, often a resident. While transport provides access to the regional referral center, this relocating of the newborn also creates social and psychological problems for parents and families.

The Professional Gap.   For the Level III transport team, a call means going out to a local hospital that is not equipped to treat difficult newborn cases. The local staff is not trained for these cases or at best is trained properly in what to do before transport arrives. Furthermore, the local hospital often does not have equipment that the team desperately needs; the radiology facilities, for example, may not even approach what the team regards as basic. And the local hospital may have more old-fashioned rules, for example, restricting mothers from seeing their babies before transport.

This difficulty, of working on someone else's turf, is compounded by the image of the "hot-shot" Level III team coming in to take away newborn patients. In some instances, there is an added complexity to the status difference—it is a "hot-shot" nurse taking an infant from a local physician.

These difficulties are illustrated in the account given to us in a western state by a nurse-practitioner who was part of an all-nurse transport team. In this particular case, it was the local pediatrician who referred the case:

> Last night—a baby, three pounds, four ounces, two months premature. The pediatrician who referred is an older man, a good person, but not knowledgeable about such cases. He was given instructions over the telephone on how better to stabilize the baby. But the instructions were not followed well and it probably made the baby worse trying to follow them. When we got there, the baby was in total shock. I had a good staff nurse with me. The physician had gone home. The [local] nurse had never told the mother. They had literally cooked the baby under the heater. I did the blood transfusion. I intubated the baby, I got him resuscitated. I knew clinically he had had an intraventricular hemorrhage. I looked at his blood gases. I knew it was a bad intraventricular hemorrhage. And the outcome usually is not good in such cases.

The Gulf Between Family and Tertiary Center. Communication between professional and client even under the best of circumstances can be problematic. Communication during a crisis is especially difficult, when professionals feel harried and often would prefer not to deal with the emotional issues, and when clients psychologically may "tune out." The transport team, while taking the baby away, is expected to explain to the family what they are doing.

At Northeast Pediatric, most of the transports were within the greater metropolitan area; a minority were long-distance, from more than fifty miles away from the hospital. Despite the relative proximity (in comparison to regions with a more dispersed population), communication with parents at time of transport was a troublesome issue. The social worker, speaking to the n.i.c.u. nurses, said:

> How can we promote bonding during transport? One of the main tasks of parents is mastery. . . . But they feel they've been unable to produce. We have to support the concept of ownership—that this is their baby even though we're coming to take it away.

The professional expectation is that physicians and nurses should inform the parents but hedge on the evaluation of the infant's condition. Indeed, this social worker, still talking about transport, recommends the omission of details.

Do not give the parents unnecessary details about the future. You do not want to give them too much of a pathological image. It is almost impossible to grieve and bond at the same time. Do not overload them.

The task of telling parents that their newborn is dying is an onerous one, but sometimes necessary for the transport team. The nurse-practitioner quoted above faced this situation on a recent transport:

> This mother had no idea the baby was so sick. I had to tell her. She was nineteen years old. I had to tell her her baby was probably going to die. So I talked and said I understand you haven't been told. She said no, the doctor said the baby had to go [to the city]. I said, "The baby is very sick." I told her what we had done. I told her simply. I didn't mention the hemorrhage. I left that out—it has so many connotations. I didn't think she needed it or would understand it. I said the reason for going [to the city] was the need for a doctor who feels comfortable with such babies. I asked her about her pregnancy. I said the baby was very sick and that we'd try, but that I couldn't promise that he'd make it. I wanted to be honest. I explained how he would look—his face—and that if he did live that wouldn't be a problem. She started crying. I picked up her hand and held it.

Dividing the Family

The transport typically divides the family. Once the baby is born, the common practice in the United States is to transport only the baby. The father (and mother if well enough) may follow using other transportation. Often the mother remains hospitalized at the maternity unit. If the father wishes to be involved, he must choose which hospitalized member of his family to be with—the baby at the tertiary center or the mother at the referring hospital.

Resistance to transporting the family stems partly from a concern for avoiding anything that might distract from the primary patient, the infant. In addition, there are emotional and legal implications, as well as the issue of economic feasibility. One transport coordinator in a southwestern state said:

> We never transport the family for several reasons. Liability insurance does not cover the family. And we don't want freaky parents along. Also, remember, we use twin-engine planes.

A lawyer affiliated with Northeast Pediatric gave this advice:

> *Practitioner:* "What about a mother who wants to come back on transport? I had a case where the doctor said she was okay, but she took up my time on the airplane."

Lawyer: "What does your protocol say? What are you set up to do? What is your specialty? If you are advertised as an infant transport team, you run a greater risk by bringing along the mother. You have a legal obligation to transport the infant and give it the best of care. Something really serious might happen to the mother during transport and then you (a) can't deal with that and (b) can't do your best with the baby. Then you may legally be in for a real whammy."

Transporting mother and child would solve some problems but create others, as Wilson noted:

The mother also is being removed from her social support system and her other children who may be very dependent upon her. . . . While she may be close to her baby, she has been suddenly uprooted from home with little preparation for such a venture. (1978:93–94)

Transport, by definition, means that families are divided or that family members are removed from their social context and familiar surroundings.

Working Conditions in Transit

Despite sophisticated transport technology, providing medical care while in transit still is difficult. One is working in a moving vehicle. There is less supervision than at the tertiary center. And there are fewer helping hands available. An infant who goes into failure in a Level III unit will immediately be surrounded by as many as ten people, but, during transport, the available team is small. Furthermore, in a two-person transport team, one person, such as a resident, often is relatively inexperienced. A Northeast Pediatric n.i.c.u. nurse commented, "The doctors don't get trained for transport. We [nurses] have to teach them. We go out on transport all the time."

The goal of the transport team is to stabilize the baby's condition and move the baby as quickly as possible to the more sophisticated center. An attending physician at Northeast Pediatric explained this policy during the orientation for new residents:

The point is to get back here as soon as possible. Some people might think they should do a workup there, do as much as they can. But in fact the point is to just do what you have to and get back as soon as possible.

She also talked of the difficult working conditions during the actual transport of the baby, which for Northeast Pediatric usually was by ground transportation:

However, if it looks like you may have to intubate before you get back here, be sure and do it at the referring hospital, because it is hard to do it in the ambulance.

Despite the sophistication of many current transport systems, neither air nor ground vehicles can provide the optimal work setting.

OTHER PEOPLE'S MISTAKES

A considerable part of neonatologists' work is perceived as correcting other physicians' mistakes. As an n.i.c.u. nurse observed, "The babies are butchered before we get them, and you can't do anything about it. The doctors protect each other." On another day at morning rounds, the physicians got into a black-humor discussion about the poor condition of the babies on which they were supposed to work. The conversation continued, with an indictment of community physicians:

> *Resident:* "Considering what we have to work with, [that twin] is the only one doing badly."
> *Fellow:* "I know, I was just giving you a hard time."
> *Resident:* "How the kids do here is no reflection on the people here."
> *Fellow:* "I know. We're at the height of sophistication, but we have no control over what those morons [in the community] do."

These mistakes are often those of the referring obstetricians, but they can be those of any person responsible for the care of the pregnant mother, the labor and delivery, or early neonatal care.

Hughes (1951) pioneered the sociological study of mistakes at work, noting both the difficulty of defining what is a mistake and the related question of who has the right to define what constitutes a mistake. He also pointed out that how mistakes are handled reveals a great deal about professional values.

More recently, as we mentioned in the discussion of training residents, Bosk (1979:37–70) developed a typology of medical mistakes based on his field observations of surgeons, including technical and judgmental errors versus normative errors. A technical error occurs when the surgeon's "skills fall short of what the task requires." The expectation is that such technical errors can be made by anybody, but not very often. A judgmental error means the choice of an incorrect treatment strategy. In contrast to these two types, a normative error occurs when "conduct violates the working understandings on which action rests." Such errors are almost always made by subordinates rather than by attending physicians. Bosk's study focused on relations between superordinates and subordinates within a service. His concepts, however, are also useful in analyzing the relationships between Level III neonatologists, with more prestige in the profession at large, and local physicians, with less prestige.

Technical Errors

At Northeast Pediatric, all of the unit staff were attuned to what constituted community physicians' errors. Any official reaction was the duty of the attending physicians, and most specifically of the unit director. But in daily behind-the-scenes conversation, physicians of all ranks and the staff nurses were outspoken about community practitioners who erred.

The technical mistakes most talked about were the clear-cut violations. There were, for example, procedures done so wrong that any reasonable and properly trained person would have done them right. Or there were preventable mistakes that could have been avoided if one had had sharp personnel and caught the problem in time.

Technical obstetrical mistakes included elective cesareans done too early and without accurate testing for gestational age, delays in delivering an infant, and iatrogenic cases of asphyxia and meconium aspiration. In one cesarean done too early, the Northeast Pediatric staff talked with derision of how it was "unmonitored for any assessment of gestational age." The fellow who did the transport described the baby as "horrible by the time we got there. Seized all the way coming back. As bad an RDSer as I've ever seen." One weekend, this infant's case was presented, as follows, to the attending physician covering for the day:

> *Fellow:* "It was an elective cesarean."
> *Attending physician:* "How much money do the parents want? . . . It's free money in a court of law."

His comments, in context, made it clear that this case was a blatant example of improper procedure. In another case of an elective cesarean done too early, the Northeast Pediatric physician said the baby was, as a result, suffering "terrible hyaline membrane disease." The physician commented to us:

> There's no justification for not doing the tests to determine age—ultrasound, level of surfactant in the amniotic fluid. This was a totally preventable disease. We think he'll be fine, but he was at risk for all sorts of things.

Delays in delivering a baby, especially after problems had been detected, were also the topic of derogatory n.i.c.u. conversation. One such case, resulting in an asphyxiated, severely compromised infant, provoked considerable discussion, especially since the mistake occurred at a hospital with a good reputation and one that had close ties with the n.i.c.u. The medical record indicated serious problems:

> Labor complicated by variable and late decelerations. Pitocin induction without success. Prolonged fetal bradycardia [reduced heart rate] noted and cesarean section done. Infant delivered meconium-stained with Apgars 0-2-2 [0 at one minute, 2 at five minutes, and 2 at ten minutes].

The n.i.c.u. director, with characteristic understatement, commented in response to our questions about the delivery, "There was some concern about whether things had been done as efficiently as they might have been." The resident was more outspoken and talked to us of "mismanagement." The resident described the resulting damage:

> Some liver damage, probably from anoxia; kidney—from anoxia; and brain. As for the seizures, I think it's very serious. I have the uneasy feeling that the baby may have serious permanent damage. The kidney and the liver probably will get better. The brain is more up in the air.

The nurse was more blunt: "The baby will be a vegetable."

Cases of meconium aspiration also provoked criticism. In about 10 percent of deliveries, meconium is present in the amniotic fluid at birth. Pulmonary disease occurs in infants who aspirate such meconium (Klaus and Fanaroff, 1979:190). The following conversation occurred during social service rounds:

> *Pediatric consultant:* "Meconium aspiration is avoidable. The obstetrician can prevent it. There are tip-offs. You need to get someone there to intubate and suction—in seconds."
> *Resident:* "Once the membranes of the mother rupture and you see the meconium, then you can do something."

The group continued talking, the general point being that if people on duty at the delivery are alert and trained, then the problem is preventable provided action is taken quickly, before the baby breathes.

Technical errors after birth were also ascribed to various community physicians. These mistakes included physicians' inability to do procedures that have become commonplace in specialized neonatal care. The resuscitation sometimes was poorly done. In one case, for example, the n.i.c.u. nurse reported:

The Apgars were 0 and 0. The pediatrician called us. He didn't know what to do. It was a case of literally describing CPR [cardiopulmonary resuscitation] on the telephone.

Errors of Judgment

In Bosk's study, the surgeons' most common errors of judgment involved overly heroic surgery or the failure to operate when they should have. In our study, the community physicians made errors of judgment in referring infants. They referred newborns who were "too sick" or "not viable," thus heroic efforts were made in cases that perhaps should have been left untreated, and occasionally referred newborns who were "too healthy" and could have been managed in a lower-level nursery.

The n.i.c.u. staff, especially attending physicians, liked the challenge of difficult cases and were receptive even to experimental cases (although they did not use the term "experimental"). Nevertheless, some nurses, residents, and fellows accepted certain referrals with ambivalence. An example is the referral of the 480-gram newborn mentioned earlier. At the end of Monday morning rounds, a physician reported the news that the infant was on its way to the unit:

> 480 grams, twenty-five weeks gestation. Born Saturday afternoon. In oxygen, 40 percent now. Apnea. Active. Arterial line in.

The reaction was as follows:

> *Resident:* "A decision will have to be made about how aggressive to be. (Paused, reflecting a moment.) Well, by accepting her it's a commitment to be aggressive."
> *Unit director:* "Just transporting her is being aggressive."

At midmorning the baby arrived.

> At 10:40 a.m. the referring pediatrician came in with the transport team and the new infant. He was beaming and joking about the challenges he brought the unit. The staff did not look too happy to see this challenge. The pediatrician had a resident with him, a young man, whom he also took to see the baby with Werdnig-Hoffmann's disease [muscular atrophy], bypassing two more ordinary cases of RDS [respiratory distress syndrome].

The problems of the new baby included apnea, bradycardia, hyperbilirubinemia, and respiratory distress. The baby died after nine days of intensive care.

A few referral judgment errors occurred at the opposite end of the spectrum, with the newborns being too healthy. For example, a community physician made a judgment error in referring a baby that was large (3,300 grams), full-term, from an uncomplicated pregnancy, with good Apgar scores (9–10), and doing well until its temperature went up. The chief problem was possible infection. This case, the n.i.c.u. staff believed, could have been managed at a lower-level nursery, especially if the local physician had taken cultures prior to administering antibiotics, thus facilitating the diagnostic process. The n.i.c.u. residents were incensed both over the technical error (not taking cultures) and the judgment error (of referral), one reason being that this admission to an n.i.c.u. was economically wasteful.

> *Resident:* "The pediatrician cost us about $4,000. . . ."
> *Another resident:* "This place costs $626 a day just for the bed."
> *Another resident:* "You don't even have to be a pediatrician to know you culture before giving antibiotics."

Community physicians and staffs were blamed for judgment errors when they failed to intervene at all. The Level III transport team sometimes arrived to find a newborn unattended, not because the local staff gave up hope but because it had not recognized the signs of critical illness. For example, a new admission of an 1,875-gram infant delivered by cesarean section was discussed at morning rounds:

> *Resident:* "The baby was literally abandoned out there. Was in a room without a monitor at the [community] hospital. . . ."
> *Nurse:* "They didn't know the baby was sick, that's the most frightening thing."
> *Attending physician:* "So it wasn't negligence, it was ignorance."

The local staff had misjudged the condition of the infant and therefore had not begun appropriate interventions.

SELF-POLICING OF THE PROFESSION

Various empirical studies have noted the reluctance of physicians to confront each other about their mistakes or to share information about mistakes. Millman (1977) observed that medical mortality review sessions within a hospital are supposed to be "cordial affairs." Freidson (1976) noted the lack of observability of many mistakes. Bosk approached the subject somewhat differently, stating that, in surgery, "superordinates tend to be tolerant and forgiving of technical error and intolerant and unforgiving of moral error" (1979:177–78).

Forgiveness, it should be noted, does not imply a cavalier attitude. On the contrary, Bosk indicated that forgiveness is a social control mechanism that obligates the physician who is forgiven. The wrongdoer is to repay this obligation and is expected to become more vigilant in the future.

Each of these three sociological studies dealt with the problem of social control within a hospital. Neonatologists' more distant relationship with physicians in the community weakens even these professional policing mechanisms and substitutes institutional requirements.

Barriers to Social Control

The main barrier to the professional monitoring of community obstetricians and pediatricians by neonatologists is the latter's dependence on referrals. Level III physicians rely on the good will of community physicians for case referrals. This dependence is a hindrance to neonatologists' confronting individual community physicians about mistakes or even discussing differences of opinion. A common theme among attending physicians, fellows, and nurses in the n.i.c.u. is that if one complains to the community practitioners, they will stop referring newborns.

> *Nurse:* "This was an elective repeat cesarean."
> *Social worker:* "Elective without labor. For all the parents' consumer savvy, they never questioned that. How do you deal with the ethics of that?"
> *Fellow:* "You can't very well. It puts us in [the community physicians'] hands. If we undermine them, they won't send the babies to us. . . . Relationships between pediatricians and obstetricians are not good. Not very good communication in either direction. It's very hard for us."

N.i.c.u. physicians often believe that feedback is futile. In the following example, the community physician had neglected to test for infection. The idealistic Northeast Pediatric resident pushed for educating him, but the attending physician resisted, citing two reasons, one of which is the futility of it all.

> *Resident:* "I think you or [the unit director] should telephone the referring doctor and say that the treatment is inappropriate. I believe, and I know [the physician-in-chief] believes it and maybe that's why I believe it, that part of the job of a teaching hospital is to educate others. I also realize that politics are involved."
> *Attending physician:* "I apologize if I seem jaded, but I've been through this so many times. There's not much you can do. If you do call them

up and complain, they'll just send the babies to another hospital. Also, if you really complain, they don't hear or maybe they don't even know how to do the culture."

The attending physician implied that the community physician, rather than improving his treatment technique, would continue as before except for making his referrals elsewhere.

Mechanism of Feedback to Referring Physicians

Despite their dependence on referring physicians, the Northeast Pediatric staff did make efforts to communicate their clinical standards to them. These efforts were relatively indirect and did not jeopardize referrals. Three types of feedback occurred: n.i.c.u. staff's communication to or about a particular community physician, interhospital committee reviews, and more generalized educational outreach.

Collegial Reaction to Individual Referring Physicians. An important issue influencing whether n.i.c.u. physicians would take some action vis-à-vis a particular community physician was whether the mistake remained a technical error, or whether it was transformed into a more serious normative error. If this transformation occurred, some sanction might be invoked against the individual physician.

What physicians at Northeast Pediatric looked for was a pattern of mistakes, but they saw the local medical community as the agent of social control for correcting such a pattern. An attending neonatologist commented as follows in the case of an elective cesarean done too early and without proper testing:

> *Attending physician:* "Someone has to talk to the obstetrician."
> *Fellow:* "The pediatrician has."
> *Attending physician:* "Does that clear our conscience? I'd call the obstetrician. If he says he's concerned then say we just wanted to give you a progress report. But if he says that's how we usually do it, then you might send a copy of a letter to the pediatrician or to the obstetrician, with a few innuendos and then it's reported out and they [at the local community hospital] can take what steps they want."

Formal Interhospital Review Committees. Another forum for feedback was the review committee. An attending physician at Northeast Pediatric described an interhospital review committee:

> Community hospitals often feel patronized by tertiary centers. Therefore we have to work in a collaborative fashion with community hospitals.

We have a perinatal committee which includes nurses, neonatologists, anesthesiologists, and social workers from the center and community hospitals. It meets approximately four times a year to discuss maternal death (God forbid), fetal death, etc. There are three aspects to the project: (1) communication, (2) use of the data for feedback so hospitals can correct themselves, and (3) follow-up information.

The function of this committee was basically educational. Its retrospective review of cases informed referring hospitals of the teaching hospital's high clinical standards. The committee meetings reinforced the authority of the Level III unit to the extent that they also implied that only local professionals have something to learn.

Group Education. A more explicitly educational approach is the preferred method among neonatologists for upgrading the quality of care given by community physicians and nurses. Continuing educational courses at major medical centers and workshops have become commonplace in neonatology. There is a double goal in this educational process. First, neonatologists want to improve the quality of care given by all local practitioners. Neonatology is a professional "segment," to use the term of Bucher and Strauss (1961), with its own sense of mission to reform practice. Much like the physician-anesthesiologists who earlier went about preaching the benefits of physician-administered anesthesia (Lortie, 1958), today's neonatologists and n.i.c.u. nurses possess a missionary zeal to spread the word about the proper care of neonates. Their goal is to upgrade skills of practitioners in general, rather than to confront an individual wayward practitioner. Second, community practitioners' mistakes also may be handled by the group-educational approach. Rather than point a finger at a particular physician, neonatologists often believe that the more effective approach is to give feedback to a group of people.

The forms of education used are several. One is the centralized conference (typically charging registration fees) to which people from many geographic areas are invited to hear experts and to exchange information. Another way is to do educational outreach, with an individual or team from the n.i.c.u. conducting a workshop at another hospital. Northeast Pediatric offered much of this kind of outreach. Educating the local nursing staff can also prevent mistakes by less-educable local physicians. Nurses can be on the alert for newborns who are cold or losing color, even if physicians are not. The n.i.c.u.'s educational outreach mission is in keeping with the general trend found in all health services to upgrade technical skills.

It can also have the effect of increasing the numbers of newborns referred to the Level III nursery as local staff members become sensitive to criteria for referral.

MAINTAINING THE REFERRAL SYSTEM

In summary, the n.i.c.u. is only as successful as are the continuous relations between the professionals and institutions involved. Professional relations can be marked with ambivalence, but this does not prevent the appropriate referral of many infants in medical need. The principal solution that neonatologists envision for inappropriate referrals or for better care of newborns before referral is educational, rather than confrontational or punitive so that the system of referrals will run smoothly. To survive as an active emergency treatment center, the Level III must maintain an open-door policy, respecting the directives of obstetricians and pediatricians who refer patients. The career of the infant patient admitted to the n.i.c.u. is the subject of the next chapter.

5

The Sanctity of Newborn Life: Aggressive Intervention

> No matter where you draw the line, you're going to be wrong part of the time. In general, the goal is to produce neurologically intact babies. But among some you let go, some would have turned out okay. And among some you save, there will be "gorks."
>
> *Attending Physician*

> It was so hard for them to think of even passive measures that would allow her to die when they had worked so hard to save her.
>
> *Social Worker*

IDEAL AND PROBLEM PATIENTS

Within the context of newborn intensive care, there are multiple rationales for treating patients with continuous maximum care. Central to all of them is the total vulnerability of the critically ill newborn, a condition which is its own imperative for treatment. There are, in addition, professional and institutional goals that overlay the obvious clinical needs of infants admitted to the Level III nursery.

Every profession envisions the ideal client who perfectly suits the expectations of the practitioner (Hughes, 1956; Shaw, 1974; Holmstrom and Burgess, 1983). In medicine, the components of that ideal client include "the nature of the illness and its amenability to treatment; the nature of the interaction between the patient in his role with the physician in his; and, finally, the effect of the patient on the physician's career" (Hughes, 1956:23). These characteristics of the ideal patient are as relevant to the situation in the intensive care unit as to other areas of medicine. In the intensive care unit, the second factor, interaction, takes on new dimensions. The severity of the intensive care patient's illness can turn professional interaction into a one-sided and reductionist estimate of the client's behavior. The good patient is one who responds physiologically, not necessarily socially. Critically ill newborns are a special instance of intensive care patient, accommodating themselves by the double convenience of their hospital birth and small size to emergency trans-

111

port and medical rescue. The newborn also presents special problems of advocacy and treatment because each infant patient is a social and physiological unknown. As ethicist David Smith commented:

> The striking thing about newborn persons . . . is precisely that they have no visible personal past. They have had no opportunity to develop a normality of their own functioning. No physical plateau, personality, character or style of life has had a chance to surface. The newborn presents himself as totally unexploited potential—if we were cynical we could say, as a field for potential exploitation. (1974:136)

If the referral of intensive care patients is efficient, practitioners receive a high percentage of "ideal" patients. These patients are critically ill (in true need of intensive care), have the appropriate, prerecognized malady (a pathology within the unit's specialty area), and respond quickly and predictably to treatment. In newborn intensive care, the first two criteria are generally well met because of the efficiency of the referral system. Regarding true need, a relatively healthy newborn is occasionally sent to a Level III nursery, usually for precautionary reasons. In one instance, we observed the weekend admission of a full-term but somewhat lethargic baby as a favor to a physician whose other referrals were more appropriate. But this kind of favor ("babysitting," the nurses called it) was rare. Equally rare was the admission of an infant with the wrong pathology. At Northeast Pediatric, the Level III nursery addressed primarily the problems of the premature newborn. Full-term babies with other pathologies, for example, major heart and neurological defects, often were referred to other hospital divisions. Other, larger n.i.c.u.'s we visited were not quite so streamlined in case selection; still, the majority of their patients were premature infants. In all n.i.c.u.'s, some proportion of referrals are inappropriate because the infants are beyond help. But the physicians evaluating these patients' needs have difficulty recognizing the futility of treatment or feel the pressure to put borderline cases under the authority of other physicians and institutions.

The third criterion for the ideal patient—response to treatment—is most troublesome for clinicians. The ideal patient in newborn intensive care is the "quick save," the infant who responds immediately and positively to the therapy offered. One experienced neonatology fellow described the more difficult long-term cases this way:

> It's hard for this unit because we're intensive and not used to long-term. . . . We're used to being instantly gratified.

The ideal trajectory of a cure is a straight line of progress that a patient traverses quickly. The "good baby," in the eyes of the n.i.c.u. staff, is admitted with a common condition, such as moderate respiratory distress syndrome, improves gradually over three or four days (Bogdan, Brown, and Foster, 1982), and is discharged to a Level II nursery or community hospital or home. In this model case, the mandate to treat aggressively, as a reflex communication from the patient's body to the clinicians, is untroubled by debate or dissension. A full 60 percent of the cases admitted and treated at Northeast Pediatric during our observation approximated this patient model.

N.i.c.u. newborns become problem cases when they disrupt the organizational routine of new admissions or the tempo of the unit's work. Problem cases fall into three categories, each of which in some way obstructs the system. The first consists of infants who die upon admission or just after. For these babies, the career as a patient never really begins. Instead, the dying infant represents a failure for the staff and demoralizes the unit, even when the referral is termed a mistake.

At Northeast Pediatric, dying infants were still given the initial heroic interventions of emergency manual ventilation, tracheal intubation, and medications. In one instance at Northeast Pediatric, we witnessed, within an hour of admission, the use of renal dialysis in a very premature infant born with a single malfunctioning kidney and other congenital anomalies and, within six hours, the death of that infant from lung and heart failure. The gross failure of multiple organ systems in a patient forces activity to a halt, leaving the involved physicians and nurses exhausted and with the inevitable feeling of having lost. Said one resident, "You can't get away from it. Every death is a failure."

The second type of problem newborn is the borderline or experimental case, the infant whose viability is hard to assess. Most often, in the n.i.c.u., the borderline case is a severely premature infant whose viability outside the uterus is questionable. Also troublesome are infants with serious congenital anomalies or puzzling symptoms or syndromes that do not respond to treatment. Borderline cases require a disproportionate amount of unit resources and engender the most discussion about proceeding with or withholding medical care.

The third category of infants whose conditions disrupt the n.i.c.u. routine are long-term cases, those infants who remain in the unit for as long as a month and sometimes as much as a year. These newborns (for example, those who remain oxygen-dependent) progress so slowly that they seem not to progress at all or their careers are marked by an unpredictable roller-coaster course of failures and revivals. Any long-term case is troubling because, as with the infant who dies at admission, it violates the staff's hope and need for quick victories and its sense of the appropriate schedule of illness and cure. The long-term case, through the continued occupancy of a bed-space, also obstructs the flow of new and challenging admissions that is so vital to the unit.

These three clinical categories can overlap. In fact, the most traumatic case for any unit's staff is the baby who is a problem in all these ways, that is, the borderline infant of debatable viability who becomes a long-term case and eventually dies. Although relatively small in number, the very low birth weight borderline cases are increasingly becoming the norm in Level III nurseries. These kinds of cases best highlight the clinical rationales for treatment and are the focus of this chapter. However, we first look briefly at the routine cases, in which decision making about the degree of aggressive intervention is straightforward and easily accomplished. These cases form the normative context within which the borderline cases are evaluated in rational terms (see Levin, 1985).

ROUTINIZATION OF THE DECISION TO TREAT AGGRESSIVELY

The Northeast Pediatric n.i.c.u. was dedicated to the aggressive care of critically ill newborns, even in the most difficult and marginal cases. In the overwhelming majority of cases, the most fundamental decision—whether or not to "go all out"—was easily and routinely made, and the answer was in the affirmative.

These routine, easily decided cases included some medically simple cases (for example, a baby with mild RDS) and some medically difficult ones (for example, an infant with severe persistent fetal circulation). Evaluating a routine case, even a medically simple one, requires processing highly complex information. Consider, for example, the case of a 28-week-old newborn with mild respiratory distress described by the nurse on the physician–nurse transport team as follows:

> The decision making was simple. The baby was 900 grams—small, but not extremely small for us. He was twenty-seven to twenty-eight weeks. If he'd been twenty-three to twenty-five weeks, then you'd question his viability. Or if he'd been around 500 grams. He was big enough to treat. . . . He was vigorous. If he'd been seizing or if he just lay there like a

lump, then we'd be concerned. Also, we looked at his blood gases—how low had his oxygen ever been. . . . And his Apgars were good.

She explained how, with experience, one becomes skilled at integrating information:

When you walk in, you can see. You get a feel for which babies are viable. You put a lot of things together—color, activity, how the baby responds, lab values, responses to treatment.

The routine but medically difficult case requires the processing of even more information. For example, a baby was admitted to the n.i.c.u. with serious but undefined problems. The bed was immediately surrounded by machinery as the physicians tried to reach a principal diagnosis:

Suddenly someone watching the ultrasound screen called out, "Right to left shunt—there it goes!" There was elation in the group because they finally had the answer. The attending physician noted with satisfaction, "We're pretty sure of our diagnosis—PFC [persistent fetal circulation]," and directed the discussion to treatment goals.

On another occasion, this same attending physician described to us the process of decision making at admission, noting that the most difficult thing was figuring out what treatment course the newborn should be on. "Once a baby is on track, then the care is relatively easy. The hardest thing is to decide which track the baby should be [on]." Medically difficult cases such as the one described above may require a great deal of discussion, but the discussion is about which course of treatment to take, not whether to treat.

Routine, easily decided cases also include badly asphyxiated newborns with brain damage. These cases are demoralizing to the staff because the chances of turning out a "good product" are low. Of one such case, an infant who was being treated aggressively with the respirator, Priscoline (a drug that dilates the pulmonary blood vessels), and gavage feeding, the nurse said, "We're hopeful we'll be able to send the baby home and not to institutionalize him." However, as long as such cases leave the unit quickly, they do not have a major impact on the mood of the unit.

Such badly compromised infants will be admitted routinely if the delivery room decision is to refer. For example, in one case, the delivery was not properly managed. After delivery, the resuscitation was prolonged, although the infant's Apgar scores continued to be low (0 at one minute; 2 at five minutes). The n.i.c.u. fellow referred to it as an "overly aggressive resuscitation." Nevertheless, by the time of admission to the n.i.c.u., the infant was breathing and therefore considered physically viable but seriously brain-damaged. There was never any question about treatment: the treatment was given. As in the vast majority of n.i.c.u. cases, whether medically simple or difficult, the decision to be aggressive did not involve long discussion, reflection, or emotional agonizing. On the contrary, such decisions were virtually automatic.

DISPROPORTIONATE IMPACT OF BORDERLINE CASES

Borderline cases constitute a small percentage of most units' admissions, but they have a disproportionate impact on the staff's attention, energy, and emotions. A minority of cases were defined by the Northeast Pediatric staff as borderline or as not viable; only 11 of the 103 consecutive admissions we studied, for example, fit this category. These cases typically led to agonizing staff discussions about the appropriate aggressiveness of intervention. In an even smaller minority of cases, the decision was reached to withdraw or withhold certain treatment; this decision occurred in only 5 of the 103 consecutive admissions (Table 5.1).

Only in the case of extremely ill infants was the appropriateness of aggressive intervention discussed. In the subgroup of six such cases in which, after discussion, aggressive care was continued, the newborns were so ill that they either died soon (in 9 days or less) or they remained a very long time in intensive care (68 to 143 days). Despite continued aggressive treatment, four of the six babies died. All six suffered from prematurity and evidenced numerous physical problems, including, in some cases, neurological damage. Five of the six weighed less than 1,000 grams; one was slightly larger, 1,070 grams.

In the other subgroup of five cases for which the aggressiveness of treatment was debated, certain therapies were selectively withdrawn or withheld. The newborn typically was either without brain activity, dying, or suffering from a known terminal condition. The one exception was a difficult long-term case. This infant's borderline condition was discussed in frequent special meetings for four months, but the n.i.c.u. staff never could bring itself to withdraw treatment in any clear-cut way. After months of ambivalence, the staff resolved the problem by discharging the infant to a Level II unit within the same hospital. They reasoned that the baby no longer needed intensive care. The staff also knew that the baby thereby would be exposed to greater risk due to less stringent surveillance.

Table 5.1. Cases from Consecutive N.I.C.U. Series Sample Leading to Discussion of Appropriate Level of Intervention (1979)

Type of Case	Level of Aggressiveness Discussed; Initial and All Subsequent Care Aggressive	Days in Level III Unit	Outcome*
1070 gm	Low birthweight, numerous physical problems, neurologic problems (grade 3 to 4 intraventricular hemorrhage, high chance of retardation)	73	Alive
980 gm	Low birthweight, numerous physical problems	3	Died
910 gm	Low birthweight, numerous physical problems, lack of progress, finally deterioration	68	Died
710 gm	Low birthweight, numerous physical problems	143	Alive
690 gm	Low birthweight, multiple congenital anomalies, chromosomal question	1	Died
480 gm	Very low birthweight, smaller than any surviving patient at this n.i.c.u.	9	Died

Type of Case	Level of Aggressiveness Discussed; Initial Treatment Aggressive; Later Treatment Withdrawn, Decreased, or Withheld	Eventual Action Taken	Days in Level III Intensive Care	Outcome
3000 gm	Dead (brain death)	Taken off respirator, mother "held baby"	4	Died
1304 gm	Dying (from lungs and brain)	Respirator turned off; DNR decision also made	15	Died
1275 gm	Dying (from lungs)	Taken off respirator; Mother "held baby."	10	Died
740 gm	A "mistake" by the unit. "A thing we created." Numerous long-term physical problems; severe neurologic problems (grade 4 intraventricular hemorrhage)	Discharged to lower level of unit, with n.i.c.u. staff understanding that surveillance would decrease	136	Died in second unit
620 gm	Known fatal condition (620 gm with respiratory distress)	Because of parental forcefulness, treatment aggressive contrary to staff wishes; staff however quickly set limits (no cardiac massage, no cardiac meds)	4	Died

*Outcome as of the end of our field research at Northeast Pediatric.

The baby died after twenty-seven days in the lower-level unit. As an n.i.c.u. nurse said afterwards, the baby's death was "predictable." (See Chapter 8 for a detailed case study of this infant.)

Cases in which aggressiveness of care was an issue forced the staff to reflect on the value of treatment. These cases put the staff members in the position of consciously making life-and-death decisions—of "playing God," as they referred to it—a position most found uncomfortable. Nonetheless, the decisions made in the n.i.c.u. have such obviously serious and controversial consequences that they cannot always be routine. N.i.c.u. technology can prolong suffering and postpone an inevitable death in ways never before possible. It can also save permanently damaged children who, in earlier times, simply would have died. In these cases, the amount of the infants' suffering and possible poor outcomes cause some n.i.c.u. staff to wonder about the long-range goals of neonatology and about treatment limits in newborn intensive care. Borderline cases exhaust their caregivers right up to the point of the resolution of the treatment decision. Yet the presence of borderline cases in the unit, like the high frequency of infant deaths, is a predictable feature of work in the progressive Level III nursery. An expanding admissions policy and professional commitment to heroic intervention guarantee this tendency. Borderline cases often dominate the mood of the unit and generate highly charged discussions that reveal the parameters of the mandate to treat. Almost all of the factors governing the treatment of these infants work in the direction of the unit's giving maximum aggressive intervention rather than limiting, withdrawing, or withholding it.

PROFESSIONAL HIERARCHY AND IDEOLOGY

The most important determinant of aggressive intervention in newborn intensive care is dual: the sense of mission of the senior physicians and the position of authority that allows them to carry out that mission via the unit team. Attending physicians have more power and authority than do the fellows or residents. Physicians as a group have more power and authority than do nurses. The staff as a collectivity has more immediate power and authority than do parents or external authorities.

At Northeast Pediatric, all the attending physicians were neonatologists committed to their subspecialty's mission of advancing the clinical frontier. Their assumption was that the clinical frontier would move in the direction of more successful treatment of extremely premature newborns whose viability would be continually demonstrated in the clinical setting. Theoretically, a borderline baby this year might not be a borderline baby if born next year. The rapidity of change in neonatology was noted in the following conversation.

> *Nurse:* "We're doing all right with twenty-four-weekers. But this baby was borderline—the eyes were still fused. You can't afford to play that game and say it's not viable. At twenty-four weeks you have to assume they may survive."
>
> *Consulting physician:* "When we were house officers back in the dark ages in 1974 there was no question—the twenty-four-weekers didn't survive. But it will get earlier and earlier."

Attending Physicians' Authority over Staff

The attending physicians at Northeast Pediatric typically used their clout to persuade the other physicians to be aggressive. Attending physicians might question whether a particular case was viable, but only if it was a very extreme case. In those rare cases when there was a difference of opinion among physicians, it was almost always a junior physician, typically a resident, who questioned aggressive treatment. A newborn with multiple anomalies is a case in point. At the staff meeting, it was a young (and unpopular) resident, who challenged the group about policy. The attending physician pulled rank on him:

> *Resident:* "I'm willing to defer to the parents [if we find out they want aggressive treatment]. But I'm bothered that you're willing to turn out a large number of failures."
>
> *Attending physician:* "I disagree. We have very few failures compared to healthy [results]."
>
> *Resident:* "But this is not one of them."
>
> *Attending physician:* "For those of us who have more experience, we feel we don't have quite enough information to make a decision to stop."

Physicians use their power and authority to gain the behavioral (although not necessarily attitudinal) cooperation of nurses. N.i.c.u. physicians are usually more committed to aggressive care in borderline cases than are most nurses. A psychiatric consultant to the unit commented about this difference, saying to us, "Nurses are more holistic," that is, they consider long-term social consequences in evaluating cases. His observation was corroborated by our observations numerous times during our fieldwork. Again and again, we heard nurses criticizing senior physicians for being overly aggressive, concentrating on clinical problems in isolation from clinical outcome. For example, in the case of a particularly small premature infant, twenty-six to twenty-seven weeks of gestation, with intraventricular hemorrhage and patent ductus arteriosus, the physicians' treatment was very aggressive. The psychiatric consultant's reaction upon seeing the baby was: "She looks 'horrendo' by my standards." The nurses agreed. As one nurse reported to us:

> When the baby was seizing and obviously had brain damage, there were some feelings of, "Why are we supporting the baby?" About operating if the baby will die anyway. These were mostly nursing concerns, and medicine was very aggressive. You get so you don't fight them any more.

This particular baby underwent surgery for her heart problem, spent fifteen days in the n.i.c.u., and died.

N.i.c.u. nurses openly stated a more comprehensive view of patients than did physicians in staff meetings, taking the position of not wanting to treat an infant just for survival's sake. Nurses also sometimes were critical of specific attending physicians whose sense of medical mission was perceived as narrow. The more biting comments were reserved for times when senior physicians were not around. For example, about one attending physician, the nurses said, in a critical tone, "She resuscitates every time." About another, a nurse commented on attitudinal and authority differences between physicians and nurses:

> This doctor would rather send twenty kids to the state institution and have them retarded than turn off a baby who has a chance. He's caused babies undue suffering. That's not my philosophy. Of course, it's easier for me to feel my way because I'm a nurse and the responsibility ultimately isn't mine.

Nurses, more often than physicians, work with mixed feelings about patients; that is, they can actively work to save a child and simultaneously hope that the child will not survive. The case of a 567-gram baby of twenty-four weeks' gestational age illustrates this difference in occupational outlook. The infant first responded well, but later deteriorated and suffered from, among other things, bowel degeneration (necrotizing enterocolitis). The physicians decided to operate to remove the diseased part of bowel, since surgery held out the only possibility of saving the child. The nurses' response, in contrast, was to pray for her death. "As she became sicker, we were down on our knees hoping that she wouldn't make it." The baby was near death at the time of surgery, and the surgery postponed the death only one day. Still, the fact remains that the responsibility for saving the infant's life lay with senior physicians, whose right it is to interpret the mandate of intensive care.

Consensus Required to Withhold Treatment

Despite the direct influence of the senior physicians, there exists a norm that the staff should collectively air case problems about withdrawing or limiting treatment. The emphasis is on reaching a team consensus. This is a highly significant professional factor contributing to aggressive care and it works in just one direction, the same direction as the neonatologists' mission. If just a single staff member speaks up and insists on continued aggressive treatment, further treatment typically is given. The advocate need not be an attending physician; it can be a resident or nurse.

It was highly unusual for a resident at Northeast Pediatric to be more enthusiastic than an attending physician about aggressive care. But if this atypical situation occurred, it tipped the balance toward aggressive treatment. If, however, junior staff members felt that care should be stopped, they had to argue against the experience and authority of their superiors. Residents disagreeing with an aggressive treatment plan were rarely confrontational at work rounds or in conferences. Nurses could voice their opposition at formal meetings or at bedside but had no authority over such clinical decisions. Moreover, once a conclusion was reached in a decision-making conference, all participants felt pressured to abide by it.

In general, the unit's staff preferred to have parental agreement before actually withholding treatment. For example, in the case of the full-term infant with no brain activity, the fellow said to us:

> We felt the decision was straightforward. . . . The history of the length of time to resuscitate was incompatible with any hope of survival, let alone intact survival. Early Friday we couldn't get any indication of any brain activity. . . . [But as for taking the infant off of the respirator], we couldn't do that unless the parents were in agreement. We wouldn't even think of doing it without that. We have to know they feel good about that being done.

If parents persisted in demanding aggressive care beyond what the staff saw as reasonable, the staff could bring enormous pressure to bear on them to change their minds. All possible professional authority was used. For example, in one case, after seven weeks, the physicians decided that the clinical situation of the infant was hopeless and they wanted to decrease intervention. They called on a consulting psychiatrist to help convince the resistant father that this was the only reasonable course of action.

If a baby clearly was dying (that is, death was only a matter of hours or possibly a day), the staff would more freely decide to limit treatment without consulting the parents. For example, in the case of one critically ill baby whose condition took a turn for the worse, the resident and two nurses met in the conference room on a Sunday afternoon to discuss the situation. The resident began the discussion:

> It's clear now that the baby's demise really is occurring and that we need a plan for two things: (1) how to handle it with the parents, and (2) what to do if the baby arrests.

The nurses agreed with his judgment that the infant's death was at hand. The resident said, "I feel we should not resuscitate. We should not give a round of medications." The nurses agreed. The neonatology fellow stopped by and, acting for the attending physician, approved the decision. The group was in agreement that the infant's lungs were so bad that there was nothing they could do; the fellow added that he had become discouraged by the infant's brain bleeds. While it is possible that other people were later consulted, the basic course of action for handling the death was laid out at this Sunday meeting, without the parents being present. In this and other instances, such decisions were communicated to the parents as the physicians' opinion.

Treatment on Transport and at Admission: Benefit of the Doubt

In the n.i.c.u. schedule, there are actually two distinct times for medical decision making: the initial rescue intervention at transport and admission, and during subsequent care. This second phase may be subdivided further for an infant whose lengthy clinical course changes markedly and requires reassessment. In both phases, the rationale for heroic treatment rests on the belief that the hospital's technology optimizes the single most important goal of the service: physical survival. The moral component of the rationale draws on the principle of patient advocacy, again, with a stress on survival. In the following pages, we first consider the staff's justifications in both phases of clinical decision making.

The treatment of newborns is unique in that the staff must concentrate on the present welfare of a patient who has no past and whose future can only be conjectured. More than with cases of adults or even young children, the n.i.c.u. staff treating neonates is clinically in the dark.

In the initial phase of decision making, uncertainty is related to the time it takes to get sufficient medical information to make an informed decision. There are many instances when it takes hours or days to obtain the relevant diagnostic information. A common n.i.c.u. staff response is to temporarily suspend judgment. The policy at Northeast Pediatric was to support maximum intervention from the moment of referral through transport. At this early point, the team felt that it did not know all the facts of a case and therefore should treat. Consider, for example, this description of a transport:

> The baby had multiple, multiple congenital abnormalities. Some type of a "trisomy," open myelomeningocele, club hand, rocker-bottom feet, cleft palate. . . . Horrible transport. The kid arrested three times after being intubated. We were down at this hospital for five hours.

The transport was nonetheless completed, and the infant died in the n.i.c.u.

The policy was also to intervene aggressively at admission, as the infant was moved from a portable incubator to a unit isolette. For example, a very low birth weight baby (650 grams, twenty-six to twenty-seven weeks of gestation) was admitted with RDS and multiple congenital anomalies: ambiguous genitalia, cleft palate, fused digits on the left foot, low-set ears. On the day of admission, the staff fished for reasons either to go ahead or to withdraw. The resident commented, "Sure, he looks funny, but you don't know if he'll be a good baby. If you can't prove zero prognosis, you're stuck with treating." The physicians were anxious to get diagnostic information quickly. One attending physician explained, "We could find a chromosomal anomaly so bad that the baby wouldn't have to be resuscitated." The thinking was that the chromosomal test might reveal a disease that would severely limit the infant's life span to, say, a few months, and this fact would justify limiting intervention.

At rounds the next morning, the unit team was still troubled by the case. After rounds, the group (four physicians, one nurse) sat down to talk. One resident confronted the group with the question of how many damaged cases they were willing to turn out in order not to overlook a viable infant.

> *First resident:* "In this case, there's a one-in-five chance of turning out a child, period—normal or abnormal. But we also have to look at other things. If a trisomy, it would be zero. But a lot of these things chip

away at that 20 percent. With three minor abnormalities, the chances of major abnormalities are high."

Second resident: "But we haven't found that yet."

First resident: "You're saying there's some chance of being normal, and you're willing to turn out a lot of unacceptable products for this nursery."

Attending physician: "We'd accept definite neurological damage as evidence. If there was a big documented bleed and exam, we'd know his prognosis is dismal. But now we don't know."

The debate continued until the second resident commented, with resignation, "I don't have a reason to not resuscitate." The basic rule was that until one has information that gives one a reason not to treat, one is obligated to treat.

The benefit of the doubt at admission was also extended to cases of sudden arrest, even for newborns with a high probability of serious brain damage. For example, one day an infant was admitted before morning rounds and a group of physicians and nurses gathered routinely around the new admission. Suddenly the baby's heart arrested. The physicians and nurses quickly began vigorous resuscitation with chest massage and a hand-held bag for oxygen. These initial measures did not work, so the team moved to more invasive steps. The resident involved explained the scene to us later:

> *Resident:* "So you go to the 'big guns,' which are intracardiac epinephrine and intracardiac Isuprel. We did this. It was the last thing done. We knew we'd coded the kid for twenty-five to thirty minutes and if you don't get back by then there is not much you can save because the head is not being perfused with oxygen. . . . Twenty-five to thirty minutes is pretty standard, especially with a baby that we knew had a destroyed brain from his delivery."
>
> *Researcher:* "Did you really know that? What kind of information told you that?"
>
> *Resident:* "We had information that he was in utero for an hour after the other twin was born, had seizures afterward, was difficult to manage, and had PFC, which is one of the most difficult things to manage."

Despite indications of severe neurological damage, vigorous attempts were made to save this infant; the resuscitation, however, was unsuccessful and the infant died.

The countering of medical uncertainty with maximum intervention is not limited to the initial phase of transport and admission. In the next section, we discuss uncertainty as a more pervasive issue in clinical care, especially in making decisions in long-term cases.

MEDICAL UNCERTAINTY AND THE AGGRESSIVE BIAS

Choice of Type of Error

Parsons (1951) called attention to the general significance of uncertainty for medical practitioners. There are various sources of uncertainty in medicine, including the level of experience of the physician and the state of the art, as Fox pointed out in her study of medical students. There can be uncertainty related to "imperfect mastery of what is currently known in the various fields of medicine" (no one can know it all) and uncertainty due to "limitations in the current state of medical knowledge" (1957:239–40).

Neonatologists at major medical centers are attracted to the concept of overcoming the limitations of medical knowledge regarding fetal and neonatal development. For neonatologists actively engaged in research, the hospital routine of patient care can be offset by explorations into organ processes and infant development afforded by basic and clinical investigations. Informally, all clinicians in newborn intensive care are involved in a fundamentally experimental approach to casework, based on the trend toward treating lower birth weight patients. In expanding the unit's services to borderline and even experimental cases, neonatologists increase the degree of uncertainty they must face in their work.

In this situation of clinical uncertainty, the question is not whether one's predictions and course of action will sometimes be wrong. Rather, it is a question of choosing which type of error one is more willing to risk. A physician can intervene aggressively more frequently and increase the risks of saving a severely damaged, nonfunctioning child. Or a physician can be medically aggressive less frequently and increase the risk of letting a viable infant die.

Scheff's classic article on decision making called attention to the fact that the medical profession has developed norms for handling uncertainty in work:

> Judging a sick person well is more to be avoided than judging a well person sick. . . . The rule in medicine may be stated as: "When in doubt, continue to suspect illness." . . . It is far more culpable to dismiss a sick patient than to retain a well one. (1963:97)

The rule Scheff described leads physicians to judge certain people to be more sick than they really are. In neonatology, the rule regarding aggressive intervention leads physicians to judge certain newborns as more viable (more healthy) than they really are. But on a general level, these two rules are the same: Do not overlook or fail to treat a case that might be helped by your care or harmed by your lack of care. The bias remains in favor of intervention.

Crane made a similar observation about the medical treatment of critically ill patients. She noted that the medical system stresses "the preservation of life at all costs" and suggested that there are widespread threats to the norm:

> The system responds to this danger by overstressing the importance of treating, even when the patient cannot benefit from the treatment, in order to avoid the possibility that the individual who might benefit from treatment will not be treated. (1977:204)

Northeast Pediatric's tertiary unit likewise solved this dilemma by emphasizing maximum intervention. In addition, the claims to success in neonatology traditionally rest on the numbers of infants who survive, which is a further incentive for unit physicians to choose the risks of treating over the risks of withholding treatment.

New Patient Populations

In the atmosphere of latent experimentation that can pervade the n.i.c.u., uncertainty about new kinds of patients and technologies is associated with an absence of reliable information about long-term outcome. Borderline, usually very low birth weight, infants constitute the new patient population. As the clinical frontier recedes, the n.i.c.u. treats new types of patients, and treats patients in new ways. Thus, at any point in time, n.i.c.u. physicians must make decisions about some patients in their units who represent types of cases for which there have been few or no survivors. Or there may be few long-term survivors or none. This lack of information was often discussed by the Northeast Pediatric n.i.c.u. staff. An attending physician talking to residents emphasized the number of years that must pass before there exists a group of survivors that can be analyzed:

> It seems eight years is the age at which you can say how they will turn out. Prior to age eight you can tell a lot. But up to age eight you still can uncover new problems.

At social service rounds one day, a fellow and a hospital lawyer also discussed the problem:

> *Fellow:* "About quality of life, for [infants weighing] 650 to 700 grams we don't know too much. We try to do a lot of things to try to prevent brain damage."

Lawyer: "So prognosis is difficult because historically you do not have children that have survived."

N.i.c.u. physicians feel they must make decisions in a certain percentage of cases even when the results of these decisions cannot be meaningfully evaluated for a number of years. Simple survival statistics, on the other hand, are immediately available.

Neurological Outcome

The neurological status of the infant is the most important outcome characteristic by which clinicians judge normalcy. There have been great diagnostic improvements, such as computerized axial tomography (CAT) scans, and ultrasound, to aid in the evaluation of the neonate's brain and nervous system. Yet despite the current availability of CAT scans and ultrasound at most major centers, most n.i.c.u. physicians emphasize the incertitudes of predicting developmental outcome. Neurological damage may be in evidence, but there still is the added factor of infant and child development that, optimally, might override or cancel out a bad beginning. Thus, these physicians consider continued aggressive intervention to be justified.

Concerning a controversial case, one n.i.c.u. nurse recounted:

> If the baby does survive, his CAT scan [of the brain] is absolutely horrible. But the doctor says some [with scans] like that . . . do walk and talk.

Neurological damage does not inevitably result in less aggressive treatment. Indeed, physicians at Northeast Pediatric often persevered in spite of evidence such as extensive brain bleeds and serious, overwhelming neurological compromise. However, neurological damage in combination with multiple medical problems could justify the rare decision to withhold treatment. A neonatology fellow described one such case, beginning with a list of the infant's other medical conditions:

> Very severe lung disease—bronchopulmonary dysplasia—a disease that follows therapy, that is caused by the earlier medical therapy. GI [gastrointestinal] gut disease. We think it is getting better. This seems to be the one area of progress. Sepsis [infection]—we think we're on top of that.

She then spoke of the neurological condition and its effect on the staff's thinking:

The most worrisome [is] the EEG [electroencephalogram]. Not as active now. Her EEG is very, very bad. Neurology tells us, very bad. . . . Did EEG again—very abnormal, very bizarre, seems very damaged. The evoked potentials show basic functions are there, brainstem functions are there. But we're not sure about anything above that. . . . When the evoked potential was flat, we began talking in a more direct way of how much more to do for her.

The staff's enthusiasm for treatment was tempered in this and other similar cases largely by the neurological situation. In this particular case, however, other factors, including the mother's close involvement with the baby, resulted in the decision to continue aggressive treatment.

Statistical versus Case-by-Case Analysis: Discounting the Odds

The literature on medical outcome has for many years supported the strong association of serious permanent handicaps (severe mental retardation, cerebral palsy of a significant degree, major seizure disorders, and blindness) with very low birth weight (Budetti et al., 1981:34–38). Statistics on the condition of infants born weighing less than 1,500 grams come from small and not always comparable studies in which follow-up selection may be for healthier survivors (Dann et al., 1964). Major pediatric journals regularly report improvements in outcome for extremely premature infants, yet these articles do not refute the fact that a high risk of death and permanent severe handicaps is correlated with decreased birth weight.

When we consider that most infants admitted to Northeast Pediatric in 1979 weighed 1,500 grams or less at birth, it is clear that physicians did not think in terms of statistical probability but of the experimental, case-by-case advancement of the birth weight frontier. In clinical practice, the focus was on the exceptional case, the "write-off" who survived against all the odds and refuted the power of statistical forecasting.

As unit directors well know, nothing is better for the morale of the staff than the reunion party for former n.i.c.u. patients, including "write-offs" who have done well. One fellow at Northeast Pediatric, enthusiastic about the success ratio and certainly exaggerating past uncertainties about treatment, emphasized to us the tremendous impression it made on him to see children returning to the hospital for one such graduates' reunion party:

We went over the records and one-third had looked so bad that there had been discussion about taking them off the ventilator. And now at age three, they're walking around normal. Or, at age three, you can't tell definitely, but still, not with major morbidity. That's why it's so hard to stop.

Another day, a nurse showed off a graduate:

Morning rounds were interrupted when a nurse brought in a child [toddler] looking well. The nurse announced, with dramatic flair, "Six shunts—a 'write-off.' "

Still another day, a nurse at social service rounds summarized the dilemma succinctly: "Everyone has seen someone you think is going to be a 'gork' but who turns out okay."

Few hospitals heavily invest in the systematic follow-up of n.i.c.u. patients and therefore few n.i.c.u. staff members have the experience of observing the consequences of the treatment they give to the newborns. It is often up to the individual staff members to create and maintain follow-up clinics. Usually one physician per unit gets involved in either clinical follow-up or in social research on former patients and their families. Often there are no particular incentives or rewards in neonatology for this work. At Northeast Pediatric, the follow-up clinic was run on a volunteer basis, with the help of a developmental psychologist, a social worker, and a female senior neonatologist. Whatever transpired in follow-up was usually not communicated back to the n.i.c.u.; if it was, there was a strong emphasis on good outcome.

As the emphasis on victories suggests, one has to look not only at what outcome information exists but also at how physicians perceive and act upon this information. Physicians talk of odds, and, in some cases—for example, cases of known fatal conditions—their decisions are influenced by the high probability of failure. Nevertheless, the tendency is to be aggressive even against the odds, on the chance that the infant will be the exceptional one that "makes it." An attending physician, speaking to residents, presented decision making as statistically balanced:

No matter where you draw the line, you're going to be wrong part of the time. In general the goal is to produce neurologically intact babies. . . . [But] among some you let go, some would have turned out okay. And among some you save, there will be "gorks." It's important to realize this fact—that you're bound to be wrong part of the time—and to not feel guilty about it.

Yet, in fact, treatment decisions were uniformly more aggressive than this quote suggests. The overriding goal was to not overlook a pa-

tient who might, against the odds, make it. The actual decisions followed what economist Victor Fuchs called the "technologic imperative":

> Medical tradition emphasizes giving the best care that is technically pos-
> sible; the only legitimate and explicitly recognized constraint is the state
> of the art. . . . . All this sets medical care distinctly apart from most goods
> and services. Automobile makers do not, and are not expected to, pro-
> duce the best car that engineering skills permit. They are expected to weigh
> potential improvement against potential cost. (1968:192)

The technologic imperative provides a rationale for discounting the
odds and for using state-of-the-art techniques aggressively for almost all neonates. Virtually unlimited medical options combined with
strong protective sentiments for newborns are two key components
promoting aggressive intervention in the n.i.c.u. The Level III unit
itself is the organizational embodiment of the technologic imperative.

DEFLECTING ATTENTION FROM THE ODDS

Four interrelated ways of thinking, each deflecting attention away
from probable odds, orient the n.i.c.u. staff toward aggressive intervention. Each is a variation on the theme of the technologic imperative in that the battery of medical resources available shapes
clinical attitudes and behavior.

Incrementalism and Turning Points

One aspect of the daily n.i.c.u. treatment pattern is its incremental
nature. One intervention leads to another, often not by any dramatic process of decision making but in small steps. As one resident
said, "You get into the morass bit by bit." A theme often heard at
Northeast Pediatric was that it is hard to intervene halfway. The case
of an infant with a fatal condition led to this discussion:

> *Social worker:* "Once you start, can you morally, ethically, stop?"
> *Fellow:* "It's hard. It's all or none. That's why it's so important to make
>   the decision about whether to put the baby on the respirator. Once
>   you put the infant on the respirator, then you're into it. Then if he
>   needs a chest tube, you do a chest tube; if one, you do the second
>   tube. One thing leads to another. There is no [definitive] evidence
>   yet about the brain. So it makes it difficult to find a reason to turn
>   [the respirator] off, except our experience."

It is hard to wage a limited battle against death and disease; the pressures in the n.i.c.u. are to escalate the degree of intervention, that is, to opt for surgery and other procedures. One n.i.c.u. physician called this the "locomotive phenomenon."

Despite incrementalism, certain procedures in the n.i.c.u. are defined as turning points. An example is the decision to put an infant on a respirator. As Fox and Swazey (1974:10) noted about the significance of starting renal dialysis—"once this was done, 'we would be stuck with her' "—so too, in the n.i.c.u., does oxygen support signal the staff's commitment to treat. Likewise, commencing intravenous feeding can be a turning point. Physicians and nurses understand the hazards of a wrong decision. Putting a newborn on the respirator is a critical turning point. One may keep alive an infant who always will be dependent on a machine. One may prolong suffering and merely postpone an inevitable deterioration. In the case of a newborn with a fatal condition, for example, there was discussion about whether to resuscitate. The unit director said:

> There's a difference between resuscitation and putting him on the ventilator. I'd bag him [manually assist breathing] and give meds, but I wouldn't put him on the ventilator.

In this case, the physician was willing to perform short-term (resuscitation) but not long-term (prolonged oxygen support) heroics.

Physicians differ in what they see as the point of no return. But it was clear at Northeast Pediatric that once the staff started aggressive measures, they got progressively more involved and found it difficult to stop.

Investment

Another rationale for continued intervention is the staff's strong sense of practical investment in a case. As physicians and nurses become professionally invested in a baby, they want a return for their work. They see their labor as a limited resource. As one fellow asked when a baby began to fail, "How much energy, time, effort should we continue to pour into her?"

The harder the staff works on a case, the harder it may be to give up. The process is like the economic concept of "sunk money"—it is difficult to admit that an enterprise has failed and so one may end up spending good money after bad. It is difficult for n.i.c.u. staff to admit that they may have over-intervened, and thus they may continue to over-intervene, even in a medically hopeless case.

Physicians and nurses themselves use the term "investment." In the case of the baby with numerous congenital anomalies described previously, physicians were anxious to get diagnostic information on chromosomes (which might have given them a reason to limit treatment) before too much effort had been invested:

> We have to go ahead with this case. We should get some information from the geneticists about chromosomal problems. And we should get it right away, because we'll have so much invested in him in twenty-four hours.

The unit's social worker reported the staff's sense of investment in another case:

> It was so hard for them to think of even passive measures that would allow her to die when they have worked so hard to save her.

The rewards of investment and the avoidance of waste are multidimensional concepts that refer not only to labor but to emotions as a limited resource. A nurse commented, "The longer babies are around, the more we invest our time, energy, and emotions in them." The ultimate waste of effort, then, is the long-term patient who dies. In the attempt to avoid this disaster, the staff often turned to yet another clinical procedure to patch up an ultimately hopeless case.

Reductionist Mode of Thinking

Medicine's emphasis on the parts of the body is still another professional factor that encourages aggressive intervention. Cassell argues that the relative absence of humanistic concern in medicine today is due to the way physicians are trained to think analytically about cases, instead of responding personally to patients.

> The analytic thought mode is, by its essential nature, depersonalizing, as each step in the explanation of the body moves further from the individuality of one person's body to the universality of biological process. (1975:2)

Highly research-oriented neonatologists at Northeast Pediatric moved easily from the discussion of a particular infant's condition to an analysis of lung development, heart pathologies, or bowel degeneration. If the patient was reduced to a set of pathologies, aggressive treatment could go on indefinitely or until the bodily system broke down. The emphasis on analytic thought, like the emphasis on technical skills and vitalism, restricted value questions about the overall consequences of medical intervention. As long as there was a treatable organ, intervention was seen as justified. This narrow focus on pathology obscured the broader view of the patient as a potentially full social being and celebrated instead partial clinical victories. At Northeast Pediatric, even multiple severe pathologies could be treated simultaneously with maximum aggression without anyone in the unit, except perhaps the nurses, stepping back for an overview of the patient's condition. A sign on one physician's wall (in another hospital) phrased the problem ironically: "If God gives you an infant but takes away the lungs, heart, kidney, and brain, maybe He's trying to tell you something."

Death from the Proper Cause

Physicians' preference for a certain kind of death also contributes to continued aggressive care, or at least selective aggressive care. Even though a patient's overall case may be hopeless, physicians do not like the patient to die of a discrete technical lack that they can fix. For instance, a consulting psychiatrist at Northeast Pediatric made the following observation:

> Doctors each have a way they like a baby to die. For example, in this case, the baby had a pneumothorax. They could put a tube in, or they could do nothing and the baby would die rapidly. They had decided pretty much not to resuscitate. But the doctor on call could not let the baby die for that reason [from the pneumothorax]. People like a certain kind of death, even though death is coming. . . .

To quote a phrase used by n.i.c.u. physicians, the child should "die of his disease." As mentioned in Chapter 2, this perspective became a bone of contention between medicine and nursing in the case of a baby with a fatal degenerative disease. The physician thought that if the infant developed an infection, he should be given antibiotics (even though death from his primary disease was imminent). The nurses, in contrast, thought that administering antibiotics was wrong because it would merely delay the inevitable and prolong the infant's suffering. The physician won out.

Furthermore, from a physician's perspective, a compromised child should not die from a mechanical problem. For example, in the case of the baby with multiple anomalies, even a resident who was outspoken against aggressive treatment said, "You're not going to let him die of a blocked tube." This resident advocated not being aggressive in this case, but nevertheless thought it important that there not be any equipment or technical failure that would bring about the infant's death. The focus has narrowed to the issue of technique, not broadened to the overall state of the patient; doing the right thing means using appropriate technical skills.

The four rationales for intervention—incrementalism, case investment, the analytic approach, and the notion of appropriate death—in their combination of reductive thinking and pragmatism are characteristic of modern medicine in general. Their repercussions have changed with the growth of acute care, hospitals, and medical specialization. All four rationales deflect attention from a broader calculation of the patient's chances for a meaningful life. Their influence on aggressive medical intervention is reinforced by the ideology of advocacy, which for the infant patient is construed almost entirely in terms of maximum medical treatment.

ADVOCACY FOR THE INFANT PATIENT

Mission of the Unit

The n.i.c.u. staff often expressed the desire to protect the best interests of the newborns by giving intensive care treatment. At Northeast Pediatric, physicians and nurses saw themselves as advocates for the patient. A fellow, discussing a controversial case with us, explained:

> Sometimes we have babies that prove to be a burden on the parents and on themselves. But you can't predict. You have to be an advocate for the child. It takes a lot for us to give up on a child.

Typically, being an advocate meant promoting the idea that a "child deserves every chance," that is, every chance to live.

Identifying with the child's life is a partisan position. The aim is to exclude from one's mind (and from decision making) any factor that might indicate less aggressive care, provided the consensus of the staff is to treat. For example, although physicians are aware that a severely damaged child has a major impact on a family, their goal is to screen out such information, especially if it is information about parental rejection.

A social worker at Northeast Pediatric with a more family-centered view attended a staff meeting held to determine whether to continue treating a borderline infant. The neonate had been very ill since birth, and her early course was complicated by severe patent ductus arteriosis requiring three operations, and bowel infection. After seven and one-half weeks of intensive care, the baby was still critically ill and had become neurologically compromised. At social service rounds the neonatology fellow summarized the case:

> Neurologically, seizure last week, poor prognosis. Not improving at all. Lungs the same, GI [gastrointestinal system] the same, neuro worse.

By this time, the resident had explained to the mother that the baby's "brain might not be too good," and the mother appeared to be accepting of this condition. The social worker, concerned not only with the mother's overt response but also with the impact that caring for the baby would have on the mother's life, shared her thoughts with us about the staff meeting:

> I was thinking of both mother and child. They [the physicians] were thinking of just the baby. The physicians' orientation is very much for the baby's life. When I mentioned the relationship of mother and child, [the unit director] said, "The ethicists tell us we can't consider this. Our responsibility is for the baby." He is absolutely committed to a neonatal unit that is keeping the babies alive.

In this borderline case, the n.i.c.u. staff continued to treat the infant. Some physicians questioned how much effort should be put into the case, but later, when the infant's heart stopped (after twelve and one-half weeks of intensive care), the staff intervened aggressively and stimulated it with cardiac medications. These had "absolutely no effect" and the infant patient died.

Personification of the Newborn

Critically ill infants are exceptionally passive patients; the majority of them are in the Level III nursery only briefly. To offset the potential depersonalization of the neonatal patients, n.i.c.u. staff members often constructed social identities for them. By closely observing neonates' behavior and responses to treatment, nurses and physicians could transform even the smallest and sickest infant into a personality with idiosyncratic characteristics and motivation. This socially constructed actor became a justification for medical heroics because the newborn had been defined as unique and irreplaceable.

An important part of this attributed personality was the will to live. As the physician-in-chief explained to us early in our research, "The baby tells you whether to go all out." In one case, an infant had multiple, severe physical problems and eventually became neurologically compromised. The infant's early "feisty behavior" was seen as a positive sign, and the staff worried when this behavior changed and the infant became lethargic. Nevertheless, the patient's ability to continually "pull herself out of sepsis" was cited as a reason to continue treatment. She died after eighty-seven days of intensive care. Another, similar infant was described to us by a nurse:

> For the first three nights, I worked on her and we were sure she wasn't going to make it. We just didn't want to resuscitate at all. But every morning, she came back, and then there was nothing we could do but continue treatment. She just wasn't going to check out [wasn't going to die]. But that other baby said, "No, thank you, I'm checking out," and died.

In other cases, an infant's staying power was perceived as creating an obligation to initiate treatment—perhaps even against the staff's wishes. N.i.c.u. staff members were somewhat ambivalent about the admission of the 480-gram infant described in Chapter 4, but the baby had stayed alive without medical support for thirty-six hours in the community hospital.

The metaphysical emphasis on the will of the neonate shifts the physician's decision-making authority to the infant and implies that the infant is responsible for what happens. Meanwhile, the staff concentrates on analyzing numerous test results as if they were messages from a real but otherwise mute persona. Good blood gas tests are interpreted to mean that the infant wants to live. Improving lung x-ray films mean that the infant is trying to survive. Conversely, an infant's failure to thrive means a failure of the infant's will.

Physicians and nurses also personify the newborn through the promotion of nicknames, clothes, toys, and personality attributes. N.i.c.u. patients now include infants who in earlier times would have been classified as miscarriages and occasionally include some who would have been labeled stillbirths. Of course, n.i.c.u. staff are familiar with the medical designations of miscarriage and stillbirth, but within the closed world of the unit, these concepts fall by the wayside. Such products of pregnancy, once admitted to the n.i.c.u., become patients and as such are expected to have human attributes.

In contrast to some traditional societies that postpone naming a child until its survival is reasonably certain, the n.i.c.u. staff usually wanted newborns to have what Goffman (1961:21) called "identity kits," names and possessions that give the infant a unique personality. The staff at Northeast Pediatric encouraged parents to name even the smallest and most ill newborn and to bring in toys and clothes. If the parents were reluctant, the staff compensated by inventing nicknames, and nurses would make or buy toys, clothes, and decorations for the isolette.

The Northeast Pediatric n.i.c.u. staff went further than did some at other Level III units in personifying the newborns. The staff prided itself on humanizing the infants in reports to parents. Some staff members took it as a measure of their professional progressive thinking that, in addition to giving parents medical information, they talked positively about the infant's motivation, coping, and personality. Consider this discussion of a 900-gram infant at social service rounds:

> *Physician* (developmental specialist): "I talked to the parents. It is the first child after several losses. The atmosphere—they'd been afraid. But the staff had personified the kid for them. They talked about him using his first name, talked about his hand swiping at the tube as being adaptive."
>
> *Psychiatrist* (approvingly): "They made him a 'mensch.' "

Parental Advocacy

Parental commitment to the treatment of the newborn is another factor contributing to aggressive care. Parents may be committed to their infant's survival at all costs because the infant is the product of a "precious pregnancy," in which there has been a history of miscarriage or infertility. Perhaps the mother's medical condition, for example, diabetes or hypertension, had added risk to her childbearing. The critically ill infants of such parents can strike a special emotional chord in the staff of a Level III nursery.

The case of an infant of parents with a long history of infertility illustrates this point. Although she was a large newborn of forty-one weeks' gestation, her condition was critical and she had been given a muscle relaxant (Pavulon) to keep her from dislodging tubes and monitor leads. Her isolette was surrounded by the attending physician, the fellow (looking very tired), residents, and nurses:

> *Physician:* "General picture very poor, obviously. Problems almost insurmountable. Pavulonized, so can't really do much to get a neurological exam."
>
> *Fellow:* "We said to the parents: 'the baby is on the borderline, terribly sick, may not survive'."
>
> *Nurse* (emotionally): "So what are we going to do, turn the baby off? I think we owe it to the parents, to ourselves, to whatever, to do what we can."

The infant was given maximum support. Later, at social service rounds, there was the following exchange:

> *Presenting nurse:* "The baby probably will not make it. A doctor and a nurse who worked with the baby all night and who are very emotionally involved—they think we have to do everything we can. Dad was in today, crying, kissing the baby. . . ."
>
> *Another nurse:* "You can see how everyone feels for that fifteen years of infertility."

The baby died after two days in the n.i.c.u.

Parental commitment also influences treatment in cases of severely brain-damaged newborns. The question is whether parents will have an accepting attitude toward such a child. Crane (1977) found that the family's attitude toward the brain-damaged child and its treatment is an important factor in the decisions made by physicians: "If the family does not define such an infant or child as socially dead, it is more likely to be treated" (1977:199–200).

At Northeast Pediatric, parents' acceptance of brain damage positively influenced aggressive intervention. As shown in previous sections, the n.i.c.u. tended to give maximum treatment to neurologically damaged children, whatever the parents' wishes were. In cases in which multiple severe physical problems included severe brain damage, the physicians' enthusiasm for aggressive care dwindled. Yet continued parental commitment could tip the scales and lead physicians to continue aggressive care, sometimes even beyond the point where they thought it even remotely reasonable to do so.

The case of a "feisty" newborn whose condition later deteriorated demonstrates such parental influence. The neonatology fellow described the multiplicity of medical problems, including an electroencephalogram suggesting severe neurological damage. The fellow then indicated the influence of the mother's views:

> When we explained to her that the baby's chances of being normal were small, that most likely she was very damaged, the mother responded in a positive way. She said she knew what retardation was and she could handle it. Therefore, we continue, we do all we can to support the baby. We're not sure what she will be like.

The fellow indicated a willingness (though somewhat reluctant) to honor the mother's wishes:

> Even if we still felt we were prolonging the inevitable, if her mother still wanted to continue, we would.

However, the n.i.c.u. physicians were annoyed by parents who presented them with what seemed to be unrealistic attitudes, whose acceptance of brain damage, for example, went further than what they themselves saw as reasonable. One resident became exasperated about the above-mentioned case:

> The mother is an extremely spacy lady. She had no idea of what the baby's condition was. I said to her that the brain might not be too good. I was trying to do two things: to indicate the status of the baby and to see what kind of commitment she had to the baby. I failed on both counts: she didn't understand and she said, "I want the baby to live. I have retarded friends."

Apparently, the mother did not understand that the infant was going to be much more than merely retarded; the physician felt she was out of touch with reality. Knowing the mother and hearing the resident's account, the psychiatrist dismissed the mother's views, saying, "This is not a woman who will help you with a reasonable approach." The mother's views, however, may have continued to affect the staff's behavior. Soon after, a resuscitation (unsuccessful) was attempted when this borderline baby had a cardiac arrest.

Parents' sheer determination coupled with their commitment to the survival of their infant also contributed to the aggressiveness of treatment in the n.i.c.u. If physicians were reluctant to treat an infant, committed parents could prevail, at least to a point. The case of a 620-gram baby of twenty-five weeks' gestation with respiratory distress syndrome and multiple anomalies provides an illustration. The combination of such a low birth weight with severe respiratory distress syndrome was regarded as a fatal condition. The parents in this case, however, wanted "everything done." The staff obliged. The baby was put on a respirator and an exchange transfusion was done to counteract hyperbilirubinemia. The nursing coordinator summarized the situation at social service rounds:

> The person on duty when the baby was born said to the mother that it was fatal apnea. The mother said, "Please put him on the ventilator." Since then we've been very aggressive. The fellow also told the parents that the condition was fatal. But the parents picked up the ball and said please put him on the respirator. So the parents are dealing with the issue of having been the ones who asked. And I'm not sure it would have happened otherwise.

A second contributing factor was the perception that this had been a "precious pregnancy" for the parents. As a nurse explained sympathetically, "The mother is a 'DES [diethylstilbestrol] daughter,' no children, miscarriage, then this one."

On the other hand, one neonatology fellow was extremely critical of the aggressiveness of the intervention and spoke up at morning rounds on the day after admission:

> Without RDS, a baby that weight could survive on room air and those are the ones that do. But in this case, with multiple problems, we are just prolonging life and medical expenses. We've done too much already. The parents want this baby, that's why we're stuck with it. Yesterday there was some hope, but today we have pneumonia. I don't know. You just keep doing it because the parents want it, not because the prognosis changes.

Despite the initial aggressive treatment, the physicians set limits very early on about how far they would go in this case. On the day after admission, the fellow talked of not resuscitating the infant. On the next day, the resident presenting at morning rounds said:

> The plans are not to put any more tubes in, not to do cardiac massage, not to give cardiac meds.

As the baby lingered on rather than dying quickly, the treatment plans became less clear-cut. On the fourth day after admission, the attending physician held out for continued support, saying:

> It would be spectacular if he survives, but we should give him every chance.

The baby died later that day.

An example of parental advocacy that better justified maximum intervention was recounted to us by an attending physician at Northeast Pediatric who defended the staff's complying with the parents' insistence on treatment. The case had occurred in 1976, several years before. The infant, of very low birth weight, was at that time regarded as too small to put on the respirator. The mother, unable to have future pregnancies, insisted that the baby be given oxygen therapy. Against their better judgment, the physicians agreed. The "little peanut" survived and in good condition, and was running around the child follow-up clinic as the attending physician told us this history.

In a case observed at another unit, the mother of an infant showing minimal brain activity insisted that the baby be kept on the respirator for twenty-one days because she had a friend whose newborn was similarly damaged but who "woke up" after just that number of days. The nursery staff disagreed, but since they could not persuade her to give permission for the withdrawal of respirator support, they had to follow her wishes. The Karen Ann Quinlan scenario that the staff had dreaded came to pass. After twenty-one days on the respirator, the infant was taken off oxygen support and survived in a near vegetative state for another three weeks.

THE CLOSED-WORLD PHENOMENON

In determining therapy for critically ill newborns, Level III nursery staff tend to deny external influences, usually selecting opinions that conform with the mandate to treat aggressively. Parents who want more medical support are listened to, but parents who are adverse to saving a critically ill or disabled newborn at all costs have a strenuous time opposing the staff's opinion to the contrary (see Stinson and Stinson, 1979, 1983).

In the same way, other external constraints on the unit's treatment policy are avoided or ignored. For example, physicians at the Northeast Pediatric n.i.c.u. felt strongly that economic costs, which are admittedly high for Level III care, should never influence decision making. Medical indications alone should determine treatment for the patients. As the physician-in-chief at Northeast Pediatric explained to us, "We believe that cost can't enter into it." An attending physician expressed the identical theme:

> I can't let the cost enter in. If the cost for these twins, both of them, is $200,000 and Medicaid paid $100,000, the other would just be taken as a loss.

The economic burden of hospital expenses on parents was similarly dismissed on the presumption that some reimbursement would cover costs. Concern about future economic liabilities resulting from an infant's handicaps was notably absent. Even in social service rounds, the focus was on the short-term management of family problems.

The influence of the law was also kept at bay, although the indirect impact of well-known court cases was admitted. For example, one nurse described the effect of a well-publicized case in which a physician was tried for manslaughter for a legal abortion after which the fetus showed signs of viability:

> After that, we had lots of cases brought in here that never would have been before and, because of legal fear, they were treated beyond reason.

In day-to-day decisions, however, the law was a remote backdrop. The staff knew that the unit's records constituted evidence that could be subpoenaed in a legal case, but the general attitude, matched by the pattern of actual behavior, was that the n.i.c.u. should make decisions based on its own normative clinical criteria. For example, discussing an infant with apparent brain death, a neonatology fellow emphasized the importance of making the treatment decision within the unit:

> We feel we should handle it among ourselves. It would be more difficult to do something in court. There are criteria for brain death in adults. There are no criteria in babies. The court would complicate matters. We don't feel the necessity of getting the legal sanction.

Not all Level III nurseries were as untroubled by legal intrusion as was the unit at Northeast Pediatric. The statute of limitations for pediatric cases often extends to eighteen or twenty-one years after a child's birth. In several nurseries we visited, the hospitals were confronted with suits regarding iatrogenic retrolental fibroplasia and other neonatal problems originating years ago. In major medical centers, n.i.c.u. state-of-the-art technology and the all-out effort to treat patients aggressively make it difficult to bring conventional malpractice suits against the staff or the hospital.

Nor did most Level III nurseries feel coercive pressure from their hospital review boards or ethics committees concerning treatment decisions. These groups, usually composed of physicians, nurses, social workers, and representatives of the law, clergy, or community, served as a forum for discussing problem cases, not for telling n.i.c.u. physicians how to treat patients (Youngner et al., 1983). With the proliferation of hospital ethics committees, fostered in part by the Baby Doe regulation, their role could change, although it is unlikely they would be less than protective of physician and hospital interests. At Northeast Pediatric, the unit staff kept its own counsel, claiming the authority to resolve difficult decisions within its own domain.

6

Where Patients Go: Death and Survival

Our whole thing is to get them in and out fast.   *Nursing Coordinator*

We could have autopsy rounds we have so many deaths!   *Fellow*

The regional Level III nursery at Northeast Pediatric had a vested interest in the fast turnover of cases. The staff was accustomed to working with quick, routine cases. Senior physicians and nurses, trained for acute care medicine, had a short-term clinical focus. Given their mandate to rescue newborns, they preferred to discharge infants no longer in need of maximum treatment and free up beds for new and sicker patients. The nursing coordinator stated succinctly, "Our whole thing is to get them in and out fast."

Like all hospital patients, n.i.c.u. patients are discharged in two ways: dead or alive. In the aggregate, the discharge of patients has an enormous impact on the staff's pace of work. At the same time, the unit team reacts strongly to individual infants' deaths. Each such event punctuates the routine admission and discharge pattern. The regional referral center experiences an exceptional frequency of death and dying because of its selection of high-risk cases. A unit like the one at Northeast Pediatric, which does not provide an intermediate level of newborn care, is particularly vulnerable in this regard. Its clinical successes, infants essentially on the road to recovery in a week's time, are quickly sent back to the community hospitals, and the beds they vacate are then filled with sicker high-risk patients.

The successful transfer of authority over the surviving patient from the Level III center to a Level II unit elsewhere is based on trust that the receiving unit will continue care. Just as they felt ambivalence about receiving referrals from local physicians, the staff at Northeast Pediatric both needed to return infant patients to local institu-

143

tions and worried that these institutions might undo the good work accomplished at the tertiary level.

DEATH: DISCHARGE TO THE PATHOLOGY DEPARTMENT

Death as an Integral Part of N.I.C.U. Work

Neonatal intensive care units, like most intensive care units, have both recovering and dying patients. The Level III nursery, because it is a unit for the critically ill, has a high death rate. For example, for the year we observed and the prior year combined, the mortality rate averaged 15.8 percent, and for the previous two years together it averaged 17.5 percent.

It is also crucial to consider the demographic context within which the n.i.c.u. exists. The infant mortality rate in the United States is low, and childbirth is supposed to be a happy, joyful event. Furthermore, the newborn is expected to live to adulthood. Ariès (1962) reminds us that in past centuries, the Western demographic profile was very different. The infant mortality rate was much higher, and women had numerous children with the hope that a few would survive. He suggests that under such conditions ordinary people did not permit themselves to become too emotionally invested in children that they might lose. In contrast, today in the United States and many other industrialized nations, the infant death rate is below fifteen per every thousand births. A child is expected to survive and usually does. Contemporary parents have fewer children and strongly identify with their infants, sometimes even before they are born (Leifer, 1980). To lose a baby in the face of these expectations is especially traumatic for parents, and the loss also affects the n.i.c.u. staff.

Even when death is not occurring in the n.i.c.u., it is an ever-present possibility. The fragility of the patients is a theme often reflected in work rounds. Consider this discussion about whether to use antibiotics:

> *Resident:* "One of the things that neonatologists are worst at is studying antibiotics. They are creating resistant organisms [through overuse]."
> *Nurse:* "But what about kids that you don't put on antibiotics who die?"
> *Fellow:* "The consequences of not starting antibiotics outweigh the consequences of starting them."
> *Attending physician* (to resident): "The consequences are overwhelming."

Those staff members more experienced with the tenuous condition of the patients—the attending physician, the fellow, and the nurse—all sided against the resident.

The high death rate, especially from some pathologies, is illustrated in the case of a newly admitted baby suffering from persistent fetal circulation (PFC). The attending physician answered a telephone inquiry about the baby's condition:

> Has PFC secondary to her meconium aspiration. . . . The mortality for this stage of the disease is 20 to 30 percent. . . . Almost certainly the effect of asphyxia. A circular problem—have to try to break the cycle. What we do is hyperventilate. But literally a quarter of these babies go.

The ever-present possibility of death was reflected in the language used in the unit. For example, in presentations they gave at social service rounds, staff members often used phrases such as "If the baby lives out the week," "He was at death's door," "I just want people to remember he could die," "She probably won't make it through the night," "This baby can't live long," and "Probably a terminal baby." In addition, there were many commonly used euphemisms: "They were waiting for her to go to heaven," "Is she going to slide out?" "The baby just went down the tubes," "The baby said, 'I'm checking out,'" and "We're losing a baby."

The daily n.i.c.u. routine also involves working with the repercussions of death and dying: autopsies, delayed burials, grieving parents, and the critically ill twins who are reminders of their dead siblings.

Trajectory of Dying

Glaser and Strauss (1968) emphasized the importance of the predominant types of death in a hospital unit and the temporal features of terminal care. They wrote of "dying trajectories," noting two characteristics, duration (dying takes time) and shape of the trajectory (e.g., a sudden plunge straight down; slow, steady deterioration; or vacillation).

In the n.i.c.u., three dying trajectories are important: the sudden death of a new or long-term patient; the prolonged, lingering death (which in the n.i.c.u. means a day or so); and the roller-coaster clinical course, with various ups and downs (comebacks and crashes) before death. Of those babies with an up-and-down course, some die and some survive.

Sudden Death. N.i.c.u. patients are so fragile that, whether newly admitted or long-term, they may take a sudden turn for the worse and die within an hour. Also, some babies arrive at the unit on the verge of death (e.g., overwhelming sepsis) and die quickly. What these cases of sudden deaths have in common is that staff members were working intensively with the patients but the patients died despite immediate and massive efforts. These patients typically died without their parents being present because there was no time to notify them. A cardiac arrest and resuscitation that was unsuccessful is the most dramatic example of sudden death. It illustrates the unit's mobilization under pressure and the teamwork and camaraderie of the staff.

9:00. A newly admitted baby suddenly arrested. People converged on the baby, and someone got the crash cart with all the medications. The baby was mostly obscured from view, but the team's conversation let one know what was happening. The resident said, "I think I should needle the heart." Someone asked for a chest-tube setup. The attending physician pressed on the infant's chest.

9:08. By chance, two people arrived from cardiology with the ultrasound machine right in the middle of the resuscitation. The main nurse involved glanced over her shoulder as they entered the unit and said, "What a great time for an echo (slight laugh)." The cardiologist started directing the group as soon as he arrived. He looked at the patterns on the monitors up on the high shelf and gave directions to the group. He said, "As long as you massage and ventilate, you have time to do everything deliberately." Various medicines—Isuprel, "epi" [epinephrine] and others—were requested.

Twelve people now were involved in the effort: the attending physician, the fellow, and two residents, a medical student, the nurse who had been working with the baby prior to the arrest, three other nurses, another nurse by the crash cart, the ultra-sound technician, and the cardiologist, who took over the direction of the resuscitation.

9:26. Nine people were still right around the baby's bed; in addition, two more nurses remained on the fringes of the group.

9:29. The code was called (i.e., a decision was made to quit) and the group broke up. The attending physician said, "Okay, I'll call the [community] doc." The cardiologist left the unit right away, and as he was leaving, the fellow and the main nurse acknowledged his help and said, "Thanks a lot." As the group dispersed, the nurse also said, "Thanks, everyone." The doctors disappeared and the nurse was left to clean up the dead baby and wrap it. The attending physician and the fellow stood talking by the coffee machine, and the resident telephoned the father.

Even though a baby dies, the daily routine must go on. At 9:40, only eleven minutes after the unsuccessful resuscitation, work rounds started. The group was a little disorganized as it began, and the transition from death to daily rounds was accomplished with a few jokes that relieved the tension.

Death in the n.i.c.u. is always a defeat. But if it must occur, death by an arrest that does not respond to resuscitation efforts fits the tempo and organization of work. The scenario is decisive and clear-cut, with few if any ambiguities. Team decisions about the degree of aggressiveness follow a relatively well-established protocol. The major decision concerns how long to continue the resuscitation effort, and this decision must be made immediately and executed within a short period of time, thirty minutes to an hour. This work lets the staff do what they do best because a resuscitation, successful or unsuccessful, is the epitome of intensive care. It is an aggressive, indeed, heroic intervention that is labor- and machine-intensive, requires precision teamwork, and focuses almost exclusively on the acute short-term clinical situation. Finally, there is no time to summon the parents, and unless the parents are present by chance (an unlikely event), the staff is free from the intrusion of the family's emotional reactions.

Prolonged and Orchestrated Death. The second dying trajectory in the n.i.c.u. is prolonged, lingering death. In most prolonged cases, there is a turning point at which the staff team both recognizes the inevitable and openly states it. Someone will announce, "The kid is dying," or "It's only a matter of hours." From the turning point of acknowledgment to the actual death typically is a matter of, at most, forty-eight hours, and often much less.

What these prolonged cases have in common is that the infants cannot be quickly removed from sight. Unlike the infant who is unsuccessfully resuscitated, the newborn dying a lingering death remains in the unit, a visible reminder to the staff that they have failed. Because the dying takes place over a fairly long time, there is interaction between the staff and the parents, either by telephone or in the unit.

What these cases also have in common is that they raise the possibility of the staff's orchestrating the death—both its pace and the social scene around it. Such cases raise the issue of whether staff should do anything to shorten the suffering and hasten the inevitable. They also permit the possibility of the parents being present. Parents typically are asked whether they wish to come into the unit to be with the dying newborn and, if so, whether they would like to hold the infant.

Among lingering cases, a particularly painful and emotion-filled death scene is the one in which both these issues are decided in the affirmative. The staff decides to withdraw medical support and limit the time of suffering by allowing the disease to take its course. The parents, knowing that, decide to hold the infant as it dies. The following is a case in point. The infant was a twin who had weighed 1,275 grams at birth, had severe respiratory distress syndrome, and had spent ten days in intensive care:

> The baby looked awful. The color was very strange, not blue or black, but dusky. The baby was not moving, although this was partly due to his having been given Pavulon [a muscle relaxant].

> A nurse was sitting at the head of the bed. She commented, "His lungs are shot, it's just a matter of hours. [The attending physician] is with the parents now."

> The primary nurse and the attending physician, who had come back into the unit, walked toward the bed. The nurse looked to be near tears— looked like her eyes had started to water. She had some metal tools in her hand to remove equipment. Someone brought a folding screen to put around the bed for privacy. A rocking chair was put on the left for the mother. The parents were brought into the n.i.c.u. The father helped guide the mother to the rocking chair, and the baby was then handed to her.

Another nurse described her feelings about handling a similar death scene with another newborn. Initially, the infant seemed viable. But as time went on, it became apparent that the prognosis was very poor. The baby had hypoplastic lungs, no left kidney, and a polycystic right kidney, fibrous to the point that it was not functioning enough to support life. He was in intensive care for six days when the decision was made to withdraw support. The nurse reported:

> I took the chest tubes out and an endotrachael tube connecting him to the respirator. I dressed him in a tee-shirt and blanket and took him to the parents [in the small room reserved for parents]. He lived about twenty minutes. I stayed outside the door and went in a couple of times to check. The parents were holding him when he died. . . .

> I talked to the [primary nurse] about it. We both felt comfortable knowing the baby wouldn't live. But you can't take all hope away from parents. There's always that hope when I take a baby off the respirator— you hope the baby will take a breath and turn pink.

The Roller-Coaster Trajectory. A not uncommon clinical course for an n.i.c.u. case is one that resembles a roller-coaster ride. At times it looks like a baby will make it; at other times it looks like the baby will not. Sometimes such a case is described as follows: "This baby has had every complication a 'preemie' can have." Some babies have a series of crises and crashes, yet rebound after each. Some of these infants ultimately survive and some do not. Roller-coaster cases that continue for a long period (twenty-eight days or over) are especially draining on staff and parents. Darlene Bourne, the subject of Chapter 8, is one such roller-coaster case that ultimately ended in death. If such a baby dies, the staff may feel both relief and a bitter sense of wasted effort.

Diagnosis and Dying. In addition to the trajectory of dying—the duration and shape—other factors influence the impact death has on the unit. For example, the primary diagnosis for the dying patient is relevant to the staff's feelings about the case and is most upsetting if it is in their specialty area, that is, lung function. Regarding a baby dying of respiratory problems, a nurse said to us:

> Feelings are running higher because he's dying of his lung [problem] and we should be able to do something about it. The [other baby dying of Werdnig-Hoffmann's disease] is different—we can't do anything about it.

Staff Members' Reactions

Staff members typically expressed some sorrow when a baby died. For example, a baby weighing about 2,000 grams died of overwhelming sepsis. The resident commented, in a troubled way, "It was a nice-looking baby and it was a shame that it died." In other cases, the prognosis was so grim that the death was hoped for, at least by some of the staff. In one such case, the nurse said about a death, "It's a relief for everyone who was involved."

At times there were interactive effects between the death of one infant and the care of another. For example, a long-term infant with a roller-coaster clinical course died. The death did not adversely affect the technical care of other newborns, but it did affect the response of some junior physicians and nurses to subsequent admissions of the same type, so that it was difficult for them to assume primary responsibility for the new cases.

Although in general each death was keenly felt, occasionally there was a somewhat different reaction. Death was so common and the pace of work so fast, that, at times, death became medically routine. For example, one day, during radiology rounds, the fellow became confused about which infant died:

> *Fellow:* "You've got the wrong x-ray [film]. That kid has been dead for two days."
> *Resident:* "No, no. It's the other baby who died."

On another day, at the conclusion of an unsuccessful resuscitation, the physician-in-chief happened to walk into the unit. The fellow explained, "We're in the process of losing a baby." The conversation continued, and at one point the following occurred:

> The fellow said, "There's nothing dramatic to show you." He paused, and realizing the irony of saying this just as a baby had died, he added, "At least not on the positive side."

Coping Strategies of the Staff

Staff members had specific coping strategies for dealing with the deaths of infants. These included gallows humor, the repression of memories, and focusing on the technical.

Gallows Humor.   As Fox and Swazey (1974:320) noted, medical students and house officers traditionally use gallows humor in responding to death. The n.i.c.u. staff made its share of jokes about death and dying, as well as about the conditions of patients who might die.
Some jokes related to the clustering or frequency of deaths:

> *Fellow:* "We could have autopsy rounds we have so many deaths!"
> *Staff member:* "This is the Memorial Bed for PFC [persistent fetal circulation]."

Some jokes related to the generally poor condition of babies admitted—the "carnage" with which the staff had to work.

> A nurse, April, was working with one problematic baby, and at the other end of the unit another nurse, Jennie, and the resident were working with another problematic baby.
> *April:* "Come help me, the baby's just lost her chest tube."
> *Resident* (working on the other baby's re-intubation): "I can't come to you right now. My loyalties are divided."
> *April:* "That's not true, you just don't care about this poor baby."
> *Jennie:* "You know, April, it's survival of the fittest."

April: "I'm not convinced that one is more fit than the other (laughter from the nurses and resident)."

Some humor, as in these three scenes, was related to the poor condition of a particular patient:

Fellow: "He has the white, near-death look."
Resident: "Don't go giving him ideas."

Regarding another baby, for whom the x-ray film and clinical condition did not match, an attending physician said (laughing):

Remember the day we had a good x-ray, and the kid looked like death warmed over?

And regarding still another baby, who had four chest tubes in place:

Fellow (in a serious tone, gently supporting a discouraged resident): "I realize [the baby] is really tenuous in terms of his outcome and may not make it. But I'm saying this to make you feel it is worthwhile doing something: [The unit director] has seen and I have seen children with more chest tubes. He's nowhere near the record for chest tubes and nowhere near the record for air leaks."
Resident (with a faint laugh): "How about the record for the number within a certain time period?"

Some jokes were about the aggressive use of technology in marginally viable cases. The humorous remarks reflected criticism, or at least ambivalence, about the unit's aggressive stance. The following two comments were made by nurses—often the group more critical of intervention—at social service rounds. Regarding a 780-gram baby with multiple problems, a nurse said, with a smile:

The baby will first have to live to go to CAT scan.

And regarding a newly admitted ultrapremature infant:

The new baby—530 grams—will go to the OR [operating room]. That's a sin (laugh).

Humor was also used to express hostility toward problem cases. One morning at rounds, a conversation about Darlene Bourne (the subject of Chapter 8) was begun by the resident's saying, "She arrested last night." This was said as a joke. As noted in the chapter on physicians (Chapter 1), humor could be used to indicate a distaste for the field of neonatology; one resident said he was going to go into a more cheerful branch of medicine, cancer in children.

To an outsider, perhaps most of all to parents, such joking might be unnerving. Yet humor is one mechanism that helps staff members continue with their emotionally difficult work.

Short Memory.　　When a death occurred, the corpse and other physical remnants of the event were quickly removed. The dead baby was taken either to another area of the unit (to await the arrival of parents) or to the pathology department. The equipment and any mess were quickly cleaned up. All that remained was an empty bed, and, in a busy unit, that was quickly refilled. Infants who died were forgotten faster than were infants who had been successfully discharged.

There can be some unsettling barriers to repressing the fact of an infant's death. One obstacle for the staff is a delay imposed by parents when an infant dies, and, for whatever reason, the parents do not arrive quickly at the unit. A nurse described such a case:

> The baby was cold and stiff when we took it to the morgue. The mother (aged seventeen) was very distressed. The baby died at 8 a.m.; the mother came in at 9 p.m. The parents came in very drunk the night before—vandalized the things out on the desk. The mother spent longer here than I would have. The baby looked horrible—tongue hanging out, cold, blue, edematous [swollen].

Another problem is a delay in burial. In one case, the mother took about three weeks to go through the right steps for burial:

> *Fellow:* "The admitting office keeps calling about when is this baby going to be buried."
> *Nurse:* "The mother goes, 'How will this baby be buried?' She asked for a birth certificate for each [twin]. She said, 'How will I get it buried?' A secretary said, 'You need a death certificate, but you can't get a death certificate until you get a birth certificate.' "

The death of one of a set of hospitalized twins also makes it difficult for the staff to put death out of sight. The surviving twin is a reminder of the sibling's death. The surviving twin becomes even more precious and the emotional risk of loss, to parents and staff, is greater. The death of one twin can be seen either negatively or positively, like a glass half empty or half full. Commenting on the pattern of losing one twin, a nurse, rather depressed, said, "We haven't turned out [saved] a complete set of twins all summer. We always lose one." In contrast, another day, an attending physician known for her undaunted optimism, said enthusiastically, "We saved one of each set of twins."

If the surviving twin is still hospitalized, the parents continue to have contact with the n.i.c.u. They too remind the staff of the prior death. While some parents immediately focus their energies on the surviving twin, a common pattern for the parents is to be torn between grieving for the lost twin and bonding (as is encouraged by the staff) with the surviving twin. Simultaneous parental grieving and bonding, to use n.i.c.u. language, makes for a more complex interaction between staff and parents.

Focusing on the Technical. Another strategy in the n.i.c.u. used when a baby died—and thus became a professional failure—was to focus on technical and clinical issues. Most often this meant showing an interest in the autopsy.

Physicians saw the autopsy as a learning experience. Sometimes they began to talk of the autopsy even while the patient was still alive. One day, the resident expressed hostility about a long-term, puzzling case:

> *Researcher:* "What caused the arrhythmia?"
> *Resident:* "Who knows? I'm a doctor and I don't know. And I'm getting tired of it. Some day she won't be here. She'll be in pathology. Maybe they can tell us what this is."

About a different baby, a fellow said, "If he dies, we've got to get an autopsy—there are so many questions on this kid." This technical focus shifts attention away from failure to a positive aspect of the work, namely, the intellectual answer to the clinical puzzle in order to avoid failure in the future.

Staff–Parent Interaction Surrounding Death

The n.i.c.u. staff not only manages dying patients but the families of dying patients. As Glaser and Strauss (1968) noted, "family handling" centers around four issues: preparing the family for their infant's death, persuading them to give responsibility to the hospital, coaching them in proper hospital behavior, and helping them to grieve.

The n.i.c.u. staff worked on all four of these issues. Staff members believed that parents should be told about the impending death of their infant. Therefore, physicians would begin to talk about the infant to indicate that the clinical course was not hopeful. Depending on the case, the parents might be told explicitly that the expectation was that the infant would die. For example, in one case, the nurse reported:

> We have told them the chances of [the infant's] surviving are zero twice. So it's a miracle the baby is still alive.

This baby eventually died, after six weeks in intensive care.

Physicians exercised discretion about the timing and explicitness of the messages about death. For example, early in the clinical course of a 780-gram baby with multiple, serious problems, physicians hedged their message. Two days after admission, the nurse reported:

> The parents are beginning to be told [about the baby's condition], for example, by words like "bloody [spinal] taps." They haven't been told flat out that the baby might die.

Telling the parents about their infant's likely death is a process, and the news often is conveyed gradually.

The n.i.c.u. staff sometimes started parents on a course of grieving before their infant died. Consider this case discussion at social service rounds:

> *Nurse:* "Probably a terminal baby. And a difficult social situation. No one has taken the baby as a primary nurse. At first no one took the baby over the weekend because they didn't think the baby would make it to the next day. . . ."
> *Developmental specialist:* "If one is going to die for sure, you should start [the social-psychological] process."

The unit staff urged parents to face facts. However, it also encouraged parents' attachment to their babies. Parents sometimes experienced difficulty dealing with these two messages. Regarding a baby with a roller-coaster course, a nurse reported:

> [The mother] told me, "You're saying hold my baby but you're also saying he's going to die." And I came back with something like, "It must be frustrating."

The unit nurses encouraged this mother to touch her baby and to become emotionally attached to him, and simultaneously they told her the chances of the baby's surviving were zero. Staff members understood why some parents started to become emotionally withdrawn, but they preferred that parents parented well even as their newborns were dying.

When an infant died, physicians encouraged the parents to delegate still further responsibility to the hospital, namely, to give permission for an autopsy. Some physicians requested autopsies more often than nurses sometimes thought proper. As one nurse, somewhat critically, explained, "Medicine asks for the autopsy—and they always ask." Another nurse described a particular case:

> [The attending physician] was trying to talk [the parents] into an autopsy. She was called away. The parents said to me, "Should we have an autopsy?" I said, "It's your decision, but you can restrict it." So the parents said just to look at the kidneys. To me, that was their decision and the doctor was trying to push them. It's not my right to urge them. I'm a nurse—my background is different from the doctor's, who wanted to further the cause of research.

Parents' responses to autopsy requests varied, ranging from refusal to grant permission to interest in the findings.

Although managing the family of a dying infant is complex, the discharge of a dead infant to the pathology department is straightforward. Typically, the autopsy is the only issue to be negotiated. In contrast, the discharge of surviving infants, who vary in their conditions and the level of care they need, often requires complicated negotiations.

SURVIVAL: DISCHARGE TO OTHER CARE-GIVERS

The n.i.c.u. is, by definition, a temporary caretaker of critically ill infants. Surviving newborns are to be entrusted to other care-givers as soon as possible. The unit's mission is defined first by the severity of the patient's condition. As the surviving patient's condition improves, the consideration of discharge becomes obligatory:

> *Nurse:* "The baby's real cute, really cute."
> *Fellow:* "As soon as they get too cute around here, it's out the door."

Likewise, size, which implies age in this context, is relevant. One fellow remarked:

> He's our patient because he's small. He's going to stop being small and stop being our patient.

The time-limited responsibility of the n.i.c.u. is accentuated in a Level III referral center like Northeast Pediatric that does not house a Level II or Level I nursery. In the multiple-level nursery, stopping maximum intensive care typically means just moving the infant from one room to another; often the same staff rotates through the various divisions. Discharge from the exclusively Level III unit is more abrupt. It usually means transport to another hospital with a Level II nursery or sometimes discharge to another unit within the same hospital. Obviously, the staff in charge of the infant changes.

At Northeast Pediatric, the clear-cut discharge from the exclusively Level III nursery had implications for both staff and family. For the staff, it often meant involvement in a complex set of interinstitutional relationships and negotiations about referring the infant to other care-givers. For the family, it meant having to adjust to a second nursery and staff. Painful though the Level III n.i.c.u. experience was for them, parents did become accustomed to this particular unit, its protocol and personnel. Some parents even resisted the transfer of their infant. The staff, in turn, resisted parents' attempts to delay a transfer, and they tried to prepare parents for such a move. A nurse summarized the staff's approach: "From day one we tell people the baby won't be here forever."

When to Discharge Patients from the Level III Nursery

At Northeast Pediatric, an infant's medical condition was overwhelmingly the main consideration in deciding when to discharge him or her. Most often, discussion focused on some specific medical condition, such as that of the lungs or heart. Almost as frequently, discussion focused on the general medical condition, whether the baby was stable and merely needed to grow.

The second criterion for discharge was availability of other care-givers to provide the level of care required. The availability of bed space in another nursery was a prime consideration.

The third prominent criterion for discharge was the pressure to free up bed space in the Level III nursery. This aspect never took precedence over an infant's clear-cut medical need, but the most propitious moment for discharge was rarely clear-cut, and in this discretionary area, bed space could be a central factor hastening or delaying discharge. For example, in two separate instances of infants nearly ready for discharge, a nurse made the following comments, which depended on the bed space available in the unit:

> We got five kids in thirty-six hours over the weekend. He might get bumped and go to another hospital for three or four days.

> We can wait a day—we have one or two spaces.

Thus, discharge decisions were influenced not only by an infant's condition but by the dynamics of the referral system, and also indirectly by the economics of the hospital, which prospers when its beds are full.

A fourth criterion was whether the baby required Level III intensive care. This concern is linked to two prior criteria, the infant's condition and creating bed space, as indicated in this physician's comment:

> The baby will be out today or tomorrow. There's no justification for him to be here for feeding. He's not an intensive case. We don't want to turn down sick babies in the community.

Again and again, the discharge discussions referred to the intensive care mandate of the unit: "We can't offer transitional care," "We have nothing else to offer," "It's getting to be a luxury to keep this baby here."

In addition to these four major criteria, cautionary thinking delayed discharge in certain cases: a "precious" twin whose sibling had died, an infant perceived to be at risk for abuse, or an infant who, if kept in the n.i.c.u., could skip a brief stay in an interim Level II unit and go directly home.

Overwhelmingly—and to the dismay of nurses—attending physicians were exceedingly cautious in discharge decisions. If they erred, it was almost uniformly in keeping a baby too long rather than discharging one too soon. The unit director, evaluating a case, succinctly stated the mentality:

> It makes me nervous to discharge him so soon. Kids can get into trouble. They don't watch as closely elsewhere as we do.

Where to Send Infants for Intermediate Care

The assumption in Northeast Pediatric's newborn referral network was that infants discharged by the n.i.c.u. would go back to the referring hospital. In most cases, the infant was transported back. In some problematic cases, the transfer was made to another speciality unit within Northeast Pediatric or to one of its affiliated hospitals. Tables 4.1 and 4.2 present data on referral and discharge patterns at Northeast Pediatric.

The overriding criterion in deciding where to send a baby was the competence of the receiving hospital's nursery, that is, the correspondence between the level of care that the baby required and the level of care that a particular hospital could provide. The Northeast Pediatric staff talked of having good or bad luck with particular hospitals and frequently evaluated their nurseries. They mentally catalogued which hospitals were good at basic procedures such as monitoring apnea, oxygen therapy, phototherapy, gavage, and general monitoring. The mission of these other nurseries was mainly surveillance. Thus, not surprisingly, none of the intermediate nurseries to which infants were discharged could match the staff-to-patient ratio or resources of the Level III nursery at Northeast Pediatric.

There was a conflict in some cases between the n.i.c.u.'s assumption that an infant should return to the referring hospital and its insistence that the hospital nursery to which the infant was returned be competent to the precise degree stipulated by the Level III staff. The solution usually was to delay discharge until the infant could get by with less care.

> Hang onto him a little longer. That hospital doesn't do so well with oxygen. We could send him back to most places but not there. He'll need a couple of extra days here.

To protect the infant and avoid offending the referring hospital, the newborn was simply kept at Northeast Pediatric longer. In other cases, the discussion focused on the fact that there were hospitals other than the referring one to which a baby could be sent.

The local hospital staff's self-perception of competence, especially the limits they set on themselves, was also relevant. Medical conditions demanding close surveillance were especially troublesome because nurse-to-patient ratios were never 1:3 as it was at the maximum-care nursery. According to Northeast Pediatric's staff, Level II nurseries often had some particular condition that they were nervous about. One hospital refused a patient prone to apneic spells because the nurses could not handle the responsibility. Another hospital refused an infant because the staff was not comfortable managing oxygen therapy. Just as referring hospitals depended on the Level III unit to manage high-risk infants, the same hospitals were reluctant to welcome the infants back until they were well enough to be managed using more limited resources.

Tensions About Discharging Infants to Intermediate Care Facilities

Discharging newborns to another facility or unit for intermediate care meant, by definition, that the Northeast Pediatric n.i.c.u. staff had to negotiate transfers across institutional boundaries. Interinstitutional relationships often are problematic, so it is not surprising that these discharge negotiations at Northeast Pediatric were complex and often frustrating.

Hospital nurseries and other Northeast Pediatric units that were potential recipients of discharged infants had their own sets of concerns, including their own cycles of admission and discharge. No matter how anxious they might be for cases in general, there were times when other nurseries were reluctant to admit particular infants. Nurses at Northeast Pediatric discussed this problem:

> *N.i.c.u. nursing coordinator:* "I'd be concerned that she's not lost in the system. The staff over there thinks it's a dump."
>
> *N.i.c.u. nurse:* "We explained she was born there. They don't want another chronic kid."

Sometimes Northeast Pediatric pressured other facilities to take infants. In one case, for example, a mixed-level nursery denied a Northeast Pediatric fellow's request to transfer an infant but later complied when the attending physician repeated the request. The attending physician joked about negotiating strategies:

> You have to tell them that either they take the baby or they get the new transports over the weekend.

Transfer to another facility means a disruption of care and raises the question of continuity. Major attention, especially by nurses, was given to writing discharge plans for infants. The n.i.c.u. staff might also meet with the staff of the receiving unit, especially if the transfer was within Northeast Pediatric. If the discharge was made to a more distant facility, the staff members still might make multiple referrals or contacts about a case within their respective occupations: physician to physician, nurse to nurse, social worker to social worker. The Northeast Pediatric n.i.c.u. also took care to avoid scheduling transfers at a time, such as on Friday, that would result in a fragile infant's arriving in the new nursery when less than the full, regular complement of staff was present.

Despite such attention to details, even the best-laid plans sometimes went wrong. Once discharged, the baby and his or her care were no longer under the n.i.c.u.'s control. One discharge case that became especially controversial illustrates the various discontinuities that can occur, the difference of opinion that may exist about what constitutes a suitable facility, and troubled relations with parents. The case was an infant with spina bifida discharged to the neurology unit at Northeast Pediatric. Problems with the transfer, plus a different routine in the new unit, caused the parents to become very upset. An anonymous letter sent to the Level III staff complained about the care the infant was receiving in the new unit. This became a focal point in social service rounds:

Nurse: "The baby was doing well so the neurology unit is where the baby ended up. The parents were upset—the baby was off the monitor, was bottle [fed] instead of gavaged. The parents started coming back up here. They complained that the baby was next to someone age fifteen, et cetera. The fellow told the mother that he would see the baby every day, which is appropriate. And, nurse to nurse, we will talk; for example, the baby should not be bottled. So the fellow helped and said the baby should stay there. Then this [anonymous] note was put under our door. So we're trying to get things together [with the new unit], doctor to doctor and nurse to nurse . . . I doubt that a nurse wrote that letter. The [baby's] father is very verbal. You're the shrink, but I think that person needs help."

Psychiatrist: "It depends on what's going on."

Nurse: "I feel comfortable that all the right things were done for this transfer."

Primary nurse: "I do think the parents' gripes are legitimate. The [neurology] floor is not set up to care for prematures. [The parents'] request to take the baby to another hospital or home is reasonable. The mother was up here yesterday. . . . She was worried about the little children turning the dials. She observed some nurses feeding her baby and, as she described it, it doesn't sound very kosher."

Nurse: "I went over all the feeding. The baby went with a very detailed plan."

Primary nurse: "But the primary nurse [in the new unit] went on vacation and obviously she didn't communicate that information to the associate nurse."

N.I.C.U. FINANCIAL CHARGES

Distribution of Charges

At the end of each patient's career comes a financial reckoning. For most of the infants admitted to the n.i.c.u. at Northeast Pediatric, additional hospitalization is required at another, though less intensive and less expensive, level of care; their time in the Level III nursery is the most precarious and most costly (Kramer, 1976). Just as most cases (252 of 344) were referred to Northeast Pediatric from community hospitals in 1979, most survivors (154 of 285) were discharged to these same hospitals for intermediate care, presumably of short duration. A small percentage (6 percent) of survivors that year went directly home to their parents. Another 17 percent died and were sent to the pathology department.

The short stay of most Level III admissions is reflected in hospital bills. We reviewed the hospital charges for the series of 103 cases we followed and, of 101 complete records found that approximately two-thirds had charges of less than $10,000 (Table 6.1) and were discharged in a week or so. At the other end of the spectrum were the 10 percent whose five- and six-figure charges accounted for one-half of the total charges and more than one-half of the total hospital bed days for this series of patients.

Between the infants who were discharged quickly and those who stayed on were still other infants who were referred to services within Northeast Pediatric. These infants were usually on the road to recovery but had persistent neurologic or cardiac problems; the idea was to maintain their access to consulting specialists while dimin-

Table 6.1. Distribution of hospital charges

Charges ($)	Number	Percent	Cumulative percent for 101 consecutive cases
1,000–1,999	22	22	22
2,000–4,999	22	22	44
5,000–9,999	21	21	64
10,000–18,999	11	11	75
19,000–59,999	16	16	91
60,000–99,999	6[a]	6	97
100,000–250,000	3	3	100

[a]Excludes one rehospitalized infant.

ishing the level of clinical care provided. The nurse-to-patient ratio in these other units was much lower than in the Level III nursery, 1:5 or 10 as compared with 1:2 or 3. Within our sample, these extra hospital days following newborn intensive care added from $2,000 to $12,000 (not represented in our tallies) to the bills for six infants. An important difference in charges between these and the Level III nursery was the bed rate. The n.i.c.u. rate averaged $600, the others $250.

In exceptional cases, the Level III staff would feel compelled to keep a patient under clinical surveillance and take on the job of schooling mothers (and occasionally fathers) in special care techniques. This was so for the two longest-term survivors on the unit who spent months in the Level III nursery (see Table 6.4, Part C). In both cases, the risks of transfer outweighed the inconvenience of scaling down care (the infants were relegated to side areas of the unit) and dealing with distraught parents. In a third, nearly identical case, the staff decided to transfer the infant to another division, reasoning that the space was needed. The complex advocacy issue underlying this decision is described in Chapter 8.

The readmission of a former Level III patient was an exceptional event. One infant (admitted before we began our serial study of cases) was discharged to a community hospital after forty-two days of Level III treatment, including surgery for patent ductus arteriosus. Ten days later, she was back in the n.i.c.u. for an additional thirty-five days of therapy, including brain shunt surgery. In this worst-case scenario, the initial charges of $61,000 were covered by commercial insurance. In the second phase of n.i.c.u. care, Medicaid was applied to the $33,000 charges.

Table 6.2. Reimbursement for 101 consecutive cases in 1979 (rounded to nearest thousand)

	Blue Cross/ Blue Shield	Medicaid	Private insurers	Government (federal and CHAMPUS)	HMO
Number of cases	41	32	17	7	4
Percentage of cases	41	32	17	7	4
Total charges	$639,000	$739,000	$389,000	$48,000	$176,000
Survival rate, pct.	88	78	88	43	75
Average case charge	$16,000	$23,000	$23,000	$7,000	$44,000
Percentage of total charges	32	37	19.5	2.5	9

Total charges for 101 cases = $1,991,000
Average case charge = $19,700

HMO, health maintenance organization; CHAMPUS, Civilian Health and Medical Program of the Uniformed Services.

For the patients we studied, Medicaid paid a large proportion (37 percent) of charges incurred (Table 6.2), more than the 15 to 20 percent cited in other studies as the Medicaid share. According to accounting officers at Northeast Pediatric, the turnaround for Medicaid reimbursement was averaging one ·full year and forcing the hospital to dip into charity funds. Nor did Medicaid fully cover all charges. From the hospital administrator's perspective, private commercial insurance and Blue Cross/Blue Shield offered more efficient and complete reimbursement, although in 1979 these organizations had begun closer evaluations of six-figure n.i.c.u. bills.

The average charge per case for Medicaid patients was higher than for infants insured by other plans, among them insurance for government employees and members of the armed forces and their families.

The Role of Birth Weight

Although birth weight by itself is only a general indication of clinical status, we found a strong association between extremely low birth weight and high financial charges (Table 6.3). Infants weighing less than 1,000 grams at birth (and in our series these included one 480-gram newborn) incurred charges averaging $57,500. One-half of these infants (eight of sixteen) were Medicaid patients, which may ac-

Table 6.3. Birth weight and charge distribution in 101 consecutive cases (charges rounded to nearest hundred)

480–999 grams (17 cases; 7 deceased)
   Total charges = $976,600
   Average per case = $57,500

1,000–1,499 grams (21 cases; 7 deceased)
   Total charges = $534,700
   Average per case = $25,500

1,500–2,499 grams (31 cases; 4 deceased)
   Total charges = $264,600
   Average per case = $8,500

2,500–2,999 grams (12 cases; 0 deceased)
   Total charges = $40,200
   Average per case = $3,400

3,000+ grams (20 cases; 1 deceased)
   Total charges = $175,100
   Average per case = $8,800

count for the higher charges paid by government. For infants in the next birth weight category, 1,000 to 1,499 grams, charges averaged $25,500. In the 1,500 to 2,499 gram birth weight range, the average charges went down to $8,500. For infants weighing 2,500 to 2,999 grams, the average charge was about $3,400 per case. The largest infants, those weighing more than 3,000 grams were not without serious problems. Their survival rate was good, and half of them needed little more than oxygen or phototherapy. The other half, although they survived, were severely traumatized at birth, either asphyxiated, with meconium staining, or having persistent fetal circulation; some had serious congenital anomalies. As survivors, these medical puzzles and victims of accident were often referred to the neurology division.

Low birth weight newborns were clearly the toughest cases and greatest challenges for the n.i.c.u. staff. Data for 1979 indicate that infants weighing less than 2,500 grams accounted for 80 percent of

Table 6.4. Economic and clinical data, selected cases, 1979

Group A
Level III N.I.C.U. Charges—$19,000 to $59,000

Case	Charges	Coverage	LOS (days)	Birth-weight (gm)	Clinical status (discharge)
1	$21,000	Private	18	1300	RDS; rehospitalized for neurosurgery
2	19,000	Private	10	1145	RDS; deceased
3	19,000	Private	22	910	RDS; apnea; infection
4	27,000	Medicaid	22	1460	RDS
5	59,000	Medicaid	46	900	PDA ligation; chronic, lung disease; apnea
6	39,000	Private	29	1300	PDA ligation; RDA; infection
7	23,000	Medicaid	18	1270	Anoxia at birth; RDS
8	26,000	Private	27	1200	RDS; PDA ligation, intestinal infection
9	50,000	Private	38	880	RDS; PDA; ? neurologic
10	30,000	Private	23	1875	Poor neurologic; seizures; RDS
11	50,000	Private	32	1700	PDA ligation; heart disease; RDS; ? neurologic
12	34,000	Private	27	1500	Brain shunt; heart disorder; RDS
13	32,000	Private	15	1100	PDA ligation; RDS; deceased
14	51,000	Medicaid	41	1200	RDS; ? neurologic
15	39,000	Private	40	920	RDS; apnea; PDA ligation? neurologic
TOTAL	$519,000				
AVERAGES	$34,600		27.2	1244	

Group B
Level III N.I.C.U. Charges—$60,000 to $149,900

Case	Charges	Coverage	LOS (days)	Birth-weight (gm)	Clinical status (discharge)
1	$76,000	Private	73	1070	Severe brain bleed; gastrostomy
2	80,000	Medicaid	66	690	PDA ligation; BPD; ? neurologic
3	73,000	Medicaid	56	3020	Heart and lung diseases; ? neurologic
4	94,000	Private/Medicaid	77	1600	Rehospitalized for brain shunt; heart disease
5	95,000	Private (HMO)	68	910	Multiple anomalies; PDA ligation; deceased
6	82,000	Private	79	1420	Brain shunt; poor neurologic
7	69,000	Private	50	1140	PDA ligation; ? neurologic; intestinal infection
TOTAL	$569,000				
AVERAGES	$81,000		67	1407	
				(1138 without case 3)	

Group C
Level III N.I.C.U. Charges—$150,000 to $246,000

Case	Charges	Coverage	LOS (days)	Birth-weight (gm)	Clinical status (discharge)
1	$173,000	Medicaid	143	710	Severely retarded (cretinism:) congenital heart disease
2	150,000	Medicaid	136	740	O$_2$ dependent; PDA ligation; brain shunt; deceased
3	246,000	Private	239	940	Severe cerebral palsy; home
TOTAL	$569,000				
AVERAGES	$190,000		173	797	

*Rounded numbers.
†LOS = Length of stay in Level III nursery.
‡Unless otherwise noted, patient discharged to Level II nursery.
RDS, respiratory distress syndrome.

all mortalities. In our series, they accounted for 95 percent (eighteen of nineteen deaths). As birth weight goes down, clinical outcome and the expense of the care given become more problematic. In Table 6.4, the twenty-five most expensive cases (accounting for nearly 80 percent of all charges) suggest that the treatment of the newborn of very low birth weight means increased financial and clinical investment, without strong guarantees of good outcome. Of the twenty-one survivors in this high-cost group, sixteen were neurologically damaged, eight of them—without controversy—destined to be severely retarded.

The clinical problems of this group of patients were evident to the staff because the infants stayed so long in the unit.

As disturbed as the unit physicians and nurses might get about these patients, they did not see or discuss actual billing charges for any of the infants they treated. This was a matter for the hospital, third-party insurers, and parents to settle, which to all appearances they did (and without conferring with the n.i.c.u. staff).

The unit staff was free, therefore, to pursue clinical goals without reckoning costs or feeling the pressure of a general limit on diagnosis and treatment. Commented one attending physician, "The hospital can't tie our hands like that." This freedom was defended as an ethical necessity, that is, as fundamental to a disinterested, purely clinical judgment of medical need. The impetus (and mandate) to treat aggressively was so strong in this unit that information on charges, even if posted, would probably have been regarded as irrelevant to treatment decisions. Whether it might have affected admissions policy is another, unanswered question.

The long-term costs consequent to clinical decisions were also a nonissue in the n.i.c.u. Especially for newborns in the experimental group, those born weighing less than 1,000 grams, rehospitalization, special rehabilitation programs, and even institutionalization were calculable deficits (Boyle et al., 1983). But these problems were external to the staff's understanding of its responsibilities.

More difficult for the staff to dismiss, as we see in the next chapter, were the infants' parents, who served as constant reminders of the larger, life-changing repercussions of the unit's authority to treat.

III

The Family

7

Parents and Newborn Intensive Care

> I can't tell whether these parents are crazy or they're stressed.
>
> *Resident Physician*

> It's important to say [to parents that] you cannot tell which way it will go. We're following kids. If someone says they can tell outcome at this stage, they're lying.
>
> *Attending Physician*

THE QUESTION OF GUARDIANSHIP

When a newborn is referred to the n.i.c.u., the parents remain the infant's legal guardians and, in theory, have control of important medical decisions. Professional practice standards in this country support this role. For example, section 2.10 of the Current Opinions of the Judicial Council of the American Medical Association affirms that:

> In caring for defective infants, the advice and judgment of the physician should be readily available, but the decision whether to treat a severely defective infant and exert maximal efforts to sustain life should be the choice of parents. (1981:8)

In addition, in a study of physicians' attitudes about the treatment of defective infants, Todres et al. noted that "the majority of pediatricians supported the right of the parents to withhold consent for the performance of surgery" (1977:200). The authors then cited the 1976 World Health Organization report concerning newborns with congenital defects, to the effect that . . . "the decision should be that of the parents, the role of the physician being to explain to them as accurately as possible the consequences of available options" (1976:16–17).

Despite these statements, American parents have little control over their newborn's referral or treatment. The referral agreements between physicians and hospitals predetermine why and where an infant is sent. Once admitted to the hospital, the newborn is treated as a patient with maximum medical needs, not as a family member. The more emphasis put on intensive care, the more parents must follow the lead of physicians in evaluating treatment, for, in this context, the problems of the newborn are defined strictly in medical terms.

As in adult medicine, not everything that can be done for a severely ill patient should be done. According to one perspective, the worth of therapy, calculated on the basis of the future ability of the patient to take on normal social responsibilities, is a vital factor in treatment decisions (Crane, 1977). Crane argued this point for infants as well as adults:

> One would expect that those newborns who have the capacity to develop normal social relationships with their families and others will be actively treated. Those whose relationships are expected to be abnormal due to severe physical disability or brain damage will be less actively treated. The willingness of parents to attempt to develop normal relationships with such children is also an important consideration. (1977:13)

The best measure of the full social repercussions of newborn intensive care is the long-term well-being of the infant and its family. Yet the organization of the n.i.c.u. service makes this difficult to gauge. Routine care for the infants is a short stay in the n.i.c.u., usually a week, involving only cursory communication between the staff and parents. When it comes to medical follow-up, the efficiency of the system breaks down; few Level III units vigorously track the aftermath of medical treatment or systematically inquire about the family's coping with the fragile, perhaps abnormal, newborn. The rare long-term infant cases elicit the most frank confrontations with the problem of moral decision making. In contrast, when a newborn dies quickly, the baby and family are forgotten in the rapid pace of the service. In our sample of 103 consecutive cases, nearly 80 percent (79 infants) were discharged alive or had died within one week. This fast turnover of cases affects how much the staff can know about the infants' parents (Sosnowitz, 1984). As Bogdan, Brown, and Foster observed in their study of a neonatal unit:

> Most assessments of parents are based on limited knowledge, derived mainly from short observations, or second hand. What is known is episodic, not informed by the context of the perinatal experience in the lives of the parents. (1982:41)

There are multiple ways in which parents are distanced from the Level III nursery. The regional referral system automatically puts geographic distance between infants and parents. The new mother of the newborn is herself a patient, often suffering complications from childbirth, and has limited access to the n.i.c.u. nursery. Parents must negotiate for entry into the unit with the staff and, because of the child's condition, must also negotiate for the privilege of touching and handling their infant. Nursery visiting rules vary; in many units, parents can visit at any time and are urged to come frequently but are not encouraged to linger for hours or stay overnight. Some nurseries are strict about visiting rights for other family members or friends; others admit the newborn's siblings or extended family as a matter of course. Whatever the rules, the tension between the need to protect frail newborns and to accede to the wishes and rights of their families permeates the atmosphere in the Level III nursery.

Temporary Guardianship

During the time an infant is a patient in the n.i.c.u., the staff has definite expectations of the parents and strategies for managing them. Though their interventions may permanently affect a newborn's fate, the practitioners of intensive care plan on having temporary autonomy to do their clinical work. Since most cases are relatively short-term, interaction with parents is based on the working assumption that the power of guardianship passes to the physicians on admission and then reverts to the parents when the infant patient is discharged. During that time of provisional guardianship, for the sake of their own morale and to ease the burden of responsibility, the staff wants approval, even gratitude, from the infant's mother and father. Once the immediate clinical goals are accomplished, the staff looks forward to passing responsibility for the infant on to caring and capable parents. The n.i.c.u. staff expects neither protracted responsibility for representing the interests of individual newborns nor prolonged and intimate contact with mothers and fathers.

Nor does the staff expect the parents to be perfectly rational and accepting of their infant's condition. At the Northeast Pediatric n.i.c.u., parents were universally upset by their newborn's illness. For many mothers and fathers, the birth itself was a sudden, traumatic event—delivery in an ambulance, difficult vaginal birth, or emergency cesarean delivery. In explaining to troubled parents what they were doing for and to the newborn, the staff had to justify treatment that, to the uninitiated, looks like torture of the innocent rather than effective temporary guardianship. Physicians and nurses and even nonmedical researchers get used to rows of premature babies with tubes protruding from their noses and lines radiating from their arms and feet, scalps and bellies, even to newborns in splints and bandages, recovering from surgery. But few parents are emotionally prepared for the sight of their infant as one among these other casualties. The dependence of parents on the n.i.c.u. staff begins with this first, sometimes devastating experience and continues through the course of treatment.

Parents as Patients

In contrast to the conventional physician–patient dyad, intensive care presumes the complete authority of practitioners over the patient's body, thereby distancing the family from the clinical setting. In addition, the diminished persona of the patient disturbs some important conventions in medicine. For example, the patient's motivation, belief about the value of care, and freedom of choice are not issues in the n.i.c.u.

Most medical professionals rely on social interaction with patients for feedback about the efficacy of treatment. Ideally, there is gratification in the patient's acknowledgement of a cure and reassurance for practitioners that the course of treatment is understood and approved. Because n.i.c.u. staff members cannot have a professional–client relationship with the infant patients, they tend to seek that relationship with parents. Complications abound in any attempt to adapt the conventions of doctor–patient roles to the n.i.c.u. staff's fleeting interaction with mothers and fathers, but, in general, the parents are amenable to being treated as a second order of patient, not demanding much attention and not intrusive or critical about clinical work.

The staff needs the cooperation of parents just as the individual physician needs the compliance of the patient. Several authors (Parsons and Fox, 1952; Szasz and Hollender, 1956:586) have suggested that the physician socializes the patient in the same ways that the parent socializes the child. Dependence is a key element in the relationship and, through dependence, the compliance of the patient is assured. The critical condition of the n.i.c.u. infant guarantees that parents will need and want medical expertise working on behalf of their child. Most parents are subdued, even passive, in their interactions with the staff, especially with physicians. Some parents deny their infant's problems simply by staying away. If too upset or angry or frightened, however, mothers and fathers pose a multiple threat to the unit. They can disrupt the atmosphere, jeopardize the care of other infants, and cause grave concern among staff about the welfare of their own infant. It takes a combination of the authority of physicians and the sympathy of nurses to manage parents.

Physicians acknowledge that parents have emotional problems, but generally do not see their expertise extending to the psychosocial arena. Rather, nurses, social workers, and psychologists are the experts in "cooling out" potentially disruptive mothers and fathers. If we examine the work of Becker et al. (1961), the medical culture of young physicians predisposes them against working with parents for at least two reasons. When their specialty is pediatrics, physicians may compete with parents for control of the child undergoing treatment. Second, new physicians dislike dealing with "crocks," those patients who do not challenge the life-and-death powers of medicine and present instead with psychological symptoms, i.e., "those patients who cannot be cured because they are not sick in the first place are worst of all" (Becker et al., 1961:317). In the n.i.c.u., the senior physician, as a hospital-based consultant, has few incentives to build good relations with parents. Referrals come from other physicians; parents ordinarily choose their obstetrician, not their infant's neonatologist. This raises the bureaucratic problem of physicians' accountability to patients and, by extension, to the patients' parents as legal guardians.

There is also the issue of status in routinely working with parents. House officers and nurses assume the daily first-hand contact with parents that senior physicians ignore in their preference for research, clinical, and administrative responsibilities. This follows Abbott's description of the modern division of professional labor:

> Within a given profession, the highest status professionals are those who deal with issues predefined by a number of colleagues. These colleagues have removed human complexity and difficulty to leave a problem at least professionally defined, although possibly still very difficult to solve. Conversely, the lowest status professionals are those who deal with problems from which the human complexities are not or cannot be removed. (1981:823–24)

Nurses, with their training in psychology and social work, do the bulk of the managing of parents' behavior. Lacking the authority of physicians, the n.i.c.u. nursing staff uses an instructional approach (Szasz and Hollender 1956:586–87; Hollender, 1958). They explain to parents what the different diagnostic and therapeutic machines are for; they explain the purpose of minor procedures. They explain the treatment plan, which, for parents, boils down to the projected date of discharge. The nursing staff continues this instructional role by explaining the behavior of parents to physicians, if and when the physicians need such information. For example, in the case of the death of a badly compromised two-month-old, the attending physician took responsibility for talking with the parents after they had seen the baby. The parents had insisted, against physicians' advice, that their extremely premature infant with multiple anomalies be given maximum care. They were afterward critical of the treatment provided in the n.i.c.u. and, finally, regretful that the infant had survived so long. The infant had had three primary physicians, so the attending physician on duty opted to take their place and also to request an autopsy. The primary nurse provided family background to prepare the physician for the discussion.

> *Attending physician:* "The Brownings are on their way in."
> *Nurse:* "The mother works at [a law firm]. She's taken the whole thing awfully hard, wouldn't come in for a while and cries a lot. The father's all right. He's steady."
> *Attending physician:* "He's been in a lot?"
> *Nurse:* "Right. They're both exhausted."

THE EVALUATION OF PARENTS

Although nearly all the parents of infants in the n.i.c.u. unselfishly supported medical intervention on behalf of their newborns, the general attitude of the staff toward mothers, fathers, and families was mistrustful. Horror stories about the ineptitude or irrationality of parents were standard fare. Late one evening the nurses at Northeast Pediatric regaled each other with stories of disastrous encounters with parents. One told this version of an incompetent parent making tremendous demands on her:

> One of the very first times I had to assist in the delivery room, I found out the mother was crazy, from an institution. She didn't want to lie down on her back because she was afraid she'd crush her wings. I had to persuade her that it would just be for a little while and that I'd help her with her wings.

A thematically consonant type of story was about the parent who abandoned her infant. In a regional unit in England, the story was of a woman who delivered a premature infant, disappeared for three months, and then showed up to take the baby home. Two years later, she was said to have delivered another premature infant and again abandoned the child at the unit. In another unit, we heard about the Stinson couple, authors of an article and a book on their negative experiences with the physicians who treated their premature infant (Stinson and Stinson, 1979, 1983). Senior n.i.c.u. physicians described them as the typical parents who try unsuccessfully for an abortion and become ambivalent about a live infant they do not want.

At Northeast Pediatric, categorical distrust of parents was further evidenced by the written evaluations of mothers and fathers in case records. These represented only the emotional reactions of parents and laid the groundwork for their being treated by the staff as psychosocial cases. Mothers typically were reported to cry, to appear distraught and shocked, while fathers were more often described as tense, withdrawn, blaming, or angry. After the admission of an infant to the Level III nursery, the nursing staff continued to jot down the emotional reactions of visiting parents.

Parents as Second-order Patients

The "illness" of parents is essentially social rather than biological, the opposite of the illness of the infant, which is purely biological and without interactive dimensions. The nurses, aided by social workers and psychologists, take major responsibility for treating parents as second order of patient, that is, as psychological cases. Their approach to parents emphasizes the therapeutic need for confronting and expressing emotions. Parents are not supposed to deny the reality of their infant's illness or abnormalities but are to admit their fear, shame, and anger and overcome these negative feelings. Yet the staff has to exercise caution in this approach because parents are visitors to a nursery where there is not much room for disruption. The lack of privacy afforded parents in an open unit makes it imperative that they keep their emotional expressions low-keyed.

Within the Northeast Pediatric n.i.c.u., the nurses were sensitive to the capacity of parents to behave in ways potentially threatening to the concentration of physicians and nurses. Several times during our research, fathers displayed anger or came into the unit slightly drunk. This out-of-control behavior was in startling contrast to the frailty of the infants and the feminine presence of the unit nursing staff (nurses usually outnumbered physicians two to one):

> Janey [a nurse] came into the lounge area looking pale and distraught. She asked where [the attending physician] was.

Margaret [the receptionist]: "He was here just a minute ago. The x-ray rounds are over, so he might be having coffee with the new residents."

Janey: "The Fitch father has been drinking. He's angry. His breath is awful."

Margaret: "That's an emergency. I'll get [the unit director]."

In minutes, the unit director came down and steered the errant father out of the nursery and to the elevator. More frequently, a mother would sit crying by an isolette, alone or with the father or a nurse. This quiet sorrow was tolerable, but the nurses at Northeast Pediatric did not like other parents to see expressions of grief or depression. Instead, the nurses preferred the presence of upbeat, optimistic mothers and quiet, gentle fathers.

Visits from other family members were permitted but not encouraged. For staff, explaining the appearance of an infant to parents was an acceptable responsibility; instructing obviously confused or surprised relatives simply was extra work. In addition, the reactions of families were potentially upsetting to the staff. The uncle of one infant visited along with the parents and grandparents but spent most of the time staring at the exposed genitals of an infant girl in the next isolette. The primary nurse felt powerless to control this behavior; another nurse consoled her by dismissing the uncle as "a moron." In units that served large ethnic populations and were mixed-level, the staff's tolerance of visiting families was greater and both staff and parents had a greater range of emotional expression. At Northeast Pediatric, the atmosphere in the n.i.c.u. was more reserved, and the infants were generally more seriously premature and ill than in many of the other U.S., European, and South American nurseries we visited. The clinical status of the newborns probably contributed to the need the staff felt to control visiting parents' behavior.

Problem Parents

The ideal parent of an n.i.c.u. patient approximates what sociologists have long described as the model patient in physician–patient interactions (Parsons, 1951:428–37). At Northeast Pediatric and elsewhere, parents who were well thought of by staff were compliant, nondisruptive, demonstrated their willingness to cooperate, and sincerely wanted to be relieved of their deviant role as parents of a sick newborn.

The "bad" parent, like the problem patient, resisted the influence of the staff. Martin's (1957) discussion of the undesirable patient, as judged by medical students, described a patient who is stubborn, refuses help, and fails to appreciate the efforts expended on his or her behalf. Fox (1957:230–32) also noted that patients who do not respond to the diagnostic and therapeutic efforts of the student physician as the physician wants are a threat to that physician's self-confidence. So, too, the uncooperative parent upset the nurses and younger physicians and made them feel less sure of their ability to influence behavior.

Parents who were infrequent visitors to the unit did not give the nursing staff a chance to confront psychosocial problems and frustrated staff members who wanted to feel personally effective. Newman, in her report on parents' behavior in n.i.c.u.'s, called this "coping through distance."

> Some infants are not visited. This may occur for various reasons. Some are being placed for adoption and for the time in intensive care are wards of the state. Others have been transported from a distance, the mother may be for an extended period in a hospital in another city and the father may be caring for other children at home. Still others may be children of single mothers who have not yet determined whether to keep the child or who wish to keep their distance until that decision is made. (1980:187)

Although they were a small minority, these parents troubled the n.i.c.u. staff because of the uncertainty that shrouds the baby's future home life. From the nurses' perspective, every infant should go home to a responsible and accepting mother and father. It is hard for the staff to know how absentee parents feel about their child.

At the other extreme were parents who tried to tell the staff what to do or who insinuated that the staff was not doing enough. These unusual, aggressive parents often had college degrees or a medical background and were successful in winning concessions (overnight visits, extra consultants, more tests and therapy) from the unit director. Their capacity to generate animosity seemed to depend only on how long their infants remained in the unit. Over a period of weeks, this type of parent became a genuine irritant to the residents and nurses who had to work closely with them. In one case, the mother (a medical technician) was convinced that the nurses were not attentive enough to her infant son, who was a very low birth weight baby and had had major surgery. She visited daily and made frequent phone calls to check if the nurses were feeding the infant on time, tending to tube suctioning, and maintaining lines and the incision area. As a result, the staff were reluctant to talk to her.

First nurse: "She has a real control problem. I think her husband does
  too. The kid's in for real trouble with them."
Second nurse: "She drives us crazy. I run when she comes in the door."

Ironically, the nursing staff occasionally were forgetful in caring for
this infant, unconsciously demonstrating the negative effect of the
mother's proddings.

The most deviant parent was the one whose behavior was erratic,
who demonstrated no apparent progression from the initial reaction
to trauma to an emotional acceptance of the infant's condition. The
prolonged instability of a parent's emotional reactions was frequently cited at social service rounds as a cause for serious concern.
The parent who reacted strongly to every clinical setback, who visited irregularly, or whose behavior varied widely from effusive acceptance to cold rejection of the newborn signaled trouble to the
nursing staff. The fault of these parents was their resistance to the
socialization agenda by which nurses and social workers intended
to turn emotional trauma into stability and strength. In the case of
one severely neurologically damaged infant, the mother went through
many emotional peaks and valleys and her ability to confront her
child's condition (which also changed frequently) varied accord-
ingly. The infant reacted poorly to being touched or fed by the mother
and otherwise failed to develop normally. After months of nursing
attention and counseling, the mother had made little emotional progress, for which she was harshly judged. As one nurse described it:

> It's been four months. She comes in a lot, too much. She still cries and
> is nervous with the feedings. She absorbs too much [of the staff's] en-
> ergy. She's like a black hole.

The golden mean of parental behavior is revealed in the typology
of difficult parents as articulated by the n.i.c.u. staff during the time
of our fieldwork: Parents who broke down emotionally at each visit
revealed parental incompetence. Parents who were enthusiastic about
their ability to handle a critically ill newborn did not understand the
gravity of the situation. Parents, for example, Jehovah's Witnesses,
who rejected certain clinical procedures were unreasonable. Parents
who demanded more intervention, for example, ligation of patent
ductus arteriosus in a baby in total failure, were also unreasonable.
Parents who showed no emotion at bedside had psychological
problems. Parents who expressed anger or frustration or despair also
had psychological problems. Educated parents thought they knew
everything; conversely, high-school dropouts were incapable of understanding medical information.

IMPROVING PARENT–INFANT RELATIONS

At the same time that the n.i.c.u. staff disparages parents' behavior, nurses try to promote parents' affection for their newborns. The thinking pervading this effort is strongly influenced by the literature on "bonding," that is, the instinctual basis for parenting that should be fostered at birth and throughout the first months of the infant's life.

> The attachment of a mother for her infant is a strong, specific, affectional bond that causes a mother to be willing to put her baby's needs ahead of her own; to make the sacrifices necessary in caring for her infant day in and day out, night after night; to protect, nurture, fondle, kiss, cuddle, talk to, gaze at, and comfort her infant; to learn its needs and signals, to resist separation from her baby and be preoccupied with its well-being, especially when they are apart. (Sugarman, 1981)

Since critical illness in the newborn forces a separation between infant and parent, the risk of disrupting physiologically programmed bonding and, consequently, the risk of "parenting failure" are high (Benfield, Leib, and Reuter, 1976). The results of this failure, argue pediatricians, psychiatrists, and social workers, are child battering and developmental failure-to-thrive in infants and children (Klaus and Kennell, 1976). Dedicated nurses at Northeast Pediatric and other hospitals sought to overcome the risk of parenting failure by encouraging visiting parents to touch, stroke, and handle their baby as the infant's medical condition allowed.

The principal goal of bedside interaction with mothers and fathers was the development of parents' identification with the infant, out of which, theoretically, comes the guarantee of special care-giving at home. The mother is the focus of maximum concern. According to the therapeutic agenda, she should be daily drawing closer to her infant, despite the distance imposed by intensive care and the regionalized service. At Northeast Pediatric, the staff viewed any parental resistance to "bonding" as deviant, although few infants could initially be held or respond to touch. For example, in discussing a mother who was holding off from visiting her newborn, the staff at a multidisciplinary conference delved into her psychological strategies. The infant was born four days prior to this exchange and weighed 1,700 grams.

> *Nurse:* "Dad came in four afternoons this week. He was touching the baby, interested in caring. He said. 'My wife is nervous that the baby will die.' I called, talked with her for forty-five minutes. Father came in

two or three times a day. Grandfather said they didn't want the mother told any of the stuff like ventilator settings. Father said the same thing. They said, 'Tell us the stuff, but just tell her the baby is beautiful.' They said that's the way they want to handle it. They said wait until the tubes are out."

Psychiatrist: "Stinks" (laughter).

Resident: "Yeah, it does. But what are you [the nurses] thinking of doing?"

Nurse: "I thought if we could bring the mother in and let her see that it's not a monster."

Psychiatrist: "There's got to be something going on. She reacted originally with denial—that's okay when one is in crisis. But the fact that she's allowing her two men to take care of her [looks bad]. (Directing his remark to the nurse) Do what you're doing. But if it doesn't work, then have a family meeting and say you want everyone here at 6 p.m. Or get more family history from the father."

Resident: "It's a red flag when the mother doesn't come in. And the question is, for how long and why? And it's related to bonding. . . ."

Psychiatrist: "There's got to be some other trauma in this woman's life— a 90 percent chance."

The parents' personification of the baby is an integral part of attachment. In a discussion of a depressed mother of an 800-gram infant:

Psychiatrist: "Is she reaching out to the baby?"

Nurse: "At first we had a problem. But now she asks not how is 'he' but how is 'Randy.' "

By stressing the individual personality of the small newborn, the Northeast pediatric nursing staff also sought to overcome parents' disappointment at seeing the premature infant. This disappointment at not having a perfect baby can be experienced as the loss of the expected normal child, equivalent to an infant's death, and provoke grieving (Solnit and Stark, 1961). The remedy sought is an acceptance of the infant as a unique and lovable person. Persuading parents to visit their baby is the first step. Persuading them to overcome their hesitancy about physical closeness to the infant is next.

Waiting for rounds, the attending physician had an informal chat with the nurse about a twenty-eight to twenty-nine weeks' gestation baby, now at day fourteen and weighing 1,100 grams. They discussed the parents' visits. The nurse reported that the mother behaves appropriately, but that the father is still hands-offish. The nurse has told the father that tomorrow she wants him to hold the baby. She is using a kind of humorous or teasing approach. She told the doctor that she said to the father, "I'm not forcing you." She also told the father, "I'll con you into it."

The conversion of such reluctant parents is a particular triumph for the n.i.c.u. staff. At one hospital we visited, an infant born weighing 700 grams was initially not visited by his mother and father, who feared making too much of an emotional investment in their small, frail newborn. Over the course of three months, the nursing staff persuaded the parents to visit and make physical contact with their child. By the end of the first month, the parents decided to give the infant a name, after which their visits and their enthusiasm for the baby grew apace. During the same time, the nurses brought in crib toys, made drawings that they placed in and around the isolette as visual stimulation, and chipped in to buy a doll's baseball suit for "the little slugger" to wear when he reached 2,000 grams.

Since the length of stay for most n.i.c.u. patients is brief, the emotional difficulties of parents disappear quickly from the staff's focus of attention. This does not mean that family difficulties cease, only that they are no longer the business of the n.i.c.u. staff. Few units, for example, are actively concerned with parents' reactions to neonatal death, even though physicians and nurses are constantly dealing with mortality rates as high as 30 percent and must frequently interact with parents whose infants die. A small study done by Benfield, Leib, and Reuter in 1976 underlined the importance of the compassionate concern of hospital personnel in determining parents' adjustment to neonatal death. Kennell and Klaus (1976) also analyzed parental grief responses and recommended that physicians meet with parents immediately after an infant's death, two to three months later, and again three to six months later. The n.i.c.u. staff's concentration on immediate clinical issues makes this consistently compassionate approach difficult for them. Even nurses who care about parents are hard-pressed to handle both clinical and psychosocial responsibilities. The emotional needs of most parents and families after the experience of newborn intensive care are addressed erratically, if at all. They either become private problems within the family, are passed on to other professionals, or are addressed in parental support groups that spontaneously arise on the initiative of social workers, nurses, or the parents themselves. The typical staff's perspective is that parents' emotional problems are temporary crises, not the reflection of deep wounds to their marriage and family life. Socialized by the nurses and social service personnel, parents should move from their reaction to the trauma to reasonable acceptance of the clinical history of their infant.

The psychosocial mission to educate the parents of n.i.c.u. patients deflects attention from the larger truth that the parents, with rare exceptions, already identify emotionally with their new-born.

> It is difficult to say when parents endow a fetus with personhood and cherish him as part of themselves, but they do this almost without ex-ception before the last trimester of pregnancy whether they wanted the baby originally or not. (Duff and Campbell, 1976:490)

The best proof of this attachment is the acute sense of loss and grief parents experience at the death of infants even of marginal viability.

In difficult long-term cases, mothers and fathers are rarely the bastions of strength the staff would like them to be. The more clin-ically difficult the case, the more complex the relations between family and staff become. For example, parents react strongly to their ba-by's medical setbacks. Their hopes wax and wane, their faith in the expertise of the staff varies, their hesitancies about the future con-dition of the hospitalized infant increase over time, and their emo-tional investment in the infant increases daily.

The longer an infant stays in the unit, the more energy the staff must put into managing and evaluating the parents. In doing this, they move from simply routine behavior assessment to scrutiny of the family structure and its guardianship guarantees. The psychol-ogy of parents remains important, but, on a broader level, the staff looks for stable family organization as a necessary condition for the long-term protection of the fragile infant. As the infant develops a lengthy patient career, nurses, social workers, and eventually phy-sicians take the long view on family resources.

FAMILY RESOURCES

Parents' resources include everything that contributes to the secu-rity of the mother and the stability of the family. These are per-ceived primarily as a mutually supportive relationship between the parents, the father's steady employment, the mother's freedom from the need to work, and secure housing. The logic of looking at fam-ily resources is simple. It relates directly to the extra care most pre-mature infants need after they leave the hospital. Normal newborns taken home soon after birth usually settle into convenient patterns of sleep, alertness, and feeding. The neonate who spends a pro-longed period in intensive care becomes oriented to continuous lights and noise, the monotony of the isolette environment, the associa-tion of pain (from tests and therapies) with human contact, and in-travenous feeding. The unpredictable responses and irritability of the infant that spent its first days in the n.i.c.u. makes one kind of demand on parents. In cases in which medical treatment must continue at home, mothers and supportive fathers should also have the stamina, technical expertise, and resolve to follow through on care begun in the n.i.c.u. On our very first visit to Northeast Pediatric, we met the mother of an eight-month-old infant whose portable respirator was being checked out by a technician. She confided:

> We just don't sleep. We both keep waking up afraid that the machine isn't working. We have to check all the time that he is still alive.

An attending physician at the same hospital commented:

> The worst mistake I ever made was sending a baby home early to a working mother who had a seventy-two-year-old grandmother at home. The grandmother just wasn't up to the special care the baby needed. The baby had to be brought back to the hospital again. It had a cold and it could have been fatal. It wasn't, but it could have been.

At social service rounds, staff members discussed technical problems and family support in the case of an infant with multiple problems, including cretinism, a heart defect, and a gastrostomy. The mother of this child was eighteen years old.

Nurse: "The mother is competent in the care she gives the child. The father is more stand back. But one thing—the grandparents—every time the grandmother is there, she criticizes the mother: 'You're going to drop her.' Or, at bath time, 'You're going to put her head in.' "

Fellow (specialist in pediatric development): "I'd say, 'I think you're doing fine.' "

Nurse: "I did."

Fellow: "I see the [baby's] going home not as an abrupt cessation of the medical services. The day after the baby goes home, she'll need about 95 percent of what we've been doing here. . . . Whenever you send a baby like this home, the mother is petrified. The care deliverer at home will need some help."

Child development specialist: "It's a shame the grandmother is so critical because she's the woman who has the power to influence. She's the one who could mother this mother."

Nurse: "That's not very feasible. We could persuade the VNA [Visiting Nurse Association] to visit twice a day and maybe the homemaker thing could be worked out."

Resident: "You must prepare them for the gastrostomy falling out. It's likely and I've known cases where it made parents upset. We could pull it out and put it back in, as a demonstration." (The group groaned at this suggestion.)

Nurse (defending the mother): "She doesn't have any reservations about caring for the gastrostomy."

Second nurse: "Your initial point is well-taken, but your method . . . (voice trails off)."

If the parents' marriage seemed unstable or if the family situation was deteriorating, the staff moved defensively to protect the newborn. In the case of a three-week-old infant with a neurologically good prognosis, a nurse, social worker, and psychiatrist discussed the family's situation:

Nurse: "Today was the first day she [the mother] spent the whole day with me. I got a very new picture. Previously I thought they were supportive, wanted the baby. Today, I found out that they are planning to separate. Their relationship is deteriorating. He goes to bars every night—for two years."

Social worker: "She told me that was new."

Nurse: "She is a very grown-up twenty-year-old. He seems appropriate. He calls. Medical insurance ended yesterday. He's out of a job. She's planning to go on welfare and get her own place away from him."

Social worker: "She told me that she and her husband were married within the last two years. They lived at their own place. Huge carpenter ants. So they moved in with the in-laws. She said he has always been lazy. He was physically abusive to her. He hit her during pregnancy—on her arm. She said he didn't have a chronic drinking problem. Their breaking up before had to do with his not helping her. She wants to get away. The mother-in-law wants her to take him along. Catch 22. She cannot apply for welfare if he's there. . . ."

Then the discussion focused on the protection of the newborn:

Psychiatrist: "This baby is at high risk. You can say, 'I think we need a fuller evaluation.' We can do it voluntarily or it will be a [child neglect and abuse order]."

Social worker: "It would have to be a soft [order] because this baby is not in that much danger."

Nurse: "I'm concerned that we make the abuse possibility a high priority. We know a baby is at risk in neonatal intensive care in general and there is cumulative stress."

The association of low socioeconomic status with premature birth inevitably brought the staff in contact with family problems associated with poverty. Since about 30 percent (32 of 101) of the patients in our sample were insured by Medicaid, the nurses and physicians who participated in social service discussions frequently confronted the destabilizing influences of poverty: unemployment, underemployment, change of residence, illegitimacy, single-parent house-holds, low levels of education, and elaborate histories of medical problems and reliance on welfare programs.

A debated question was whether economically disadvantaged parents could provide the same protective security for the prema-ture infant as could those who are more financially well-off. Several times, the staff discussed some well-known studies suggesting that parents of low economic status abuse their premature babies (Hunter et al., 1978). The n.i.c.u. staff at Northeast Pediatric, like those in other units, knew practically nothing about parents' finances or what happened to the infants after discharge. Instead, the nurses drew on their own solidly conventional notions of marriage and family life to estimate family resources. More than a little guesswork was involved. According to admission records, some 75 percent of the mothers were married; the marital status of the rest was single, am-biguous, or unidentified. The fast turnover of cases made accurate judgments about families nearly impossible. Only in long-term cases did families become known to the staff and subject to the full weight of social evaluation and to possible professional intervention. The nurses were most approving of the nuclear family organization, in which a married couple seemed committed to each other and in which the husband was steadily employed. There was ambivalence about the role of the extended family; for example, in-laws should support the couple's relationship, not intrude on it. Deviations from the nuclear family model presented the problem of how the baby would be cared for after discharge. Can an unmarried teenager or a divorced woman or a grandmother take care of a fragile newborn? From the staff's perspective, a strongly committed, stable couple was the best insurance that an infant would be safeguarded after leaving the n.i.c.u.

In combination with an infant's severe medical problems, an un-stable family situation registered as more of a threat than did the emotional instability of parents. There was always hope that par-ents could psychologically adapt, if they had each other. If the mother's morale was good (even though the family situation was less than ideal), at least some staff members would feel positively about their own commitment to care of the marginal infant. Those unmarried mothers who seemed emotionally well-adjusted and whose own parents were supportive had their champions among the nursing staff. Yet on several occasions, the staff had difficulty interpreting the attitudes of single, black mothers and perceiving the supportive role of their kin. In one instance, an unmarried black woman in her late twenties told the staff that she was not ready to tell the father of her baby about the birth.

> *First nurse:* "She knows who the father is but says she isn't telling him yet."
> *Second nurse:* "Her sister has permission to visit. She was in yesterday. I can't figure it out."

If a parent showed promise of neither an appropriate emotional attitude nor family stability, the staff's willingness to treat the severely compromised newborn could falter or treatment might continue as a matter of unit policy. In short, a bad medical prognosis was counted as one strike against an infant. A parent's poor psychological profile was counted as a second strike. An unstable family situation was counted as a third. The three-strike situation hit all levels of failure—biological, psychological, and social.

COMMUNICATING WITH PARENTS

For communication with parents, the stated policy of the Northeast Pediatric n.i.c.u. staff was frankness. The educational directives of senior physicians, the professed ideology of nurses, and the practical instruction of new residents all stressed the staff's responsibility to be open with parents about the condition of the infant. Parents were encouraged to phone in at any hour to inquire after the newborn and there were no formal restrictions on visiting times. Parents who did not keep in daily contact were called by either the primary nurse or the primary physician. At least part of the rationale for frankness was to avoid parents' anger. If a baby went into failure during the night without the parents' knowing it, they were bound to feel shut off from caretaking and question the staff's competence and honesty.

Consistency in communicating with parents was another of the staff's goals. Like parents who were kept in the dark, parents who heard one version of their newborn's medical condition from a physician and another from a nurse were bound to be frustrated.

Parents wanted clear answers to simple questions. They wanted to know if their baby would be coming home before or after Christmas, if the baby was retarded or not, if the baby would live or die. The answers to these simple questions, however, were based on physicians' interpretations of complex information. The policy of consistency required that nurses listen carefully to physicians' statements about a given case and translate highly technical discussion into the language of the parents. For example, physicians (attending physician, fellow and residents) at work rounds would frequently discuss and authorize multiple tests along with plans for oxygen therapy. For an infant receiving 30 percent oxygen with quickly resolving respiratory distress syndrome, the experienced nurse could calculate that extubation would be attempted in another day or so and, barring complications, could arrange discharging the infant to a community hospital before the end of that week. When parents asked about a baby's progress, the nurse could suggest a reasonably accurate schedule for discharge.

Obstacles to Communication

In the daily life of the unit, the obstacles to both frankness and consistency in communicating with parents were formidable. These obstacles divide roughly into professional and structural categories. Among the professional impediments are paternalism toward parents and the technicality of medical language. A less familiar obstacle is the physician's notion of clinical progress as it conflicts with the broader concept of the infant patient's total well-being.

Paternalism. The physicians' attitude that parents should be protected from harsh realities takes several forms. One we found common, not just at Northeast Pediatric but among other n.i.c.u. physicians, was that they, not parents, should assume the responsibility for withdrawing support, even when infants were near death. Presenting parents with the decision that treatment should be stopped was considered humane and, more, the responsibility of the n.i.c.u. physician. As we saw in Chapter 5, prolonged aggressive intervention at least partially relieves clinicians of this painful task. They prefer that all therapeutic options are used, after which they can point to the massive failure of organ systems as the cause of death, not that any individual disconnected a respirator. Whether the infant's biology fails or the physicians' clinical arts prove ineffective, the staff's intent is to protect parents from the guilt presumably resulting from the decision to cease treatment.

In a parallel way, some physicians choose to "lay the crepe," that is, to communicate information about the clinical status of the newborns so as to diminish parents' hope for their baby's survival. This, too, is a common attitude.

Many of the physicians we approached thought that giving parents optimistic outlooks in the first hours after birth of their premature infants was dishonest and misleading. They thought that if a mother is prepared for a death, she will go through the experience with less emotional upheaval. (Clyman et al., 1979: 722)

This approach contradicts (and perhaps antedates) the theories of bonding and grieving, which advocate parents' consciously investing their emotions in the sick infant to resolve psychological problems (Klaus and Kennell, 1976:209–39). Which approach is in the best interests of parents is hard to say because so little is known about the reactions of the mothers and fathers of deceased newborns. Physicians are bound to judge subjectively and may not even have a consistent personal or professional orientation toward death (Cassell, 1972).

The other bad news communicated to parents is that their baby is permanently brain-damaged or disabled. Paternalism heavily colors the interaction when physicians try to play down the severity of the problem. The stock phrases are "We can't promise he'll be first in his class," "She'll be slower than other children," and "A good loving family will take this baby a long way." Unfortunately, trying to protect parents from understanding the degree of injury suffered by their infant leaves them unprepared for future hardships.

Technical Medical Language.   Several studies have described the barriers to communication inherent in medical jargon (Belknap, 1956; Rapoport, Rapoport, and Rosow, 1959). Communication between physicians and clients can suffer when the nature of the illness and its remedies are not effectively relayed (Playa, Cohen, and Samora, 1968). Medical language can be used to protect the status of the professional group and to control information (Quint, 1965). Like other specialized areas, neonatology relies on a shorthand of initials, acronyms, and slang that is difficult to translate for the lay public. Take this linguistic example of a resident presenting the specifics of a case during work rounds at Northeast Pediatric:

> This is a new player. Stable, twenty-six to twenty-eight weeks, 720 grams. A twin; the other twin died of IVH. The Apgars were unremarkable, 2 and 6, I think. Umbi line, fluid management, not hypernatremic. PIE worsened. Pneumothorax on right side—two chest tubes. Not draining at present; pneumo resolved. Transferred her from the community hospital for PDA. LA/AO at 1.35. 3-over-6 murmur; maybe even a 4-over-6 murmur. No evidence of VSD, but the data looks inaccurate. The chest x-ray looks benign. I gave "dig" and Lasix. 36 percent oxygen; she was 30 percent there [at community hospital]. She looked crappy, the lower body was gray. We got 7.79, 19 PCO, 130. She crumped. The family

walked in as the baby bottomed out. They wanted to sit and watch. I asked them to step out for a minute.

The informational bases of the staff and of parents are so different that this case description was translated to the parents as "a temporary difficulty with the heart."

Despite the heavy preponderance of premature babies in Level III nurseries, few efforts are made to inform parents about the common problems afflicting infants born before term. For example, in 1979 at the Northeast Pediatric unit, 69 percent of all admitting primary diagnoses were respiratory distress syndrome or heart and brain conditions related to prematurity (Table 7.1). Yet there were no pamphlets or charts to illustrate and explain lung disease, or patent ductus arteriosus in the premature heart, or the fragility of ventricles in the brain. Parents were discouraged from looking at other babies in the n.i.c.u. and from comparing cases or progress. In one

Table 7.1. Primary admitting diagnoses on the Northeast Pediatric n.i.c.u. in 1979

	Total	RDS	Heart/brain pathologies	Asphyxia/meconium aspirations	Sepsis/ Other	Multiple anomalies
Admissions	344	188	47	37	57	15
Percent	100	55	14	11	17	4
Deaths	59	36	9	7	2	5
Percent	100	61	15	12	3	8

RDS, respiratory distress syndrome.

large unit, this staff control of information broke down when computer terminals were installed within the unit, near the isolettes. Some parents quickly learned, by watching the physicians, to call up their infant's records on the terminal screen. The staff was particularly aggravated when several parents discussed and compared computerized medical records, including progress charts.

The Notion of Clinical Progress. Immersed in a specific battle against newborn pathologies and measuring success on the basis of minute physiological changes, the n.i.c.u. staff sometimes misconstrues what parents want to know. A typical exchange is the following:

Parent: "Doctor, how is my baby?"
Physician: "He's doing just fine. Progressing nicely."

The parents want to know if the baby is becoming normal, like the baby they expected. The physician, focused on clinical data, is thinking that this infant was born weighing 700 grams, was started on 90 percent oxygen therapy, and now, two days later, is receiving 70 percent oxygen. For this birth weight, given the usually grim outcome in small babies, such progress is indeed good. As for the overall health of the newborn or chances for its normal development, those are other questions, central to the mind of the parent but peripheral to the clinician's view at this stage in treatment and perhaps throughout the entire course of intensive therapy.

As we observed in discussing aggressive intervention, the capacity of neonatologists in Level III nurseries to immerse themselves in the immediacy of clinical work can also function as a denial of the long-term consequences of their treatment decisions. The survival of an infant with serious damage can mark a clinical victory for physicians but spell personal tragedy for the family. The quest for narrowly defined clinical success can also undermine the physician's responsibility to inform the parents about their infant's general health. Physicians do not intend to mislead; often they feel pressed by the enormity of their mandate to rescue critically ill newborns and by a lack of clinical victories. Said one senior physician at a Midwest unit, "We can't turn straw into gold. Parents don't understand what we're up against [in treating extremely premature infants]."

Since residents are less experienced and less committed to the n.i.c.u., they find the task of telling parents about setbacks especially difficult. Attending physicians and fellows often assumed the responsibility of conveying to parents the news of an infant's death. However, the hardest chore for the n.i.c.u. staff was telling parents about the problem of serious permanent damage to the newborn. Retardation was the first question on many parents' minds but it was the last question that physicians of any rank wanted to discuss. Their usual defense was that neonatologists cannot predict long-range outcome; the service best handles immediate medical emergencies. This is so, although with the increasing use of sophisticated ultrasound and other diagnostic technologies, the precision with which neurological damage can be evaluated is increasing. The longer the history of newborn intensive care, with premature infants as the mainstay of the patient population, the harder it becomes for physicians to discount the long-range consequences of treatment. The following conversation, about an infant born weighing 820 grams, shows how a senior physician at the Northeast Pediatric n.i.c.u. argued for hedging statements about the long-term prognosis:

> *Attending physician:* "I don't think you should use the word 'retardation.' "
> *Resident:* "This kid has a grade 2 intraventricular hemorrhage."

Fellow: "Maybe it was grade 3 [that is, even worse]."

Attending physician: "With the word 'retardation,' you make it a self-fulfilling prophecy [because parents will react to the child as if it were retarded]."

Fellow: "Intraventricular hemorrhage correlates with it. It's important to tell the parents."

Attending physician: "You should say that some have 'developmental problems.' "

Fellow: "I'd want to know."

Attending physician: "It's important to say that you cannot tell which way it will go. We're following kids. If someone says they can tell outcome at this stage, they're lying."

Resident: "I've said there are problems—but I think the time to wrap it up is when the baby goes home."

Fellow: "This baby will make it, one way or the other. But to involve families, I think they have a right to know what's going on here each day. I don't think it's fair not to tell them the importance of an intraventricular hemorrhage. They have to sign a consent form for [brain] surgery—and informed consent means knowing. It's important that they get an accurate idea of what's going on."

Attending physician: "I think that's right. You have to tell both sides. And you have to tell them that you can't tell now [what outcome will be]. And it's very important to be positive to parents. If your attitude is negative, parents will pick that up. Parents always assume the worst, uniformly."

Fellow: "I have yet to get in trouble with parents, over a long time [i.e., working with parents long-term]. They may have a problem dealing with honest approaches in the acute phase, but in the long run they respect you for it."

Resident: "It's important to not take away hope."

The attending physician's claim of clinical uncertainty suggests a defense of experimenting with extremely small newborns, about whom less is known. One interpretation of the attending physician's argument, therefore, is that physicians should be positive with parents lest the parents trouble the physicians' pursuit of progressive medicine. Another is that they want parents to be accepting of their newborns.

Organizational Obstacles to Communication

Structural impediments to communication with parents are a function of the bureaucratic organization of newborn intensive care and the efforts of staff members to protect that system of care. The three obstacles we noted reflect the behavior of the n.i.c.u. team as a managerial group. They also reflect the educational goals of the teaching hospital and the corporate dynamic of n.i.c.u. referral systems.

Administrative Secrecy.   Administrative secrecy fits the general category of what Hughes (1942:18) called "protecting the secrets of the temple," those facts and processes that professionals in complex organizations prefer their clients never know. In the same vein, one could argue that the proponents of the service benefit from parents' lack of understanding. As sociologists Moore and Tumin put it:

> Ignorance on the part of a consumer of specialized services (for example, medical or legal advice) helps to preserve the privileged position of a specialized dispenser of these services. (1949:788–89)

Yet it would be a mistake to think that a professional conspiracy controls communication between staff and parents. Rather, a combination of professional attitudes and bureaucratic imperatives protects the inner life of the unit. Like individual physicians, the staff team can use paternalism or technical jargon or organizational imperatives to manipulate information.

Essentially a professional team (see Goffman, 1959:89–92), n.i.c.u. physicians and nurses nonetheless act like administrators when they deliberate and rehearse what information to convey to parents and how. Bok's descriptive comment on administrative secrecy is apt:

> In order to create a pattern out of chaos and avoid haphazard choices, administrators must be able to consider and discard a variety of solutions in private before endorsing some of them in public; the process of evolving new policies requires a degree of concealment. (1982:175)

Similarly, the application of a fixed policy to a changing patient profile requires the elaboration of some of the secrets of the temple. For instance, the serious medical condition of the newborn in intensive care certainly justifies the staff's separate deliberation. However, in view of the ultimate responsibility of parents for the welfare of the infant, the substitution of behind-the-scenes decision making for discussions with parents raises guardianship problems. Exclusive staff conferences at Northeast Pediatric occurred at virtually every clinical crisis. Important treatment decisions were reached and then communicated to parents. For example, in consultation with a neurologist, the n.i.c.u. senior physicians would decide that a severely premature infant needed a brain shunt. They would set the time and date of the operation and then call the parents in for a conference to explain the need for the procedure. The parents would then consent to the surgery. Or, having reached a critical juncture in treatment where a DNR ("do not resuscitate") order seemed necessary, the staff would hold a closed conference to make the decision, drawing on their evaluations of the family as well as medical indications. Then a physician would ask the parents to come in, ostensibly for a second discussion but actually to tell them what the physicians had decided was best to do.

The n.i.c.u. version of administrative secrecy is also used to keep parents from knowing about medical mistakes. In one instance, a resident on transport discovered a poorly placed tube that had caused a newborn to asphyxiate. The infant turned out to be the child of one of the n.i.c.u. physician's neighbors. Two other physicians discussed the case:

> *Psychiatrist:* "It raises an interesting ethical question. What do you tell the parents? The tube was in the esophagus. What is the system of payment? If you tell the parents, they'll sue [the original hospital]. If you don't tell the parents, they'll personally have to bear the cost of iatrogenic [error]."
> *Fellow:* "Is that true? If the illness is defined as perinatal insult, then it can be covered by the state."
> *Psychiatrist:* "The more basic question—is your obligation to the individual patient? If so, then you would suggest to the parents that something is improper."

This was a purely academic discussion. The matter of error was not investigated and the parents were left uninformed.

Educational Goals. The major conflict between a hospital's educational goals and the n.i.c.u.'s service mission is in the short-term rotation of residents. At Northeast Pediatric, parents depended on the primary physician (a resident) for authoritative interpretation of clinical facts. For short-term cases, the six-week rotation of residents should not have been a problem. Yet on any single day when three new junior physicians took over, every case on the unit changed hands. All the parents then had to find and identify their child's new physician.

Over the course of a six-week rotation, occasionally a resident would develop good rapport with parents. Several residents returned to the unit after their rotations were over to check on infants they had been covering, and some house officers expressed a real sympathy for parents. Even if a primary physician was remote or did not relate well to parents, families still depended on him or her as the most credible source of information. In clinical terms, the residents at Northeast Pediatric learned their cases well, but they frequently had to check with the nursing staff about which visiting parents belonged to what baby, and in no sense did they compete with the nurses in interpreting parents' emotions or social situation.

For parents to lose a primary physician after weeks of close interaction and be confronted by a new and perhaps disoriented replacement added to their anxieties, especially if they were intent on making daily visits and expected to be well-informed. In the following exchange, the parent is expected to learn better, not the staff.

> *Nurse* (to attending physician): "Mr. Jackson is furious that he can't find [the primary physician]. I told him that the new residents came on yesterday and were just getting their cases. He blew up. He wants to see [the director] right now."
> *Attending physician:* "I'll handle it. But he's got to get used to talking with the right physician [i.e., the primary physician]."

In very long-term cases, those extending over months, primary physicians came and went two, three, and more times. Added to this were the rotations of neonatology fellows on a staggered six-week basis and the shifts in senior physicians. While physician authority was paramount in the unit, the provision for a steady source of physician–parent contact was lacking.

The worst repercussion of the physicians' rotations and shifts was inconsistency in treatment. For example, the course of treatment for a borderline case could be reversed not because of new data but because of the appearance of a new team member. As we noted in the chapter on aggressive intervention (Chapter 5), it took only one staff member to effect sustained heroic efforts for an infant. With every change in physician, the possibility existed that the team would modify, in a major or minor way, the infant's course of treatment and that a revision of prognosis would be communicated to the parents. Maybe another test would be made, maybe not; maybe an operation was worth risking, perhaps not. Unknowingly, parents had to adapt to this subtle repercussion of staff rotations and teamwork dynamics.

The Referral System. The modern hospital system has been described as an open system, with inputs and outputs of services and patients, and as a negotiator with other organizations (Ver Steeg and

Croog, 1979:308). As part of that organization, the n.i.c.u. referral system weakens contact between parents and staff members while it reinforces communication between and among professionals and institutions. This situation is not unusual for some hospital-based specialties, such as radiology, anesthesiology, or pathology, whose practitioners do not actually have patients. Neonatologists have referred to them only incompetent patients, so that, organizationally, parents are incidental to the service and to the entire system of admission and discharge, except as the parties responsible for payment.

In following their infant from one hospital and nursery to another, parents are expected to navigate a complexity of forms and bills, of institutional rules, and of physicians' authority and advice. At Northeast Pediatric, efforts to educate parents about the referral system were nonexistent. Perhaps the bureaucratic differences between community and central hospitals made it difficult for the hospitals to publish a brochure containing an overview of forms and organizational procedures. Or perhaps the personalized nature of contact between physicians on the local level and those associated with the n.i.c.u. resisted systematic description. In either event, the transport of an infant through as many as five different service divisions, including several nurseries and special surgery, could create all sorts of confusion for parents. Sometimes parents received enormous and complicated hospital bills from several sources, with duplicate charges. Other parents were unsure about the extent of their insurance coverage, whether they had to pay the bills or a third party would pay. One couple's private insurance had limits on hospitalization coverage for their newborn. The mother of this infant, whose billing charges had just reached $80,000, sat in the corner of the Northeast Pediatric unit, holding her child and crying. She said (to the researcher):

> My husband is furious. I think we're going to lose the house. I don't know how we can pay for this. (Pause.) Maybe I can write my representative in Congress.

This family eventually qualified for Medicaid.

Educating parents about bureaucratic forms and requirements, about admission and discharge processes, about reimbursement and hospital insurance was given a low priority in the n.i.c.u., which is understandable. But it was also given a low priority in the hospital. The great majority of parents got through the referral system and their infant's patient career by complying with what physicians told them to do and by responding as best they could to the demands of administrative offices. Occasionally, an emphatic note to parents from the hospital accounting department would be affixed to an infant's isolette, a hint that there were costs to reckon.

For an unhappy few, the impersonal nature of the referral system produced direct, immediate catastrophes. One father was escorted in by a nurse to see his premature, newborn son, who had multiple congenital anomalies. The nurse did not know and could not tell from the admission sheet that this was the first time the father would be seeing the child:

> I thought he had seen the baby before, at [the referring hospital]. He took one look and bolted out of here. He looked angry. I can't blame him. The baby's a mess.

For an unknown number of other parents, the confusion surrounding n.i.c.u. referral had consequences that never surfaced and were never identified in the unit. The referral of an infant with a slight chance for survival changes the context and the parents' experience of death, complicating the inevitable with panic and hope. Certainly the less well-educated and inexperienced parents were confused by the transfer of their newborn from one kind of service to another and, for many infants, to yet a third hospital service, the Level II nursery.

PARENTS AS RATIONAL DECISION MAKERS

For their critically ill infants to reap the benefits of a large hospital's nursery, the parents have to endure temporary separation from their infants and the drawbacks of an impersonal bureaucratic system. How much of this separation and disorientation is necessary? It takes tremendous effort for the n.i.c.u. staff to stand back from their work and ask this system-level question about the families whose lives they affect so deeply. Instead, physicians and nurses tend to see the parents as traumatized and, in that state, as obstacles to the protection of the infant's well-being. They view parents' highly emotional behavior as something between a basic deviance and a more commonplace vulnerability that reveals itself under pressure. Said one physician during the discussion of problem parents, "I can't tell whether these parents are crazy or they're stressed."

The emphasis on parents' emotional reactions obscures the extent to which the service itself exacerbates the parents' pain with poor communication and then uses psychosocial labeling to keep parents under professional control. There is as much (if not more) consistency in the strong identification of parents with the interests of their infant as in the medical solutions offered by neonatology. As two well-known clinicians noted:

> . . . we have encountered far more pessimism and cynicism about the human condition among members of the helping professions (law, clergy, and medicine) than in families of sick persons or defective infants. (Duff and Campbell, 1976:489).

Yet the irrationality of parents, as the staff sees it, precludes their participation in decision making. With its highly professional and technologic orientation, the intensive care unit relies on management of the parents to isolate the newborn as a patient and keep the family at bay during the most important episode of the infant's life. At present, institutional and professional management of families in the n.i.c.u. is secure. But there is no particular guarantee that the interests of newborns are better protected when parents are prevented from playing a more active role. To the contrary, the staff's diminished sense of accountability to other responsible adults fosters a narrow focus on the infant's survival and can give greater latitude to latent experimentation and even neglect. In most instances, there is no conflict between what the n.i.c.u. service wants and what the families want for the newborns. In some cases, however, neither staff nor family remain consistent, effective advocates for the infant. In our next chapter, we look at this worst-case scenario as it actually happened at Northeast Pediatric.

8

Darlene Bourne: The Patient as Social Problem

Are we prolonging death? Would we do anything different in two or three months than we are doing now with this baby?
Neonatology Fellow

This child probably cannot care for this baby.   *Social Worker*

THE CENTRAL DILEMMAS

The biography of Darlene Bourne began in mid-July with her birth to a fifteen-year-old black mother. She weighed 740 grams. Along with a twin sister who survived only one day, Darlene was transferred to the Level III nursery at Northeast Pediatric. The birth was a repeat cesarean for Darlene's mother, whose first child, a boy, had been born when she was thirteen.

Darlene's time as a hospital patient exemplifies the central dilemmas that the n.i.c.u. staff faces in treating extremely premature infants. Uncertainty surrounding treatment issues was a key factor. Changes in staff personnel was another. Professional attitudes varied according to the number of deaths and severity of cases in the n.i.c.u. Finally, the staff's evaluation of the infant's family eventually influenced Darlene's course of treatment.

We will look at the major phases of Darlene's life from three vantage points. The first is the professional assessment of her clinical status on a daily basis. The second is the composition of the n.i.c.u. team and its influence on medical decisions. The third is the staff's evaluation of the family. Our narrative emphasizes critical junctures in the patient's career at which a consensus was reached and crucial decisions were made. In general, Darlene's case represents what Fagerhaugh and Strauss (1977) describe as the "accumulated trajectory," a case history in which, through no one person's fault, hospital care develops its own momentum apart from the ideals of professional service or the patient's interests.

198

TREATMENT PHASE ONE: THE BEGINNING OF THE CLINICAL HISTORY

The first week of Darlene Bourne's life constituted an important phase in the staff's classifying the infant as a survivor and perceiving serious family problems. Initially, Darlene's condition was diagnosed as severe respiratory distress syndrome and patent ductus arteriosus, two problems common in very premature infants. Upon her arrival at the n.i.c.u, she was receiving 100 percent oxygen and, because of jaundice, was placed under phototherapy lights. The staff maintained the high oxygen level for the first day but expressed fears about its causing blindness or chronic pulmonary disease.

On day four, Darlene suffered cardiac arrest and a serious lung collapse just before morning rounds. The staff could not find the infant's pulse but succeeded in inserting a tube in her chest and inflating the lung. The baby's life was saved. Subsequent nightly "crashes" followed, but Darlene always "bounced back." Early on, she was characterized as a "rock" who held onto life tenaciously.

TREATMENT PHASE TWO: THE HEART OPERATION

By the end of the first week. Darlene's condition was still poor, but she was alive and her condition was stable. The attending physician predicted that she would live only a few months. Nonetheless, like other patients in the unit she received maximum support therapy and her case was routinely reviewed by consulting physicians. A neurological consultant who examined her on her fifth day in the n.i.c.u. suspected brain bleeding, and asked that spinal taps be done. The rationale for the request was that the staff should know if there was brain hemorrhaging so that treatment options (for example, surgery) could be considered.

Various institutional and staff influences worked toward Darlene's undergoing surgery for the patent ductus arteriosus. The operation was frequently performed at Northeast Pediatric, even on very low birth weight patients, and the staff felt there was little risk attached to it. At the time, the hospital was part of a major national study designed to test the efficacy of surgery versus pharmaceuticals in treating the condition and two non-unit physician researchers were actively recruiting patients for the study. Still, the weekend substitute attending physician in charge of Darlene's care on day eleven was not enthusiastic about her having the operation. At Saturday morning rounds, he argued with the primary physician:

Primary physician: "They [cardiac surgeons] are willing to take her to surgery. I think we should send her to surgery today, even if she's questionable, to get her duct tied."

Attending physician: "What you would gain is a couple of percentage points, as far as the risk of getting BPD [chronic lung disease]. What you're risking is sudden death."

By the next day, persuaded by the surgeons, primary physician and the researchers, the attending physician had changed his mind:

This is the time to tie her duct, today. From the baby's point of view we have to get the duct tied today. The baby is allowing us a little bit of health today.

Arrangements were made for the operation to take place the next day.

An important influence in this decision was the infant's primary physician, a young black woman who acted as Darlene's champion for the first month of her life. This resident was consistently optimistic about the child's future and argued that her family situation should have no bearing on the decision to treat. She persisted in her advocacy despite a gloomy medical evaluation that included, for example, on day fourteen, bloody (burgundy-colored) spinal taps, unimproved respiratory distress syndrome being treated with 70 percent oxygen, a heart murmur, and feeding problems.

Perception of Social Problems

In the early days of Darlene's crashes and recoveries, the unit staff began to take notice of the family problems reported by various social workers. The psychological problems of the mother were the most troubling. According to the unit's social worker, the death of Darlene's twin had provoked highly morbid reactions in the mother. A school-appointed psychotherapist, who visited the unit to confer with the social worker and nurses, explained that Darlene's mother was suffering from a lot of guilt about the twin's death. Handling the practical details of funeral arrangements seemed to be beyond her. Three weeks after the baby's death and autopsy, Darlene's mother went to the cremation at the funeral parlor with a camera to photograph the deceased infant. She then tried to display the photographs at her mother's (Darlene's grandmother's) household, but the grandmother resisted. The nursing staff was also troubled by the mother's youth, possible sexual promiscuity, previous illegitimate child, her erratic school attendance, and the fact that she was not living with the grandmother but seemed to be on the street a lot. In the first week, she told the primary nurse that she was living with a friend and would not give the phone number. As the nurse described it:

> The mother says, "I'm at a friend's and I can't give the number out." We ask, "Does your mother know where you are?" She says, "Oh, I call my mother every ten minutes." I confronted her. I said, "I don't think you're telling the truth."

There was also confusion surrounding the identity of Darlene's father. The first story to circulate in the unit was that the father was present and involved. The second was that the father was a married man in his forties who had other children by his wife. From where, then, the nursing staff asked, would support for the mother and child come? The thirty-two-year-old grandmother was the legal guardian of the mother's first child. Would she also take on the responsibility of this unhealthy infant when she already had three other young children of her own to care for?

In the first two weeks of Darlene's life, the n.i.c.u. staff learned that her mother and grandmother each had a cadre of social service professionals; the arrival of Darlene would add more to the group. Darlene's mother had the special therapist at school. Her grandmother received payments from Aid to Families with Dependent Children (AFDC) for her own children and for her daughter's son. Darlene's arrival raised the question of whether the mother ought to apply herself for family welfare assistance. The family also had a community social worker, a black woman, assigned to it. Instead of relieving the nurses' misgivings about Darlene's family situation, the complex social service ties confirmed for them a history of social pathology. On day seven, an experienced unit nurse commented wearily after social service rounds, "It's already a depressing assignment."

The mother's distracted behavior while visiting the unit did nothing to allay the staff's concern and prompted discussion of foster care for the infant. The mother told the unit social worker that she was eager to see Darlene, but when she visited, the primary nurse reported that "her attention was everywhere but on the baby." In her defense, the primary physician noted that she was "confused" by the change in physicians and nurses occurring at each shift. Despite her dismay at the mother's "flat affect" and inability to communicate, the primary nurse expressed her willingness to work with Darlene's mother. Unfortunately, the first major expression of emo-

tion by the mother turned out to be anger. After the patent ductus
arteriosus ligation, she was told that the baby had developed a heart
murmur. She blamed this problem on the operation which, as she
saw it, damaged the baby's heart. The house officer on duty when
she visited made no headway with his argument that the murmur
and the operation had nothing to do with each other. His frustration in communicating with the mother spilled over into his case
presentation at work rounds the next day.

> *Fellow:* "Mom and Daddy okay?"
> *Resident:* "Definitely not. Mom is fifteen and dumb."

Reassessment

By the third week of Darlene's life, the nurses were openly expressing their sentiments that, while they felt sympathy for her, they had
no hope for her survival. The female primary physician held out for
treatment despite objections from the two other house officers. Thus,
Darlene continued to receive vigorous resuscitation when she went
into failure and, in the attempt to "wean down" her oxygen, as many
as six blood gas tests were taken each day.

On the twenty-seventh day, a set of computerized axial tomographic (CAT) scans of Darlene's brain arrived in the unit and
changed the staff's attitude toward treatment.

> *Attending physician:* "What about the CAT scan results?"
> *Resident:* "They're hardly something we can talk about in public."
> The record book was brought out and the photos looked at. They showed
> severe hydrocephalus [water in the brain] and a grade 4 bleed.
> *Fellow:* "There is some cortex left but not much. Severe bleeding on right
> and left."
> *Resident:* "I guess there are kids who walk around with CAT scans like
> that."
> *Primary physician* (slightly amazed): "There's hardly any cortex you can
> see in these photos."

A conference on Darlene's case was called the same day. In it, the
physicians and nurses tried to hammer out a medical plan for the
infant and a way of approaching the family.

The attending physician, the fellow, two residents, and two nurses
quickly reached the consensus that the infant's feeding plan should
remain the same. They agreed that if their management of oxygen
therapy caused the baby to develop a pneumothorax they should
correct it. They also concurred that blood gas tests should be limited

to only two per day to curtail the frequent resetting of oxygen level, pressure, and flow. Then the discussion turned to resuscitation:

Primary nurse: "Do we resuscitate or not, that is our next question."
Fellow: "No, I don't think so."
Primary physician: "I think that's fair. Last week I would have said something different."
Fellow: "Are we prolonging death? Would we do anything different in two or three months than we are doing now with this baby?"

The primary physician made reference to another small baby who had died after three months. The mood of the conference became grim.

At this impasse, the group turned to social issues:

Fellow: "What are the social issues here? What kind of baby will this look like in the future?"
Primary physician: "I don't believe that makes any difference at all. (With emotion) I will take personal responsibility for signing a [custody order] if this baby survives, so that the baby can be put in a good, loving home."

The attending physician asked the nurses for their opinions:

Attending physician (to primary nurse): "How do you feel?"
Primary nurse (her face reddening and her eyes filling with tears): "More than anything else I want a definite plan of caring for this baby. If the baby arrested, I would like to give it one round of meds and just leave it."
Primary physician: "I would go so far as giving no meds. I think we have to support her up to the point where we just can't. It may turn out that she'll die [while receiving] 100 percent oxygen."
Attending physician (to second nurse, scheduled to take over from the primary nurse when she went on pregnancy leave in two weeks): "How do you feel?"
Second nurse: "Personally there are times when I'd just like to leave the [ventilator] settings and walk away. But then I ask myself, could I live with it in a week?"
Primary nurse: "If this baby lives we have another problem. And that is how much deficit the treatment we gave it caused. I think the baby has a chance. I think it's small and I think we should support it."

The male house officer questioned the attending concerning the probabilities of survival:

Resident: "What are the chances in this weight range, relative to [another case] born at 650 grams?"
Attending physician: "There are few if any survivors in this weight category."

Resident: "It's very important that we find out what the statistical prob-
    abilities are here. I know that [in the hospital's pediatric general care
    nursery], given a baby two months older, they would not be turning
    up the dials the way we are."

(This comment about the pediatric nursery's less heroic standards
of care later proved to be prophetic when the staff began consider-
ing transfer plans for Darlene.)

The group then discussed communicating with the mother:

Primary nurse: "We've got to change our messages to the mother and
    grandmother. I've been telling her [the mother] simple things. We've
    got to change them and really inform them it's a really serious con-
    dition."
Primary physician: "I've already begun to do that. I told the mother today
    there was a good chance the baby would die. I don't think the mother
    understood, but how different is this from any other case? It's de-
    nial, like in [another case]. The mother understands English, if not
    the technological vocabulary."
Resident: "She's not with it enough to tell us what to do with the baby."
Primary physician: "But I told her if [the baby] survives this, she's not going
    to be 'right upstairs.' Now that was the expression I used, 'right up-
    stairs.' And I think that's pretty clear."
Primary nurse: "But does she know that the baby won't be able to feed
    or dress herself? It's not just a matter of the baby being slow in
    school."
Fellow: "It would probably be cerebral palsy."

The attending physician had the final, somewhat ambiguous, word
on the treatment plan:

Primary physician: "Do we make this a DNR [do not resuscitate] or do we
    not up the respirator?"
Attending physician: "To the best of my understanding, this baby has a
    negligible chance of survival. Yes, it's legal not to resuscitate. It's al-
    most impossible to give halfway intensive care. If you're just pro-
    longing death, then I have no problems with withdrawing support.
    What we have to give is responsible support and since this baby has
    chronic, not acute, trouble, then I don't think we want to 'hop' on
    the gas changes. But we do want to keep an eye on her. If there
    were a respiratory arrest, I wouldn't run fast because her chances
    are poor for recovery."
Primary nurse: "If she arrests, do we resuscitate?"
Attending physician: "This baby probably isn't going to arrest. She's too
    hardy."

The quick call for this conference on Darlene had excluded the social worker. Later, she queried the nurses about the staff's approach. The nurses said that they stick strictly to medical factors in their conferences. One nurse, Helen, was very emphatic: "This is a medical decision on how we're going to continue treating this infant." The group's decision was to limit blood gas tests to two per day, with no radical increase in oxygen therapy but with full resuscitation planned in the event of failure.

Two days after this conference, new residents replaced the old, and Darlene's primary physician, her principal advocate, left the unit.

ENTERING TREATMENT PHASE THREE: THE BRAIN SHUNT

Darlene lost her resident physician advocate but her case came to the attention of the pediatric neurosurgeons at Northeast Pediatric. By focusing on her brain hemorrhage as a single and remedial problem, the neurosurgeons persuaded the senior neonatologists that a brain shunt was necessary. Curiously, Darlene's own biology cooperated in this decision; except for her brain, her general physical condition improved.

At first, the attending physician was wary of incursions into the n.i.c.u. by the neurosurgeons and warned the novice primary physician "to keep the 'neuros' at bay." The attending physician wanted the surgery decision to be made at the discretion of the neonatologists.

Difficulties with the new primary physician emerged at once. On the first evening of his service, while the primary nurse was off duty, he increased Darlene's oxygen level from 80 to 85 percent. The resident had not carefully read the sign-off notes nor had the night nurse explained to him the policy of only dialing down the oxygen percentage for Darlene. Curiously, this error in oxygen maintenance began an improvement in the condition of Darlene's lungs. Significant progress was made in reducing the infant's oxygen dependence. Between days thirty and thirty-five, her oxygen level was reduced from 85 percent to 76 percent. By day thirty-eight, Darlene's oxygen level was down to 62 percent and she had doubled in weight since birth. An ultrasound test revealed continued bleeding in her brain, and consultants urged brain shunt surgery. The unit director gave approval with the remark: "The kid looks all right and that's about it." The primary nurse put this ironic juxtaposition of comments into her notes on Darlene's thirty-fifth day:

Mother more trusting of staff. Reinforce information on baby's neurological status: to mom. Possible shunt might be mentioned to family. Neurosurgeons to decide on the timing of shunt.

Darlene's condition was closely monitored by the staff and several neurosurgeons. A CAT scan taken on day forty-two revealed a worsening of the bleeding in the brain, so the infant underwent brain shunt surgery two days later. The mother, after the previous operation (for patent ductus arteriosus), had sworn that she would never allow another operation, but the brain shunt had been explained to her by nurses and physicians as essential to saving the baby's life. Later the staff would find out that the mother and grandmother understood this decision as a strong vote of staff confidence in the infant's potential for normal development.

Tough and Ordinary Cases

The day after Darlene's brain shunt operation, while she was slowly recovering from anesthesia, the physician-in-chief of Northeast Pediatric visited the n.i.c.u. and enthusiastically suggested a presentation of the baby's case at grand rounds. The unit director preferred another case, one of a girl born weighing 900 grams who had weathered a very difficult medical course and was now a healthy toddler. The head of the hospital argued for Darlene's case, "which will represent the kind of problems you have to deal with ordinarily in this unit." The attending physician, who was worried about the infant's slow recovery from surgery, countered, "We could pick a case which would really show us at our best." Replied the hospital head, "That's not the point. If anyone wants to see us at our best, they can refer to the [prestigious journal] article." But the plan to present Darlene's case was dropped, and instead, the choice was made to present the success story of the child who had done well.

This request to go public with an exemplary case came at a bad time for the unit. There had been a rapid sequence of deaths in the previous month; four very low birth weight infants who had survived initially had died in either the second or third week of care. Now, the unit had on hand eight cases, including Darlene, who fit the same pattern. Each had survived their first week and yet their prognoses were poor. Over the next three months, the unit staff held on to its difficult long-term cases; the most deaths would be those of infants who had survived three days or less.

TREATMENT PHASE THREE: TREATMENT REVERSAL

After her brain operation, Darlene's recovery was slower than expected. Her oxygen level remained at about 65 percent. Her weight fell to 1,050 grams. A new, loud heart murmur developed. Two days after the brain shunt surgery, a new neonatology fellow arrived for his first stint of service at Northeast Pediatric; he opposed the group's decision to limit respirator support.

> The primary nurse told [the researcher] that she was really furious with the new fellow, who had drawn five blood gas tests on this baby today. Four gases after the first one were bad, so he had consistently bumped the oxygen up for each reading, from the 60 percent range. Now the baby is at 86 percent oxygen. The primary nurse indicated that the resident who was on board at the time "should have known better." She said she was upset with the new fellow because he disagreed with the existing plan to not take frequent gases and not dial up [the oxygen level]. He wants another meeting. The fellow said that the baby's chances for survival are real. She had retorted that the baby's lungs were deteriorating.

On this, the fifty-second day of Darlene's life, the neurologist's report read: "Generally depressed, does not open eyes—will only respond to painful stimulus—hypotonic—full anterior fontenal—question of shunt [being] operational. Suggestion: increased ICF [intracranial fluid, that is, the shunt operation may not have worked]. Continue to keep head propped up. Recall neurosurgery. Get [x-ray] film of shunt."

On the same day, with a sense of renewed crisis, the staff called a conference to discuss Darlene's case. This time, the social workers were included. In the first part of the hour-long session, the unit staff precisely formulated its treatment policy. The director was supportive of the primary nurse's argument that they should return to a restricted plan. She got everything but an apology from the new fellow, whose attempt to reinterpret the case was essentially vetoed. Specifically, the group agreed to "wean down" the oxygen level two degrees if the blood gas tests, to be taken only once a shift, looked fairly good. As one nurse put it, "The problem here is making the baby move." In the case of failure, the infant would get limited, manual oxygen support. If the baby extubated herself, that tube would be replaced, but nothing more would be done. The fellow said, "It's really a matter of our taking our chances with this baby since what we're doing to her in terms of a cure is also creating its own problems. We're not doing her any favors."

When the medical treatment plan was settled, the physicians (the

attending physician, the fellow, and two residents) became quiet and
left the discussion to two social workers and four nurses.

> The primary nurse touched on what to do about letting this baby go home
> to a fifteen-year-old mother with a grandmother who, every time she is
> in the unit, states clearly that she'll take no responsibility for caring for
> the baby. The nurse said, "How am I going to explain to the mother how
> she's going to give the baby meds, how she's going to handle fluid, how
> she's going to deal with follow-up?"

This nurse also said she got conflicting messages from the grandmother. For example, the grandmother talked about buying a bas-
sinet or crib for the baby's homecoming, her only question being
how big the baby would be at the time of discharge. The nurse was
confused by the question because she saw a serious delay in the baby's going home. The grandmother displayed this optimism at the
time the mother was signing consent forms for the brain shunt surgery. The hospital social worker commented:

> The grandmother can't afford an expensive bassinet or crib anyway. What
> she was probably trying to express was hope and to hold onto the baby,
> since they really didn't have much choice but to hope, with the baby going
> in for an operation.

The discussion then turned to the mother. The community social
worker, who was close to the family, described the mother's guilt
about giving her first child over to the grandmother, about losing
Darlene's twin, and about now having a sick baby. The unit social
worker pointed out that there were other things going on in the
mother's life. The girl's therapist at school had left that position. The
mother disappeared for a while after her boyfriend "had thrown her
out." Now she was back at the grandmother's but "not acting as if
she belongs there." The community social worker reassured the
group that the mother, despite her troubles, was talking about returning to school and getting her life in shape.

This social worker also commented on the grandmother's denial
of her responsibility for Darlene.

> She has her own ambivalences about caring for yet another child since
> she already has the first child of [the mother] to care for. What she is
> probably doing is trying to make it clear to [the mother] that this baby is
> her responsibility and that she's not going to take care of it. She did the
> same thing with the first child, but she wasn't forceful about it. And [the
> mother] was much younger at the time—thirteen.

The primary nurse did notice that the grandmother came in as often as the mother and did touch and hold the baby. She also noted that the mother seemed progressively more attached to the child and perhaps could be more serious about it. Yet the primary nurse tested the community social worker with this question: "What do you think about putting this baby in a foster home?" The social worker replied, firmly:

You'd have to present the reasons clearly. You'd have to go through the grandmother to convince the mother. [The mother] is probably not coming home, so you have to look at it from the point of view of the grandmother. The grandmother is really reluctant to let go of those around her. She's fairly possessive and a fairly strong woman. She lets go but only with difficulty. In addition, she has good support from family and friends and from me.

The primary nurse doubted that the mother understood the important aspects of Darlene's condition. The community social worker explained that the mother had "a learning disability in verbal processing that has improved somewhat with instruction." She added that transitions were difficult for the mother and that she had to learn to trust caretakers. "It doesn't come naturally to her." On a final, optimistic note, the community social worker said that AFDC was available to the family, with homemaker services for the mother. She affirmed her belief that the baby would be well taken care of, mainly because the grandmother "has taken such good care of the other children." She also attempted to explain to the all-white staff that Darlene's family was not that unusual in the black community where the mother and grandmother lived.

These assurances buoyed the staff's spirits. The nurse about to take over the primary nursing role expressed how much better she felt "since there's an increased possibility of a good home and the baby will be taken care of." The neonatology fellow added, "I feel better. You try not to let this social stuff enter your mind or to influence the kind of care you're giving a baby. But knowing all this makes me optimistic." Even the unit director was affected. He had earlier in the conference painted a dark picture of the infant's "survival capacity":

We want to be very frank about that. There isn't really very much that we can promise. . . . The baby's chances for survival are poor in terms of what we know now about infants born in her condition at her age and weight.

Yet at the end of the conference, he painted a more hopeful picture:

> The baby has a chance of survival—even if it's on oxygen up to the age of eight months. It can still do well. At one year this baby would probably still not be out of the woods because of its lungs. However, after that point she might have a good chance, just to be average. That's the condition of the lungs, problem number one. Problem number two—the kind of injury which has been done to the brain is the kind which results in a degree of brain damage. [He referred to the case presented at grand rounds, a 900-gram infant now one year old.] She was our smallest and now she's almost normal. She didn't have to be institutionalized. It's also remote as a possibility that this baby would have to be institutionalized. It's also remote that the baby will be fully normal. It's somewhere between the two.

The director then made the conference's closing pronouncement: "Let's assume the baby will live. It's the only way we can continue."

For the next three weeks, Darlene's condition neither improved nor degenerated. She became the baby who "doesn't move" and consequently one of the least satisfying patients for the staff to care for. Her primary physician's efforts to wean her off the ventilator were unsuccessful. Oxygen levels varied from eighty-three percent to ninety percent, then, by day sixty-two, went down into the 70 percent range. The primary physician reported, "She looks better." But this was a relative assessment. On day seventy, Darlene had progressed to gavage feeding, but because of severe abdominal swelling, she had to be put back on intravenous feeding. Tests on the seventieth day showed no eye focus or response to voices. On the seventy-sixth day, the primary physician who six weeks before had inadvertently bumped up Darlene's oxygen level summarized her case for the new set of residents entering the unit. Underplaying the clinical condition of the infant, the resident stated:

> The main problem is his [sic] social situation. The mother is sixteen, the father's forty-five, but out of the picture. The mother's young child is taken care of by the grandmother. The mother has a learning disability of sorts—does better with pictures. I can't imagine this mother taking care of the baby. This baby will need a lot of care.

TREATMENT PHASE FOUR: TRIPLE AGENDAS

On day seventy-six, with the arrival on the unit of a new set of residents and a new attending physician, contrasting interpretations of

Darlene's condition became evident. The senior physicians, especially a new female attending physician, believed in continuing medical care right up to the point of massive medical failure. The nurses complained about senior physicians' "compulsion" with regard to this case and instead emphasized the parental problem. They wanted the infant on a course that would ensure that she would be discharged from the unit to a reliable caregiver. Troubled by the family situation, the nurses were finding it difficult to continue to care for Darlene. The residents agreed with them because they found the case professionally unrewarding.

Not familiar with neonatology, the unit social worker focused on the resolution of the caregiver problem: either the family would take Darlene or an agency would. In either event, several social workers would keep the baby's mother and grandmother as clients.

On day seventy-six, along with the new residents, a highly optimistic attending physician rejoined the staff after a leave of absence for research. She expressed the most pioneering values regarding the difficult cases in the unit, including Darlene's. The physicians were eager to "wean down" Darlene's oxygen and end her dependence on the respirator. The nurses resisted because an early extubation could put them in the position of having to make sudden resuscitation decisions if the infant went into failure. At the nurses' urgings, the extubation was delayed.

The neonatology fellow, once enthusiastic about treatment for Darlene, had kept to the policy of restricted intervention and was not overjoyed at the infant's prolonged oxygen dependence.

Fellow: "There's no premature extubation on this baby."
Attending physician: "I've seen worse."
Fellow: "Have you seen worse that have made it?"
Attending physician: "Sure. The baby doesn't look bad for three months, really."

On the same day, the nurses, the unit psychiatrist, and the unit social workers discussed the family's and the nursery staff's problems.

Psychiatrist: "We're up to where the grandmother wants to give the mother a chance. Where we were last week was to build up the daughter's self-esteem as much as possible and use the grandmother as backup."
Nurse: "We have a new group of residents this morning. [The departing primary physician] on rounds this morning presented the social [situation] as the biggest problem. For an intact family this kid would be tough. She will need a lot of care and fairly complex care."

Second [non-unit] *nurse:* "What kind of care?"

Nurse: "Chest physical therapy, medications, big-time meds that can make a difference. Lots of appointments—neuro. Eating—hasn't had a bottle yet. Close observation of her [is being done]."

Psychiatrist: "What's the usual approach?"

Nurse: "With a more normal family, you'd say we need to start making plans. Then you'd get into the concrete. But a lot of people, myself included, did not make an investment in the baby. We thought it would die and had questions about the medical management of the child. And also the social situation was so horrendous. The primary nurse has started to have nightmares about this kid. [The baby] has worn everybody out. So there just aren't a lot of reserves. [The primary nurse] is getting married. The baby's initial primary nurse is pregnant and has left the unit. For whoever works with this baby it takes a lot of work and the outcome doesn't look that hot."

The unit nurse speculated that Darlene could be discharged in two weeks to a month. She resisted the participation of outsiders in the planning.

Second nurse: "A month is not that much time if you're thinking of the child['s] not going home. So the only way we can do it is start testing the mother."

Unit social worker: "She's an emancipated minor. But have [the hospital attorney] come and see what the next step is. This child probably cannot care for this baby."

Nurse: "Medicine and nursing have to get together first—[she named the primary nurse, primary physician, fellow, and attending physician]."

Psychiatrist: "Should someone from multidisciplinary be involved?"

Nurse: "Eventually."

Largely because of the attending physician's optimism, the commitment to treat the infant remained strong for several weeks. Darlene progressed from a respirator setting in the 60 percent range to a 50 percent oxygen level under a hood. Darlene's primary physician tried to turn the staff's attention to discharge plans, but a temporary euphoria prevailed. On day eighty-three, for example, just after the group, at rounds, had finished rejoicing over the good condition of three new arrivals, the primary physician suggested, "We should decide on [Darlene's] course. We should commit ourselves for the duration or send her to [a mixed-level unit in a nearby hospital]." The primary nurse responded, "I'm afraid they'll intubate over there [i.e., put her back on the respirator]. We'll tolerate more out of her than they will." The point being made here was that the close surveillance available in the Northeast Pediatric Level III unit would allow better, permanent weaning from oxygen therapy.

The next day, however, the staff went directly to the issue of the commitment to treat.

> *Fellow:* "She's reaching a [respirator] setting where we put her on a nasal cannula and she goes 'a la casa' [home]."
>
> *Nurse:* " 'A la casa.' Are you crazy?"
>
> *Fellow:* "Should we send her to [mixed-level unit in another hospital]?"
>
> *Primary physician:* "The social setting is as great a problem as the rest. There's no dumping her home."
>
> *Fellow:* "And [neurology division] is no good because they need the mother there to help. What about [mixed-level unit]?"
>
> *Nurse:* "They wouldn't know how to take care of her over there. I guess we are committed to this child. Am I right in saying that?"
>
> *Fellow:* "It sure looks that way."
>
> *Attending physician:* "I'd say yes."

In contrast to other staff members, this attending physician had a clear vision of Darlene's and the unit's future. She believed that four new intermediate-care beds were going to be added to the unit and that Darlene would be the first to occupy one. The attending physician said that she was trying to work out something so that the pulmonary follow-up people would help with the case. That way, Darlene could stay in the unit indefinitely but not as an intensive care patient.

The nursing staff was especially resistant to this plan and began pressing for Darlene's discharge. Four days later, the question of what to do with Darlene was extensively discussed at morning work rounds.

> *First nurse:* "The mother doesn't want this kid."
>
> *Primary physician:* "Well, there's ambivalence about long-term chronic care. The grandmother has been up and down on this. She's waxed and waned. The last I heard the grandmother was interested."
>
> *First nurse:* "I spoke with her two or three times last week."
>
> *Second nurse:* "The baby wasn't going home to either of them a month ago."
>
> *Attending physician:* "The possibilities we have to consider have to do with how much attention and care the baby will get. There is another kid and the grandmother is older."
>
> *First nurse:* "She's thirty-two. She has the same history as her daughter."
>
> *Resident:* "Maybe we should get the great-grandmother in. She's probably only forty-five."

Attending physician: "What about foster care?"
Resident: "Who would take this kid?"
Attending physician: "There are a lot of people who could take this kid."

The primary physician then made an important point about the infant's vulnerability to problems during transfer:

Primary physician: "What's really too bad is that she'll be ready to go home just at the maximum possibility of disease onset. At four months the possibility of bronchitis is high. And her chances of survival decrease 50 to 75 percent just because she's going to [a low-income] community."
First nurse: "I think that Social Service is very naive about this case. They find my judgment [of the family situation] harsh. They asked if I'd feel the same if the baby were going to a family in [an affluent community]. I said, 'No, I wouldn't.' "
Primary physician: "But their assessment may be realistic."

The attending physician then made a strong argument for protecting the infant by keeping her in the Level III unit.

Attending physician: "This kid has to be more well than other kids we send home."
Second nurse: "So she stays?"
Attending physician: "Yes. We'll have an extra four beds and she'll be our first candidate. There may be a new plan to switch her over to pulmonary [division]. We can't send her to [the general pediatric division within Northeast Pediatric]. She'll catch every virus."

The attending physician also cautioned: "The parents feel it's a dump when the baby is moved [i.e., transferred]."

While not directly contesting the attending physician's dream of providing prolonged intermediate care in the unit, the nurses and residents informally discussed where Darlene should be sent. The initial alternatives appeared to be either the affiliated hospital with a combined Level II and III unit, or the neurology or pulmonary divisions within Northeast Pediatric. These junior members of the staff were more pessimistic about Darlene's poor neurological condition than was the attending physician. They also were more reactive to changes in the unit's patient population. Just as Darlene reached her three-month birthday, the unit admitted four premature infants whose low birth weights and brain bleeds rivaled hers. The staff's approach to Darlene was marked by increased frustration and hostility. On her ninety-eighth day, she ceased breathing and was given an emergency resuscitation. This respiratory failure and revival was recounted with black humor, laughter, and jeers at work rounds.

As the primary nurse got ready to take her honeymoon leave, the rest of the staff teased her that Darlene would go with her. "She'll swim right out to the boat. There's no escape," joked one nurse.

The Family Conferences

The next week, Darlene went into respiratory failure and had to be put back on the ventilator at 60 percent oxygen. This clinical setback, coupled with reduced contact with the mother, worried the nursing staff. A special conference was called to evaluate the resources of Darlene's family.

The day of the conference was also the primary nurse's first day back from her honeymoon. The junior staff, with the neonatology fellow, gathered at Darlene's bedside.

> *Primary nurse:* "This baby is indestructible. You could have a ball on a chain come crashing through the isolette and she'd survive. She's a mini-Kong."

When the primary nurse raised the subject of the meeting to be held today, the fellow said he could live with any decision. The residents laughed and told him that he could re-intubate the baby when the time came.

> *Primary nurse:* "No re-intubation. That's over, even though we're used to her."

One resident begins to hum the song, "I've grown accustomed to your face." (laughter)

Confronting the Family

On Darlene's 100th day the staff made its first concerted effort to confront the mother and grandmother about the question of future care. The staff wanted their doubts about the family settled. The primary physician intended to pull no punches in his description of how much care the infant would need. The nurses had little confidence in either the mother or the grandmother. The social worker, in contrast, assumed that the meeting was to negotiate caregiving, either by the grandmother or by some combination of the mother and the grandmother's efforts. The social worker's intent was constructive, but she had little understanding of the severity of the infant's medical condition. Nor did she understand that only junior staff would be at the meeting and that none of them believed the baby should ever go home. What staff members wanted was a confirmation of their own belief that the baby was too ill to be taken

care of by this family. In this they succeeded. The mother was intimidated by the discussion and the grandmother clearly stated her
reluctance to deal with a baby too sick to leave the hospital.

> The mother sat with downcast eyes, fiddling with her gloves and the
> border of her skirt. The grandmother took the initiative in talking by say-
> ing that she would take responsibility for caring for the baby, that she's
> been waiting a long time for the baby to come home, and that she's look-
> ing forward to that. When the grandmother asked, "When will the baby
> come home?" the mother burst into tears. She cried silently; there was
> no halt in the discussion. The primary physician, leaning toward the
> grandmother, asked how much work she thought the baby would re-
> quire. She answered, "The less the better. I have other children to look
> after, too. The baby should stay in the hospital until she's healthy enough
> to come home." The primary physician stressed that the care of the in-
> fant would be a tremendous amount of work, that it would be round-
> the-clock, and that it would be needed for at least a year. He said that
> she wouldn't be able to go home for several months, perhaps not until
> next spring. He pointed out that she gets a lot of medical attention, that
> feeding her is hard work, that she gets many medications and will have
> to get those daily even when she is ready to go home. The primary phy-
> sician said firmly, "In no way is this a normal baby."

At this point, the mother started sobbing. The unit social worker
asked her, "What is it? Is this difficult for you to hear? Did you think
Darlene was coming home all right?" The mother sobbed and nodded yes.

With nothing resolved, the social worker suggested another
meeting in a week's time. After the conference, she told the researcher that the primary physician had laid it on "pretty heavy"
and that she hadn't known herself how bad the baby's condition
was. "I should have met him for a few minutes before this meeting.
I didn't know he was going to come down so hard."

From the primary physician's perspective, no one had been honest with this family. He commented bitterly, "There is no way the
nurses are going to let that baby go home. They're not being honest
with the grandmother and the mother in not telling them the baby
is a disaster."

The Unresolved Caregiver Problem

If the intent of some of the staff members at the first meeting was
to frighten Darlene's mother and grandmother about the prospect
of caring for the infant, their effort backfired. A week later, the two

women came to the second meeting with renewed determination to take responsibility for the child. The day before, the fellow had put pressure on the social workers to have an investigatory home visit paid to the grandmother's house, as if in preparation for receiving the infant. In reality, the nursing staff was interested in seeing hard evidence that the family situation fully justified the decisions about treatment and transfer that it would reach independent of the family. Attempts to find even the vestiges of a conventional and stable family had failed. The staff could not come to terms with anything but an intact family and a committed caregiver, nor could they deny that Darlene had continuing serious medical problems.

The unit director came to this second meeting, along with the primary physician, who took an out-of-the-way chair in the conference room. The mother and grandmother came with the mother's two-year-old son and with the community social worker. The unit social worker began the meeting by asking the mother how she felt about the last meeting. The mother reacted shyly to the question and, with some stumbling, asked how long the baby would be in the hospital, indicating she knew it was not just days or weeks.

> *Primary physician:* "It's just as you said. It isn't days or weeks, it's months. It's hard to be accurate because there's a lot we don't know, but we're talking about past the winter."
> *Unit social worker* (to mother): "Does the baby look to you as if she should spend a lot more time here?"
> *Mother:* "No, she looks just fine to me."
> *Unit social worker* (to grandmother): "What do you think?"
> *Grandmother:* "I want the child to get the best possible care and if she has to be here, I want that for her. When the baby comes home, if she's ready, then it's a question of my skill. I understand about her needing oxygen and her breathing problems. I know you can't say how she is mentally, how damaged she is. But the best for her now is to grow up to be an adult and that's what's being done now."

The unit social worker then began a line of questioning to get the mother to compare caring for her first child with caring for Darlene. The mother gave the impression that the grandmother had done a lot of the work. She said that her son cried a lot and when he did she would hand him over to the grandmother, saying "Take this baby." Then the grandmother would quiet him down. The grandmother smiled and laughed during this description. The mother said that she thought Darlene would be more quiet and easier to care for.

This comment cued the primary nurse and the two physicians to reinforce the point that Darlene would be a very difficult baby to care for. The nurse went through the difficulties of gavage feeding, special formula, eight medicines, and the physical therapy needed every three hours. During the description, the grandmother and the daughter nodded and smiled. Then the primary physician added more compelling details:

> *Primary physician:* "Other babies can regulate their temperatures, but Darlene can't. You've probably noticed there are some babies who are not in the little cake boxes like Darlene's but are in open cribs wrapped in blankets. Well, they can take some changes in temperature. Darlene can't. For the baby born prematurely this is a real problem. They can't get a cold, and changes in temperature, like in the winter, are dangerous for them. If [your son] gets a cold, it probably passes by in a few days. If Darlene gets a cold, she would have to be hospitalized. Her extremities also have a tendency to stiffen. Did you notice that? (Mother and grandmother nod.) She'll need physical therapy. They could stiffen and not bend back."
>
> *Grandmother:* "She doesn't kick like a regular baby. Is that from lying so quiet or because of her head?"
>
> *Primary physician:* "It's related to her head. (Nervous laugh.) She's like a little board."

The unit director then emphasized the baby's lung problems, which he said would require "years of returning to the hospital." The primary physician added, "I know how frustrating it is to hear us say we can't say for certain about many things. But that's the way medicine is. It's unlikely Darlene will be a normal baby."

When the unit social worker directed questions to the mother and grandmother about caregiving, the mother responded first, "I want to take care of her by myself." Then the grandmother began talking about how she had taken care of the son and was concerned with the mother's being more responsible.

> *Unit social worker:* "Have you and [the mother] talked about sharing responsibility for Darlene?"
>
> *Grandmother:* "Most of the time my talking with [the mother] is over the phone because she isn't home that much. Maybe she gets tired of hearing me talk 'cause I'm always talking about the baby. (Said with a big laugh and mother laughs too.) It's an important experience to raise a child and I want [the mother] to feel that."

The meeting ended with a vague consensus to meet again the following week. After the meeting, the primary nurse spoke to the mother, grandmother, and the community social worker about a visiting nurse home inspection.

Primary nurse: "The visiting nurses do home assessments to check for special things like where the baby would go and where the oxygen would be stored if it's needed."

Grandmother: "She'll come out to the house?" (Looks surprised.)

Primary nurse: "We do it for all the babies."

Community social worker: "Why so early?"

Primary nurse: "Well, the nurses want to know what we are shooting for. Some things might be well handled and others not. As the baby gets bigger, she'll be transferred to another unit in the hospital, not this one. And with that imminent, we want to plan long-term care. She has to have a nasal cannula plus any needs you feel have to be taken into consideration. It's better to start early to get in shape. That way we have a better hold on the situation."

Having missed this conversation, the unit social worker heard about it from one of the nurses later in the day. She observed:

It's a transparent move. It's setting the grandmother in the expectation that the baby will go to that home. I don't think anyone will allow that. A [child neglect and abuse order] would be filed if the grandmother and the mother don't go along with plans for institutionalization or a foster home.

Three days after this conference, the grandmother was in the unit. Nurses' notes on this visit described her as "bonded" to Darlene. The notes indicated that the nurses were concerned that the mother did not want to visit or talk about the baby.

THE FINAL PHASE

Giving Up: The Institutional Solution

On the same day that the grandmother visited, day 109, a consulting neurologist examined the baby. His summary read:

Formulation:

Way behind true three-month-old—no reach, no follow, no smile, no laugh or squeal, no arms and chest support—this child is really much younger than apparent age [almost two months]. Nevertheless, exam abnormal even for 1-½ month old, no follow, smile, decreased responsiveness. I think baby is not regressing, but appropriate progress seems missing. Brainstem functions appear intact but higher cortical function probably quite abnormal.

At this juncture, the staff began to consider transferring Darlene to the general pediatric division at Northeast Pediatric. Because of

the decreased level of care there, this plan had been explicitly rejected before, when hopes were higher. Now it began to emerge as
an institutional alternative to a "do not resuscitate" order.

Conflicting attitudes about the case were expressed by the unit's
staff. For example, a nurse exclaimed, "This kid is not worth saving," and a resident commented, "It's useless." Yet the written records stated: "Medically doing well. Sensitive." On day 112, Darlene
came down with a temperature of 106 degrees. She had had a series
of infections; now it appeared that she had an infection resistant to
at least two of the principal antibiotics used in the unit. Darlene now
posed a threat, as a source of infection, to other infants.

This development precipitated a strong reaction in staff members.
In conference with the other nurses, Darlene's primary nurse decided that she couldn't manage Darlene by herself. In this retreat,
she joined the primary physician, who the same week had announced that the unit director would be taking charge of the case.
To help the primary nurse, a core group of nurses volunteered to
share the responsibility.

At this time, day 119, the nurses met with the social workers at
weekly social service rounds but avoided the details of discharge
plans. The primary nurse presented the report of the visiting nurse
who had assessed Darlene's grandmother's home:

> The visiting nurse from [the community] went into the home. She's done
> a lot of work with unwed mothers. Home—four babies sleep in one room,
> appropriately. [The mother] has one room. Children dressed nicely. [The
> mother] was there. Asked the little boy who his mother was and he said
> [mother], but he calls the grandmother "mother." [Mother] had her coat
> on the whole time. She left the apartment several times while the nurse
> was there. The nurse felt the mother was not capable of taking any child
> home, not even a full-term [baby]. . . . The home has problems like all
> homes in the area. For example, one missing step, but nothing unusual.
> But the nurse was very adamant about thinking that the mother can't
> take care of the baby.

The psychiatrist asked about the infant's medical condition. The primary nurse emphasized the infant's clinical progress, for example,
that Darlene was in 48 percent oxygen under the hood and could
now be fed by mouth.

Interpreting the nurses' report optimistically, the social workers
then discussed child abuse and custody forms, and the importance
of sharing plans about intended moves with the family. The unit
social worker emphasized that the infant was top priority, not

launching an attack on the family: "You don't file a [child abuse form] against someone—you file it on behalf of a baby." The discussion closed with the social worker asking, "Are decisions being made?" The primary nurse responded, "No. No major decisions are being made now that I know of."

The Transfer

In truth, the staff had been moving quickly in the direction of transferring Darlene to the pediatric unit within the hospital. This transfer would guarantee that Darlene would not be treated as a critically ill infant. By not sending her to the nearby hospital with a combined Level II and III unit, the staff forestalled a reenactment of their own dilemma; this patient would have had easy access maximum intensive care if her condition had worsened at the mixed-level (Level II and III) unit.

Was Darlene critically ill or not? Despite the positive description offered at social service rounds, the house officer at work rounds described her as "suffering from lung disease, [respiratory] failure [during the night], and pneumonia." Five days later, Darlene suffered a cardiac arrest but was revived. Two days after this episode, the staff decided to transfer her to the pediatric nursery at Northeast Pediatric.

On day 127, the discharge plan for Darlene was announced to the mother as she visited the unit. As recorded in the nursing notes:

[Mother] appeared relatively receptive but certainly not overwhelmed. Told [mother] transfer would be [in six days]. Called [grandmother] and also explained and discussed . . . (she felt good about transfer: "I'm sure they have good doctors all over Northeast Pediatric.") Called [unit social worker] and told her [Darlene] was being transferred on Tuesday. Said she would get in touch with the new social service. Also said she would explain transfer to [community social worker].

On the day of the transfer, the primary nurse went to social service rounds with a rational discharge plan that hedged the caregiver problem:

Darlene is going to [general pediatric] nursery at one o'clock today. We met with the nurse. The primary physician from [the pediatric nursery] was up and examined the baby with [a resident here] and he wrote a very nice transfer sheet.

Later in the day, the primary nurse went home and Darlene was moved to the general nursery. Her clinical course there was rocky from the beginning. After four hours, she was in respiratory failure because her oxygen hood had not been reconnected after the transfer.

Two days later, a joint conference of concerned Level III and general pediatric staff members was held. New tests showed more problems with Darlene's heart and brain, and the new staff found her neurological status "unpromising." The general unit primary physician had wanted "do not resuscitate" orders but the nurses disagreed, asking him to wait until they knew the patient and the family better. Hence, the conference was called, which covered more about the mother's street life, learning disabilities, and inability to care for her first child than about Darlene's clinical background.

Ten days later, members of the two staffs met again, this time with the mother and grandmother and the community social worker. The new primary nurse explained to them for the first time the differences between the Level III unit and the general unit, for instance, that the general unit had fewer nurses (a 1:10 nurse-to-patient ratio instead of the 1:3 ratio in the n.i.c.u.) and the mixed ages of the patients there. The mother was distracted and uncommunicative; she left the meeting early.

The community social worker raised the touchy issue of what the transfer meant in terms of the baby's future health. The new primary physician adroitly fielded her question by asking the grandmother what she thought about Darlene's condition. The grandmother replied that she knew there was lung and brain damage, and added, "Maybe by next summer [in six months], the baby could come home." Not contradicting her, the physician remarked vaguely that they would not discharge the baby until she was off oxygen support. This continued the pattern of giving the family hope that the infant had a future with them at home.

THE AFTERMATH

Within a month, after 160 days as a hospital patient, Darlene Bourne died of viral pneumonia. The Level III staff had mixed reactions. Said one of the residents drily, "That's just what we expected." The nurses, several weeks later, informally discussed the case.

> *Primary nurse:* "I was very upset. I cried. Actually, I didn't cry but my eyes filled with tears when [the primary physician] told me. I was angry that she died. I felt angry with [the n.i.c.u. director] and the whole program for starting this whole business, all the conferences. . ."

Researcher: "All the energy put in. . ."

Primary nurse: "And she died on Christmas Eve."

Second nurse (fixing coffee): "That was just like her."

Researcher: "What do you mean?"

Second nurse: "Everything was a big problem, a big statement."

Primary nurse: "It took me three weeks to calm down. Just after that we had a lot of small babies, 600- and 700-gram babies, and all sorts of things were being done to them: PDAs, intubations, transfusions. It was awful. But I got over it."

The community social worker reported that the mother and grandmother were quarreling about the infant's death. The mother, in particular, was angry at the n.i.c.u. staff for transferring the baby to the general pediatric nursery and telephoned the n.i.c.u. primary nurse to tell her so.

Asked by the researcher why the infant had been transferred, this same nurse replied, "She was taking up a bed needed by thirty-two and thirty-three weekers with good chances—good babies." The unit director only shook his head and called it "a troublesome case."

Treatment Decisions

The staff's loss of will to continue treating Darlene was based on a combination of factors. The family situation was central. The mother's troubled psychology and grandmother's ambivalence about assuming responsibility were crucial to the transfer decision. In the Level III nursery, at the same time that Darlene was there, there were two other infants in comparable clinical conditions (see Chapter 6, Table 6.4, Part C), but both of them received prolonged maximum care. One of these infants stayed more than six months; the other stayed more than four months. The main difference between Darlene and these infants had to do with their families. The other two babies' parents were married, and although distraught, the parents maintained a stable relationship. The couples were also highly accepting of their infants. The teenage parents of one infant (who suffered from cretinism) were seen as too enthusiastic, "unrealistic" in the staff's opinion. Supported by a large extended family, these parents resisted physicians' advice that treatment should be witheld when the infant was discovered to have a major heart defect. The parents wanted and got the first of a series of surgical remedies. In the other case, the twin of the infant had died soon after birth at home, due to the inexperience of the mother with childbirth. The surviving twin was a girl; the deceased twin had been a boy. This added to the mother's guilt because the family was Mormon and the father had especially wanted a son. The mother came frequently to the unit, dutiful and distraught. Her infant had no birth defects, only the symptoms of severe prematurity, so that no single yes or no decision on treatment ever had to be made.

In still another case simultaneous with Darlene's, a 910-gram newborn with multiple anomalies, was not considered viable by the physicians. But the parents, especially the father, insisted that maximum efforts be made. The infant lived sixty-eight days. At the time the decision was made to transfer Darlene, this infant had become a "no move" patient whose condition had been stabilized by high-oxygen respiratory support. His professionally employed parents struck up a friendship with the Mormon couple, forming an alliance that put pressure on the staff to commit itself to their two infants.

There were four additional long-term survivors in the unit during the time of Darlene's treatment. (See Fig. 3.1.) Some of their families were relatively remote from the unit. In one case, the parents did not visit for weeks; in another, the parents lived out-of-state. Still, none of them presented the unstable image that Darlene's family had. The prognosis for each infant was about as unpromising as Darlene's, but the staff remained committed to treating these infants.

The presence of these other long-term cases, all of them very low birth weight newborns, made it practically impossible to opt for a no-code (i.e., no resuscitation) decision for Darlene, a comparable case. To withdraw treatment would have implied that these other infants might also lose the staff's commitment to treat, on the same grounds of poor outcome.

In addition, decisions to stop treatment were usually based on a physicians' consensus, which in Darlene's case was never clearly evident. The unit director was often ambivalent and the optimistic attending physician persisted as a general advocate for difficult, even hopeless cases. Even if the senior physicians had all agreed that further treatment would not be beneficial, there were complications in the communications with the family. Darlene's mother and grandmother were perceived as volatile and not open to reasonable argument. A further, though unacknowledged, complexity was the social welfare personnel and their potential reactions to such a decision. The social workers and therapists surrounding the family knew little of Darlene's actual medical status. The black community social worker (who was suspicious of the transfer) had tried unsuccessfully to interpret the mother–daughter household and its place in the black community to the white n.i.c.u. staff. Direct withdrawal of care might have caused her to raise questions about racial discrimination.

Overloaded with long-term cases, uncertain of the course of clinical treatment, fatalistic about the family situation, and intimidated by potentially strong reactions on the part of the mother and grandmother, the n.i.c.u. staff opted to relegate responsibility for the infant's care to another institutional division. How they were able to persuade the pediatric unit to accept Darlene we do not know. What Darlene's case does demonstrate clearly, however, is that a policy for reevaluating difficult cases did not exist in the n.i.c.u. On a structural level, there was literally no place to put an infant who was not benefitting from medical intervention. The standard referral-to-discharge trajectory did not accommodate the reality of infants who, like Darlene, were treated but who eventually no longer responded to treatment. Most important, Darlene's career as a patient shows how a critically ill newborn can become lost when all advocacy—family, professional, and institutional—falters. In nurseries that are larger and more impersonal, in situations where parents are absent, even a more healthy infant would be in jeopardy.

IV

The National and International Context

9

Newborn Intensive Care in the United States

> Every patient we admit to this unit gets absolutely the best we have to give. We don't give up on anyone. We don't have the right to do that.
> *Physician Director,*
> *U.S. Level III Nursery*

> You can't get away from it. Every death is a failure.
> *Pediatric Resident*

The Level III nursery at Northeast Pediatric presents one example of newborn intensive care in a specialized teaching hospital. Newborn intensive care can be structured in other ways, with mixed-level treatment centers, with less regionalization, and in the context of the general hospital.

Nonetheless, even when structures vary, the basic premise of newborn intensive care brings uniformity to the enterprise. The mandate to rescue newborns as victims of medical emergencies and then to amplify treatment under the aegis of neonatology is fundamental to all Level III units. Flowing from that mandate is the widespread movement to regionalize n.i.c.u. services or perinatal services (care for both pregnant women and newborns). The rise of neonatology as a subspecialty has depended on the development of the n.i.c.u. at the same time it has helped achieve that development. The claims of neonatologists to improved results in treating newborns weighing less than 1,000 grams have been widely accepted by other physicians, namely, obstetricians who refer sick newborns to the n.i.c.u. and pediatricians at community hospitals who manage Level I and II nurseries.

Perhaps most important, positive public sentiment about newborn medical rescue underwrites the n.i.c.u. enterprise. Unlike in the abortion controversy, there is little ambivalence surrounding the care of critically ill newborns; the life in question is undeniably a person's. Where ambivalence crops up is in the issue of the long-term consequences of treatment, an area which practitioners and the public have thus far been able to divorce from the mandate to rescue. Conceptually, there has been great consensus—public, institutional, and professional—about the benefits of maximum concentration of acute hospital care to address newborn pathologies. As a service institution, the Level III nursery is the ultimate expression of the value placed on infant life.

Table 9.1. Mortality rates (per 1,000 infants) in selected countries (W.H.O. sources)

Country	Mortality rate	Year
United States	10.4	1986
United Kingdom	9.1	1987
The Netherlands	6.4	1986
Brazil	70.0	1986

Outside the United States, professional and public forces vary in their influence on the special care for newborns. In this chapter, we review the varieties of neonatal intensive care in the United States as we saw them during our site visits. In the next chapter, we consider three national approaches different from that in the United States, those of England, the Netherlands, and Brazil. While recognizing the hazards of comparing cross-national data, we were equally aware in our research that newborn intensive care has become an international phenomenon, occurring in a variety of health care contexts and in countries with different rates of infant mortality (Table 9.1).

THE UNITED STATES

Sites Visited

To gain a comparative perspective on our work at Northeast Pediatric, we visited a total of fourteen other major n.i.c.u.'s during 1979–1983. Following the suggestions of physicians, nurses, social workers, and hospital administrators, we aimed for regional and institutional variation in choosing the sites to visit. Our site visits covered one to three days of work rounds and interviews with physicians, nurses, and, where possible, social service staff. In a few cases, we were able to extend our stay for a week to ten days. In one instance

Table 9.2. American n.i.c.u.s by hospital type and locale

Hospital	Region	State	City	Type	Major linkage	Level	No. of beds
A	NE	1	1	General P	No	Mixed	20
B	NE	1	1	Maternity NP	Yes[a]	Mixed	30
C	NE	2	2	General NP	No	Mixed	25
D	MA	3	3	General PR	No	Mixed	70
E	MA	3	3	General NP	No	III	25
F	MA	4	4	Pediatric NP	Yes	Mixed	28
G	SE	4	5	Pediatric NP	Yes	Mixed	30
H	SE	5	6	Pediatric NP	Yes	III	40
I	NC	6	7	Pediatric NP[b]	Yes	Mixed	28
J	SC	7	8	General P	No	Mixed	100
K	SC	7	9	General NP	Yes	Mixed	30
L	SW	8	10	General NP	No	Mixed	20
M	W	9	11	General NP	Yes	Mixed	20
N	W	9	12	Pediatric NP	Yes	Mixed	40
Northeast Pediatric	NE	1	1	Pediatric NP	Yes	III	15

P, public; NP, nonprofit; PR, private; NE, northeast; MA, mid-Atlantic; SE, southeast; NC, north central; SC, south central; SW, southwest; W, west.

[a]Linked to Northeast Pediatric.

[b]Non-teaching hospital.

(at Hospital D), regular contact was maintained for a three-month period.

The regions represented in our overview are shown in Table 9.2, along with the hospital types. Some of the oldest examples of newborn intensive care nurseries and some of the most complex institutional coordination of services, in the context of traditional medical schools, were found in the Northeast. Outside the Northeast, intensive care nurseries were newer, but were essentially variations on the same technological theme. All the units were focused on the premature newborn. Four of the hospitals we visited were pediatric teaching hospitals. Five were general teaching hospitals. In addition, four special hospital types are represented. One was an inner-city public hospital. Another, in a different city, was an elite private hospital. A third was a new, non-teaching pediatric hospital. The fourth was a maternity hospital affiliated with Northeast Pediatric.

Comparative Dimensions

At Northeast Pediatric, the admission of extremely low birth weight newborns with no formal or informal limit on prematurity was the norm. Also, the use of maximum resources, both diagnostic and therapeutic, was pro forma for all admitted patients. This approach was essentially the same in the other units we visited. The unit directors and senior physicians controlled admission and treatment, and held to the survival mandate, with few or modest restrictions on borderline cases. Some neonatologists, for example, drew the line at accepting compromised 600-gram newborns, but this was a rare categorical prejudgment.

A second generalization is that the participation of parents in decision making was negligible. Medical specialization in consort with regionalization made for considerable distancing of the families from the n.i.c.u. In some units, class and culture differences widened this communication gap even more than was usual at Northeast Pediatric. In still others, individual nurses and social workers or psychologists were single-handedly trying to overcome this distance. Still, the basic structure of the service, with its emphasis on the individual infant patient, denied an active role to parents.

These are the two major generalizations. Let us turn now to the finer points of comparison.

The Organization of the Professionals

Physicians.   In major medical centers, the standard n.i.c.u. staff organization was the physician hierarchy already described for Northeast Pediatric, with the same heavy reliance on skilled nurses. Depending on bed number, the staff size was equal to and usually greater than at Northeast Pediatric; the high professional-to-patient ratio remained constant. The only place the labor of residents was missing was in the non-teaching pediatric hospital. There, four senior physicians were in what one of them described as a "state of permanent residency." A visiting family practice intern gave minor assistance, but physicians and nurses agreed that these aspirants (the interns) should be allowed little hands-on work with patients. The physicians in this unit also mourned the absence of neonatology fellows "to give us a sense of generation."

In the teaching hospitals, there was variation in the program offered to residents, although no indication that they or neonatology fellows had much influence on admission or treatment decisions. One hospital had, for example, a joint obstetrics-neonatology program that allowed obstetricians and pediatricians to alternate rotations in each service. More typically, pediatric residents were the only ones to gain experience in the n.i.c.u., over a four to eight-week service rotation. The high labor demands of the Level III nursery have led to the overuse of the resident service in some pediatric programs, prompt-

ing the American Academy of Pediatrics to issue a cautionary statement (AAP, 1980). The many disgruntled and often unenthusiastic
comments we heard from residents might have been due to this
phenomenon or to the immediate demands of n.i.c.u. work.

Unlike the Northeast Pediatric n.i.c.u., five units sponsored ethics rounds for the discussion of difficult cases. These were, in four
instances, led by physicians; the exception was Hospital E, which
had hired a philosopher to guide discussion. The relationship between these forums and the treatment of infants was difficult to
judge. In the several meetings we attended, physicians either ex-
pounded with authority or used the groups as part of the team consensus process. That is, diverse problem perspectives—moral agency,
social justice, the fate of the handicapped—were expressed, unbur-
dening individuals of their subjective feelings and demonstrating that
the group was aware of issues. The discussions were never intended to lead to policy conclusions. After an hour or half-hour session, the staff would return to their clinical duties with policies un-
altered. Most Level III team members had no time in the workday
for sustained ethics discussions, though ethical issues were on their
minds.

Generational differences among physicians seemed more obvious
to us when we were short-term visitors to other units than when
we were long-term observers at Northeast Pediatric. In other units,
residents were more open about their preference for community-level
rather than Level III nursery careers. Several directors expressed a
need to move away from clinical work, in somewhat the way older
bench scientists may grow weary of their laboratories. Still other attending neonatologists were open about their feelings of burnout.
The area of neonatology is so young that it is difficult to predict how
these attitudes will affect future career choices and what the institutional determinants of those choices will be. Many senior n.i.c.u.
physicians are in their late thirties and forties, their careers already
strongly tied to recent developments in the United States in the organization of hospitals. Having started as hospital-employed physicians, they appear likely to remain so.

Nurses. There were variations in the organization of the nursing
staff, though not in the nurses' position in the unit team hierarchy.
The primary nursing model plus participatory management of n.i.c.u.
nurses at Northeast Pediatric proved to be relatively unique. Most
nursing staffs were under the leadership of a chief nurse who took
responsibility for scheduling and other internal matters. Several units

relied on primary nursing. One large (seventy beds) unit subdivided its staff into two working groups and, under a head nurse, instituted a cadre of nurse-clinicians as an intermediate part of the team structure.

A close working relationship with the unit director and senior physicians counted as much toward maintaining nurses' morale as did opportunities for career advancement. In the large unit mentioned above, nurses' career opportunities **were** optimal and there was primary nursing. Yet nurses' morale was low and there was overt conflict between nurses and senior physicians. One reason might have been the attitude of the unit director, who was remote from clinical work but excelled in representing the unit to the hospital and the community. The nurse-clinician positions he promoted increased the competition among ambitious nurses and opened rifts between them and nurses less interested in "professionalizing" their occupation. Nor was nurses' input in clinical decisions welcomed:

> The three nurses sat together on the large couch in the director's office. The director sat behind his large desk. To his right was a neonatology fellow who remained silent and neutral. The nurse who took the spokesperson's role said that the "baby was just not moving, wasn't growing at all" and that the latest CT scan indicated severe brain damage. Her voice cracked as she spoke and the other nurses looked tense. She then fell silent.
>
> *Director* (in stern voice): "Do you mean to say that this is enough reason to stop treatment?"
>
> *Nurse:* "The parents don't understand what bad shape the baby is in."
>
> *Director:* "One thing has to be clear. Every patient we admit to this unit gets absolutely the best we have to give. We don't give up on anyone. We haven't the right to do that. And certainly not in this case."

The infant who was the subject of this discussion died two weeks later, despite continued maximum care.

In contrast, the physicians and nurses in the non-teaching hospital unit worked closely and with ease. The clinical severity of cases was, if anything, worse than what we saw at other hospitals; several infants weighed less than 700 grams and were failing. Yet the nurses were undaunted. In an extra effort, they volunteered their time to a parental support group "because it helps us understand our work better." The expansion of the region served by the unit was documented by a large map placed in the center of the nursery. The head nurse and others were enthusiastic about their progress in reaching remote areas of the state.

In the two units (Hospitals A and E) that were not regionally expanding, the n.i.c.u. nurses were relatively passive. Both these hospitals attracted residents interested in front-line work with poor communities. They tended to upstage the nurses and social workers with their knowledge of family problems. In decreasing the range of tasks for these nurses, the residents also curtailed the nurses' capacity to speak up authoritatively.

The more authority nurses had, formally or informally, the more they participated at rounds and made their presence felt in the unit. The large size of some units, however, diminished nurses' participation. Small units, even without self-management, seemed to foster the participation of their nurses in clinical discussions. In larger units, nurses either were absent from rounds or were relatively unresponsive. In these units, some physicians had trouble remembering the names of the full-time nurses.

At Northeast Pediatric, nurses could upgrade their clinical and administrative skills. In other units, where nurses could similarly explore career opportunities, the hazards of these new responsibilities were emerging. The head of the all-nurse transport team at Hospital L put it this way:

> Last night's case made me do a lot of thinking. Why are you in this business? I'm reaching a burnout point. I've been on transport two years. I don't sleep well when I'm on call. I'm responsible twenty-four hours, seven days a week. I try to be available to help. I have to have sessions quite often now with [attending physician] to keep going. I want to do some other thing in neonatology. I'm too crisis-oriented right now.

Social and Psychological Staff. The variety in social work and psychology staffing for the various n.i.c.u.'s was extensive. Units in hospitals serving large inner-city minority populations had greater investments in social service than did the Northeast Pediatric unit. Hospital H, for example, had a full-time psychologist who ran parental support groups. Hospitals A and E employed social workers as liaisons to local agencies and the community. In these and other settings, the social workers described themselves as having considerable authority over court and adoption decisions, to the point of using guardianship claims as a means of attempting to control parental drinking, drug, or behavioral problems: "Either the parents behave or they don't get the child."

The institutional investment in social work with parents far outweighed the group or individual therapy commonly offered to physicians and nurses. When therapists were available for staff members, it was for the nurses. The presumptions were that nurses were more vulnerable to the strains of n.i.c.u. work, that for residents the n.i.c.u. was a temporary and educational experience, and that senior physicians were too highly committed to be troubled by their work. Somewhat to our surprise, and perhaps because we were nonthreatening outsiders, several directors and attending physicians expressed real dissatisfaction with their jobs and a wish to leave the field—if not immediately, certainly within a few years. Feeling overwhelmed by administrative responsibilities and dismayed by the lack of variety in clinical work, the director of a 100-bed unit commented:

> Maybe if I were doing more active research, I'd bounce out of bed in the morning the way I used to. But now that we're big time, the pressure is on. How long does anyone do this kind of work?

Whatever the feelings of physicians, experts in social and psychological problems are not encouraged to see these professionals as clients, at least not in the hospital setting. Nurses, as (mostly) women and farther down in the staff hierarchy, are considered to be more appropriate patients.

The Expansion of Referral Systems

In nearly every unit we visited, evidence of the expansion and upgrading of services was striking. In many places, regionalization was in full swing, with posted area maps (like the one mentioned above) documenting new referral sources. Part of this expansion effort included joint programs, like the one at Northeast Pediatric, between the Level III nursery and maternity services at other institutions.

These cooperative arrangements between service divisions in different hospitals are not as legally complex as the corporate consolidation of entire hospitals presently taking place in the United States (Starr, 1982:420–441). The creation of joint neonatology programs and the integration of maternity and newborn services across institutional lines does, however, reflect the same competitive atmosphere and the same concern with economic efficiency that is motivating the trend toward corporate mergers. Rather than affecting the independence of the prestigious teaching hospital, cross-hospital relationships between maternity and infant services look more like professional relations between obstetricians and neonatologists writ large in bureaucratic script. Just as the two specialties depend on each other for professional survival, this interdependence makes formal institutional arrangements inevitable. Local obstetricians still have the established relations with patients that make them invaluable to hospital-based services, especially referral units. For them, neonatologists still offer the maximum level of resources as a haven from clinical and legal hazards. The current trend, however, is toward formal contracts between local hospitals and central hospital nurseries, that is, toward a more stable and depersonalized basis for referral.

Pediatric and General Hospitals

Pediatric hospitals play a special role in this development of interinstitutional cooperation. As at Northeast Pediatric, Level III nurseries in pediatric hospitals tend to link up with maternity services in general hospitals that want to promise parents the ultimate in specialized newborn intensive care. For the pediatric hospital's n.i.c.u., linkage with the obstetric division of a major hospital complements the regional recruitment of patients from community hospitals. For the general hospital, the pediatric hospital's n.i.c.u. offers special services that the hospital lacks, services requiring a major investment in personnel and technology. For example, a major general hospital in one city had a Level III nursery, but its case load and investment in surgery did not justify its treatment of surgical cases. Therefore, infants requiring surgery were referred from that hospital to the pediatric hospital (Hospital H in Table 9.2). This pediatric hospital Level III nursery received as many as one-half of its cases from the general hospital. At the same time, as the n.i.c.u. director explained, the general hospital and the pediatric hospital competed openly for cases from community hospitals.

The new pediatric hospital mentioned above (Hospital I) inaugurated (three years after its opening) a joint arrangement with the perinatal center in a nearby general hospital. The perinatal center emphasized the transport of high-risk maternity patients and advertised its affiliation with the pediatric hospital as an additional guarantee of protection against medical risk. As another example, Hospital N in 1979 started a cooperative arrangement between its intensive care nursery (mixed-level) and a nearby general hospital. The first patients in this program were a set of triplets. The event was written up in the pediatric hospital's magazine, with emphasis on the presence of two neonatologists and a pediatrician at the cesarean delivery, "with a nurse and equipment to transport the infants. Each newborn had three people assigned to its care."

The other pediatric hospital units we visited had similar relation-ships with the obstetrics divisions of one or more major general fa-cilities. In some instances, these links between major institutions were described as a hedge against the declining number of maternity beds in community hospitals and the closing of community clinics. As obstetric care has centralized, pediatric hospital–based n.i.c.u.'s have moved to contract with flourishing perinatal centers as one kind of referral strategy.

General hospitals with both high-level maternity services and in-tensive care nurseries appear to have the competitive advantage if the recruitment of patients can economically justify the investment in a top-level n.i.c.u. General Hospital D, for example, was not as-sociated with any pediatric hospital. Its Level II and III nurseries served both infants born in the hospital and those from a constel-lation of suburban hospitals. A dense population, even in the sub-urban communities, and excellent emergency transportation ex-panded this unit from fifty to eighty beds between 1980 and 1982.

Two general hospitals (A and E) presented a different picture. Al-though each accepted infants from outside hospitals, these patients were only a small fraction of the total number admitted. Instead, Hospital A, a public hospital, served an inner-city and largely mi-nority community. Residents in pediatrics did service rotations in community maternal and child health clinics and were encouraged not only to gain a perspective on the local population but also to follow cases through pregnancy until after birth. Although not a public hospital, Hospital E promoted much the same relationship with its local and predominantly minority community. Neither of these hospitals was intent on regionalizing its n.i.c.u. services. Both had, in essence, no opportunity to do so, since other, more presti-gious teaching hospital units had already captured the suburban populations. These two hospitals received the poorest inner-city people, hence their broader social medicine focus. Both hospitals made attempts to unite obstetric and neonatal care, with joint rounds and resident exchanges. Physicians in both hospitals expressed sup-port for preventive medicine, especially when confronted by infants suffering from fetal alcohol syndrome or drug withdrawl and in cases of teenage pregnancy.

Two other hospitals we visited, Hospital G in the Southeast and Hospital L in the Southwest, were strongly affected by the rural hinterlands they served. Both units received many of their cases from rural areas and were highly reliant on long-distance emergency transport. The Level III unit in Hospital L served an entire state.

Since it was a general hospital, obstetric and neonatology services were well coordinated. In yet another general hospital, Hospital J, located in the south central United States, there was a heavy commitment to a large rural area that spilled over to another state. The unit director explained that the recent expansion of the tertiary unit to 100 beds was in part justified by the lack of competition from other comparable units. However, around the time of our visit, campaigners in the neighboring state had convinced their legislature to fund just such a competitive unit so that their critically ill infants would not have to be transported across state lines to receive care.

The more n.i.c.u.'s that are created, the more important it becomes for them to be able to compete successfully. Formal contracts to fortify referral relations are one strategy. Cooperative programs are another. Still another is more efficient management, for example, using computer technology. Computerization is a fast-growing aspect of newborn intensive care for record-keeping and research, and nowhere is its use more impressive than in promoting regional referrals.

For instance, in California, referrals by computer were used relatively early. Since 1978, the state has had two Infant Medical Dispatch Centers, one in the north at Stanford and the other in the south at the Los Angeles County–University of Southern California Medical Center. The centers rely on a computer program to process all information relating to beds, staff, and transport team and carrier availability, as well as weather conditions.

> Babies have been transported from as far south as Santa Barbara, as far north as Crescent City, and as far east as Reno, Nevada. The longest out-of-state transports thus far have been from Butte, Montana, . . . and from Hong Kong. (Hackel, 1978:11)

Casting the net this wide assumes that there are only technical obstacles to referral and treatment. This is probably an accurate conjecture, since no policy restraints on admissions appear to be in effect in any regional system.

Admission and Treatment Policy

Despite some variety in professional staff organization and in hospital type, the unrestricted admission of extremely low birth weight infants and other borderline cases was almost universal. Pursuit of the 500-gram newborn survival goal was commonly acknowledged as the current direction in neonatology. Furthermore, physicians of all ranks saw the subspecialty progressively improving outcome for smaller and smaller infants, thus justifying the admission and treatment of extremely premature newborns. The perceived momentum of the field itself, rather than any systematic investigation of treatment and results, prompted this optimism. That is, neonatologists felt that their patient survival rates were getting better and that this improvement was in line with the general progress of other units.

A wide variety of research activities characterized all the teaching hospital units and contributed to the atmosphere encouraging progressive medicine. Some physicians had projects in biochemistry, others in clinical care, still others in computer technology. In the non-teaching hospital, the director of the n.i.c.u. spoke of eventually compiling follow-up data on unit "graduates" and publishing the results. His research ambitions were overshadowed by the goal of providing service to parents and the community. For example, his staff treated a newborn baby weighing 525 grams for the sake of parents who had had repeated reproductive failures and had, exactly one year before, lost an infant of about the same size.

Technology

The scope of medical care available affects how an infant is treated in one hospital versus another. In basic support technology, such as respirators, monitors, and radiology and laboratory facilities, there was hardly any difference between one American Level III unit and another. Some units were brand new and huge, others were housed in obviously older buildings, and some encompassed adjoining rooms to cut down on noise or just to accommodate the floor layout. Four units were moving toward the extensive computerization of clinical data and had terminals on the floor. Several units had yet to procure portable ultrasound equipment, but such diagnostic equipment was already perceived as necessary.

One indication of a unit's general level of aggressive care was the availability of surgery. Hospital E, for example, did not have surgical facilities suitable for newborns in the n.i.c.u. or a pediatric surgeon interested in doing patent ductus arteriosus ligations or any other kind of surgery. Patients in this unit, therefore, were not provided a full range of surgical options. In the most comparable unit, Hospital A, serving a local and largely minority community, surgery was available but was not, according to the director, an option frequently used. The question raised here is whether the almost exclusively minority communities these two hospitals served were receiving the level of care customary for infants in other units. The experimental nature of most, but not all, newborn surgery makes this a difficult question to answer. What was clear was that neither hospital unit serving the poor had the resources to invest in surgery. The brunt of this restraint, of course, was felt by premature n.i.c.u. infants; full-term infants with surgical needs could be referred, if necessary, to a pediatric hospital.

In contrast to these two general hospitals, the units in elite pediatric hospitals had become regional surgical centers, and were nationally and internationally renowned for dramatic surgical interventions (Hospitals F, G, K, and N). Two general hospitals, by their unit directors' definition, were regional centers for newborn surgery. Still another unit, with a rural population to serve (Hospital J), had an observably close and perhaps uncomfortable relationship with surgeons. Infant surgical patients recuperated in the Level III unit as the patients of the surgeons, not the neonatologists. The other surgically oriented units were more in control of their patients.

Medical Case Types

The kinds of cases we observed at Northeast Pediatric were also typical of other Level III nurseries. Most infants were admitted for conditions related to prematurity; most infants were discharged quickly. The extremely small premature infant was no rarity. The belief that newborns weighing less than 1,000 or 900 grams could be successfully treated was evidenced by the presence of many such small newborns in Level III nurseries.

Virtually every unit, either at the secondary or tertiary level, had lingering patients whose stay was long and whose prognosis was poor. At Hospitals D and J, there were infants several months old with severe hydrocephalus, their heads the size of footballs. In Hospital G, a severely retarded one-year-old was chronically dependent on oxygen therapy. The child's parents had abandoned him, but the unit did not feel it could. In these and other hospitals, long-term cases that were no longer benefiting from intensive care were placed in side rooms, away from the main Level III area, moved to rooms occupied by more healthy infants (called "growing rooms"), or transferred to adjoining Level II units. The non-teaching pediatric hospital unit was able to choose another and more innovative option. Two nurses, described by the unit director as "saints," had opened a small clinic, based on the hospice model, for terminally ill infants. At the time of our visit to the hospital, a hydrocephalic newborn for whom no treatment was judged beneficial was about to be transferred to the clinic. By a curious twist of circumstance, the new 100-bed unit at Hospital J found itself becoming a repository for long-term cases for which community hospitals had no room or inadequate facilities. One such patient, born prematurely and with multiple defects, was a returnee; initially treated in the Level III nursery, he was referred back to the community hospital, only to be returned six months later to the Level III nursery as an oxygen-dependent infant suffering from "failure to thrive."

All Level III units are faced with borderline cases that are often treated but that do not show quick positive results. Hospital units like that at Northeast Pediatric can invest maximum resources in a marginal patient but be structurally unable to handle long-term survivors or infants who are dying. Mixed-level units enjoy more options for shifting patients from one type of care to another. But no intensive care unit is geared to handle terminal cases, even though these infants are bound to be admitted. In the large private hospital (Hospital D), an infant born without a brain was not treated, yet he was kept in the unit for six weeks until he died. After two weeks, the head nurse had trouble finding nurses willing to give the baby perfunctory nipple feedings or to change his wrappers and bed linens. It was not that the nursing staff favored treatment for this infant; rather, the nurses were against the suffering caused by such prolonged dying. Said one nurse, "We do better by animals."

The decision to stop treatment is always a difficult one for n.i.c.u. physicians. Some units in the western United States appeared to have evolved an approach different from those in other parts of the country. Some physicians at Hospitals M and N espoused a two-step approach to the evaluation of an n.i.c.u. infant. After giving the baby the benefit of an all-out rescue attempt, the neonatologists allowed themselves to reassess the case, usually after twenty-four hours. They felt committed to treat aggressively at first. Said one, "You have to give the baby every chance even though the literature on prognosis is grim." Though they felt it was difficult, the senior physicians claimed the right to cease treatment if they felt the infant was too damaged. The difference between this attitude and that of physicians at Northeast Pediatric and other units is slight. All rely on obvious physiological failure rather than evaluations of long-term prognoses or the complexities of family life.

Attitudes Toward and Relations with Parents

The distance between parents and the n.i.c.u. staff is determined first by the emergency atmosphere surrounding treatment of the critically ill infant. The newborn has the highest-priority, even exclusive, claim to the staff's attention.

Other factors can influence the marginal role given parents, but none more certainly than the regionalization of newborn intensive care. If a tertiary nursery becomes part of a regionalization effort, the staff's relationship to families will, predictably, change. The degree of change is probably more radical for a general hospital that switches its focus from the local community to suburban and rural clients. If the two hospitals (A and E) integrated with inner-city clinics were to regionalize, the existing links between prenatal care, delivery, and postnatal and even pediatric care would be weakened. Because they exist side-by-side with major medical centers that have already expanded into the suburbs, neither of these units could successfully mount such an effort.

For the hospital already geared to the tertiary level of care, regionalization is just a more systematic way of recruiting the worst cases to the source of maximum treatment. Major pediatric hospitals (and here we count Hospitals F, G, and K, along with Northeast Pediatric) are accustomed to having complicated cases referred from all parts of the nation and the world.

These same hospitals have accomplished an increased degree of vertical integration of services. For example, the expansion of ambulatory services has grown along with the development of acute care divisions. In the pediatric hospital, of course, service expansion is limited to children. After treatment in the n.i.c.u., the infant patient may go on to use other services at the pediatric hospital. There is certainly no conscious intention on the part of n.i.c.u. practitioners to create a new pediatric patient population, yet extremely premature infants do have a marked tendency to be rehospitalized and the pediatric hospital is the obvious source of continued acute care and ambulatory care as well.

Is the potential marginality of parents to the Level III unit strictly a function of referring the infants to a pediatric hospital? That is possible, but the childbirth experience of parents in large general hospitals should not be idealized. The large scale of major medical centers, the professional divisions between specialties, and the passive role commonly ascribed to many obstetric patients all conspire to reduce the parents' participation in n.i.c.u. decisions and to fortify the autonomy of physicians. On the positive side, the coordination of contact between mother and n.i.c.u. infant in the same hospital should be less difficult than visits to a distant hospital. Some general hospitals (A, E, H, and M) evidenced great concern for parents, a concern shown by continuity of social work staff, the existence of parental support groups, and the amount of time nurses spent with families. These were hospitals in which 50 percent or more of the n.i.c.u. infants were from in-hospital births. Yet the social service approach to family problems, as we saw in Chapter 3, can be another kind of patient management. Social workers at units serving minority and poor communities seemed much more aggressive in intervening legally to resolve child care problems than were the social workers at Northeast Pediatric.

The strong association of premature birth with poverty increases the chances that an n.i.c.u. will serve a low-income population. Some units serve more economically disadvantaged patients than others. The proportion of n.i.c.u. patients receiving Medicaid is becoming a vital issue for hospitals since the coverage for care is restricted and the turnaround time for reimbursement can tax a hospital's budget. Some hospitals, like Northeast Pediatric, have cultivated suburban referrals, which tend to be privately insured. Private Hospital D's unit also sidestepped the problem of Medicaid patients by solidifying contract relations with suburban hospitals. For Hospitals A, E, and C, the local population is lower-class, predominantly black, and reliant on Medicaid.

Still other hospitals serve populations that are ethnically diverse and economically disadvantaged. For Hospitals M and N, the local community is a mixture of Hispanic, Oriental, and black families. In the Southwest, the unit at Hospital L serves many Hispanics and American Indians. In these culturally mixed settings, the staff has to go some distance to communicate with parents. For example, a transport nurse at Hospital L commented:

> We get quite a few who only speak Spanish. We get quite a few who speak only Navajo. With the Spanish, I don't do anything differently. With the Indian babies I feel extremely inadequate. The Public Service hospitals are dilapidated and depressing. I go in and nine-tenths of the time the mother does not speak English and there is no translator.

Sensitive to these communication problems, some units have made policy decisions to encourage the presence of parents. The parents of severely damaged and dying infants get special consideration in most units and the provision of overnight facilities was advertised at two regional centers. But if there is sympathy for the parents of n.i.c.u. infants, there is also a growing sense within the hospital that these parents can pose a threat, legally and to the good reputation of the service.

The unit at Northeast Pediatric was relatively immune to problems with discontented parents during the time of our work there. This was not true for other units. In 1981, Hospital D had to pay millions of dollars in damages to a victim of retrolental fibroplasia who, decades before, had been adversely affected by an experiment in oxygen support at that hospital. Although an old instance of neglect, the court case brought negative attention to the contemporary n.i.c.u. The local urban community served by Hospital N had recently become stirred up by the difference between infant mortality rates for minorities and those for white infants. An activist group demanded better access to prenatal care for minority women as well as newborn medical treatment. Hospital F was the scene of the Stinson and Stinson case (see Chapter 5) which, though the institution was not identified, made the n.i.c.u. staff here acutely aware of the risks of poor communication with parents.

At the same time, there is ample evidence that many parents are profoundly grateful for the care given in high-level n.i.c.u.'s. Bulletin boards with pictures of graduates and notes from parents are common in most units. Like the annual graduates' party, also a common custom, renewed staff contact with patients who have survived in good health can affirm the value of the unit's work. This affirmation, however, is on an emotional level; it is a morale booster rather than a clear-eyed look at the clinical condition of all survivors or the appreciation of how families cope with premature or defective infants.

CONCLUSION

In the diversity of geographic contexts of U.S. newborn intensive care, the service is highly valued for its expertise and efficiency. The Level III nursery that selects the most difficult cases is usually integrated into a regional system of hospitals or is linked to other intermediate care nurseries within the same hospital. There is, however, no frequent or necessary coordination between prenatal care and neonatal units. Although some joint programs advertise perinatal services, these tend to emphasize medical management at birth with the option of n.i.c.u. referral. As with other innovations of medical technology, in the United States, newborn intensive care has developed without a rigorous effort to integrate it into the broader health care system, whether as a limited resource or a fundamental part of maternal and child health planning. Instead, the service has to be evaluated after the fact of its enormous expansion and, if possible, shaped to better justify the resources and funds invested in it.

In the next chapter we present three other examples of newborn intensive care, in England, the Netherlands, and Brazil. In these cases, the service emerges as a universally appreciated instance of progressive medicine, but also as an innovation with its own dynamic that, if not contained by comprehensive health care planning, can become an item for conspicuous consumption.

10

International Comparisons of Newborn Intensive Care

> One week ago three babies out of eleven were on respirators and that seemed like a lot to us.
> *Attending Physician, Netherlands n.i.c.u.*

> We resuscitate all, because of ethics, because we don't know the outcome.
> *Physician Director, Brazilian n.i.c.u.*

Intensive care for newborns is an international phenomenon that has taken root in hospitals all over the world. Wherever they are found, hospital bureaucracies, advanced medical technology, and specialized medical training have been generally conducive to expanding this service. In the United States' free enterprise system, hospital services have been underwritten by the government, and yet these health service institutions also exist in the open market of the medical and hospital supply industry. In other industrialized countries, the budgets of hospitals and health professionals have been more stringently controlled by government, though they hardly are immune to the buildup of costly services and technologies.

West European welfare states offer a case in point. To provide universal health insurance, these countries have used a mix of government and private plans, of state-employed and private-practice options. The populations served and the funding levels are small in comparison to those in the United States. Furthermore, as we look at two European examples of special medical care for infants, England and the Netherlands, we find newborn intensive care set more firmly in the context of long-range planning than in the United States. The goals of reducing newborn illness and death rates are much the same, but the programmatic means are different.

Our third national case is that of Brazil. A Third World state in transition, Brazil has overcome some of the economic and health problems of less developed countries but is still in the process of assimilating medical care solutions from more industrialized nations (Roemer, 1977:17–18). High rates of premature birth and infant mortality, if taken at face value, indicate an enormous need for newborn intensive care. But the scope of this infant survival problem and the high cost of newborn intensive care force the consideration of other solutions. As in the United States, medicine can be the most conservative alternative to economic and health care reforms that frontally attack the effects of poverty. In developing nations, medical services such as newborn intensive care are usually most available to the wealthy. The question arises, then: Is newborn intensive care a benefit being denied a disadvantaged population or does it divert resources from basic health planning?

Finally, in countries with socialized medicine, the issue of the cost of newborn intensive care is more directly addressed than in the United States. This is in part because socialized medicine (however it is implemented) demands rational cost planning on a cradle-to-grave basis, a comprehensive approach that we Americans have preferred to avoid. Rather than calculating the investment in medical care appropriate to an individual over a life span, our tendency in the United States is to see competition between groups at a single point in time. Are we today spending more for children than for the elderly? Should we withdraw support for renal dialysis and put more money into rehabilitation for stroke victims? Regarding children alone, we have even found it possible to expand newborn intensive care while reducing support for the handicapped survivors of medical intervention (Children's Defense Fund, 1984). The approach of socialized medicine to these funding problems emphasizes the needs of individuals over a lifetime and equity in structuring care at each age grade. Thus, expensive procedures are likely to be denied because they drain the entire funding system, or, if they are permitted, they must be available, at least in theory, to all.

The international medicalization of childbirth has increased people's awareness of the infant as patient and has identified newborn intensive care as the most progressive solution to critical illness in this population. Even when many governments and people cannot afford the service, recognition is accorded its benefits. Less well understood is the conservative use of high-level newborn intensive care to solve maternal and infant health problems that are rooted in poverty. In fact, when social inequity is perceived as an incurable ill, medicine can be presented as a paradigm of efficiency and morality: act quickly and save innocent babies' lives. Combine this with the public's belief in the power of medical science and at least temporary relief from the frustrations of larger economic and political problems is guaranteed.

NEWBORN INTENSIVE CARE IN ENGLAND: ALLOCATING RESOURCES

From a United States perspective, there are two unusual characteristics of health care in Great Britain. One is the government-imposed budgetary limit on health care expenditures. The British National Health Service is designed to give universal medical and hospital care, but it does so by limiting tax-supported services and sharply curtailing private professional activity. The second noteworthy characteristic is the decentralization of decision making about progressive medicine. As a result, when it comes to high technology, the English reject some expensive therapies, such as coronary bypass operations, while supporting other innovations, such as radiotherapy treatment for cancer (Aaron and Schwartz, 1984). Transposed into the English context, neonatal intensive care is, like other hospital services there, controlled by multiple tiers of government policy-making bodies. At the highest level, the Department of Health and Social Security (DHSS) sets broad priorities and determines general funding for health services. At more local levels, regional, area, and district health authorities decide more specifically how to allocate resources.

For instance, in 1971, the DHSS published the report of The Expert Group on Special Care for Babies. This report recommended referral to neonatal care units for all sick infants, especially those born weighing less than 2,500 grams or by difficult births such as cesarean, forceps, and breech deliveries (DHSS, 1971). However, on the regional level, there was no consistent response to this policy suggestion. For one, British physicians disagreed about the criteria for referral. For another, the referral units—special care and intensive care nurseries—were without (and remain without) specific criteria:

> In 1980, the Social Services Committee recognized that intensive care was difficult to define. The most usual definition is that it includes such techniques as "prolonged mechanical ventilation, total parenteral nutrition and the use of advanced monitoring techniques." (MacFarlane and Mugford, 1984:144)

Intensive care also takes the form of very close observation, whether or not any equipment is used. In contrast to the 1:3 nurse-to-patient ratio often found in United States Level III nurseries, both the British Paediatric Association and the Royal College of Obstetricians and Gynaecologists recommended a 1:1 ratio as a necessary additional criterion for Special Care Baby Units (SCBUs) (MacFarlane and Mugford, 1984:144–45).

In addition, local health authorities face competing financial claims from other services, especially those for the elderly. Campbell (1984) found that clinical needs (based on infant prematurity and perinatal mortality rates, by region) were not strongly correlated with nursery admission rates. Rather, the availability of cots (infant beds) and physicians' attitudes were better predictors of admission to special care. If the regional and area authorities vote to support a given number of special or intensive care cots, the likelihood is great that the cots will be filled. If the authorities vote for limits, then the service will be limited.

This regional variation, reported for other health services, allows for the existence of nurseries virtually identical to Level III units in the United States. Teaching hospitals have special claims and often provide services for especially difficult (and medically interesting) cases from beyond their immediate region. While many smaller hospitals (with fewer than 3,000 births per year) have twenty-bed special care nurseries, these are mainly surveillance units. Major medical centers house high-technology units and there is a trend toward efficient regional use of these intensive care nurseries. In the four Thames regions (Northeast, Northwest, Southeast, and Southwest) serving the greater London area, an Emergency Bed Service was established in 1979 to match newborns in need with available intensive care cots (Gamsu, 1983). Four major units (one in each region) accept infants from eighty or so smaller hospitals, most of them district general hospitals. Each of these major units has backup from lower-level nurseries. In 1979, there were 176,000 live births in the four Thames regions and these infants were served by a total of only twenty-nine maximum care cots and thirty-four intermediate cots. In rough comparison, a state such as Massachusetts, with 74,000 births in 1981, supports seven high-level n.i.c.u.'s of fifteen beds or more each.

Gamsu reported that from November 1979 to October 1980 only 40 percent to 65 percent of the infants referred to the intensive care units could be admitted. The severity of the conditions of the referred newborns demonstrates two important facts. One is that referring physicians in England have much the same clinical standards as do their colleagues in the United States. The other is that the English system does not uniformly support these standards. Of infants admitted between November 1979 and May 1980, over half weighed between 1,500 and 1,001 grams; nearly one-quarter (21 percent) weighed 1,000 grams or less. The clinical differences between the admitted newborns (246) and those rejected (152) were not great. The mean birth weight of the admitted infants was 1,742 plus or minus 808 grams, of those refused, 1,776 plus or minus 780 grams. Thus, clinical condition was not correlated with admission.

This referral trend, combined with service limits, was made clear to us on our visits to one of the Thames regional units, two of the intermediate nurseries, and another regional unit serving Oxford and environs.

At the Thames teaching hospital unit offering care comparable to that available in United States Level III nurseries, practitioners were both optimistic about the prognosis for very premature infants and dismayed at the number of refusals they had to make because their twenty-five–bed unit could not accommodate all referrals. Their interest in improving survival rates for low birth weight newborns was publicized by a chart on the staff lounge bulletin board that read "Congratulations to All" and then presented the 1977 and 1978 outcome statistics for infants born weighing 1,500 grams or less. In 1977, eighteen infants weighing 500 to 1,000 grams were admitted and 33 percent (six) survived. In 1978, fifteen infants in this birth weight category were admitted and 60 percent (nine) survived. Small numbers of cases and good survival statistics characterized the group of infants weighing 1,001 to 1,500 grams: thirty of thirty-five admitted in 1977 survived and forty-seven of fifty-five survived in 1978.

Despite their commitment to such expensive experimental efforts, practitioners at this nursery talked freely about the costs of special care and the problems of scarce resources. Commenting on one premature infant finally admitted to the unit, the head physician said, "We had to refuse her three times, but this is a problem of resources we live with every day." He went on to describe how physicians do not influence admissions policy, only the norms for treating the admitted patients. In truth, the willingness of neonatologists to treat extremely premature newborns does influence referrals, but not necessarily how many infants are admitted.

At the hospital serving the Oxford region, the shift from treating large numbers of full-term infants to a new emphasis on premature infants is illustrated in Figure 10.1, which shows the case selection,

Inborn and referred admissions to S.C.B.U.

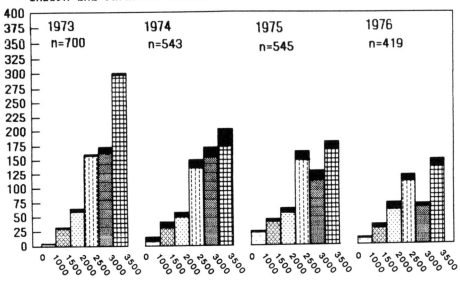

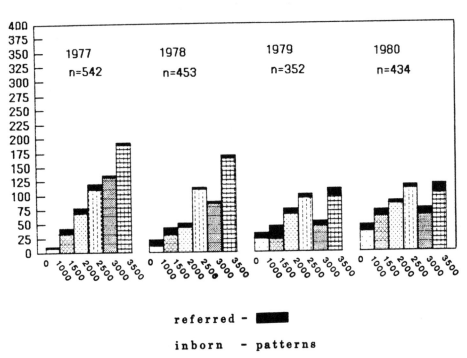

referred - ■

inborn - patterns

Figure 10.1. Central hospital and local referred admissions to special care nursery by birth weight, 1973 to 1980.

by birth weight, from 1973 to 1980. Two-thirds of the patients in this SCBU used to weight more than 3,000 grams; today, less than one-quarter are in that category. With approximately thirty beds, a dozen or so at the maximum treatment level, practitioners in this unit have experienced a tremendous rise in the percentage of infants weighing less than 1,500 grams referred from the community and from within the hospital. The increased tendency for in utero (pre-birth) transfers and the early hospitalization of high-risk pregnant women were the explanations offered for this change; infants who might have died at local hospitals now become patients at this kind of center. The same trend was noted by Gamsu (1983) for the Thames regions.

As in the United States, one of the results of this changing case selection is the presence of difficult long-term patients like Darlene Bourne. In 1983, for example, the Oxford area unit admitted a 730-gram infant born by emergency cesarean at an estimated gestational age of thirty-one weeks. After seven and one-half months of treatment, the infant died in the nursery of bronchopulmonary dysplasia, heart problems, and infection.

Another infant born weighing 2,570 grams at an estimated gestational age of forty-one weeks had trisomy 18 syndrome and tetralogy of Fallot (a combination of heart defects). This infant died at eight and one-half weeks, but not in the unit. Helen House, a new institution for terminally ill children, accepted the infant and counseled the grieving parents. In an interview, the physician at Helen House doubted the appropriateness of accepting similar cases in the future since the institution was intended to help parents whose children required years of care at home and who had no place to board them for temporary stays. Created by private donations, Helen House and institutions like it speak to family needs not addressed by the state.

While concerned with parents' perspectives and interested in follow-up studies, the senior physicians we interviewed maintained their authority over the process of treatment decision making. After stating that the staff was heavily influenced by what parents wanted, one London SCBU physician went into further detail:

> *Physician:* "We don't involve parents in the decision to turn the ventilator off, but we would take their views into account. We would sound them out. They may say, 'You won't give up' or 'You won't be unkind and go too long.' On whether to withdraw life support, doctors decide."
>
> *Researcher:* "If the doctors treat but the parents want less, what do you do?"

Physician: "Never happens. We talk and we come to a consensus with parents."

Meanwhile, SCBU pediatricians continue to pursue the low birth weight frontier. At morning rounds at the Oxford unit, one resident listed a series of vital signs, describing each as "normal" for a 640-gram patient. Countered another resident, "How do we know what's normal for a baby like this? We've never seen any to speak of." This same resident, however, when later asked about her reactions to treating such small infants, remarked resignedly, "Well, we have the technology, don't we? So the best we can do is manage cases for optimal outcome."

Referring to an infant patient born weighing 720 grams, a resident at a Thames region SCBU expressed the commonly espoused resolution of the treatment dilemma:

I've gone full circle from thinking you only help perfect babies. Now I believe you should intervene at birth in almost all cases. The decisions I feel most badly about are cases where I did not intervene and where the baby survived anyway—cases where you hope the baby will die, but the baby doesn't. Because by not intervening then you lessen the baby's chances. So now I think it's better to intervene at birth and then you have more time to assess what you're doing.

Welfare, Health, and Public Attitudes

Prenatal care under the National Health Service is universally available and used by practically all expectant mothers. The service relies on general practitioners and midwives, including those who make home visits. Unlike in the United States, a pregnant woman need not be treated by a specialist, because hospitals staffed by general practitioners are approved for childbirth. Yet there is a marked trend toward the increased use of obstetricians on the institutional level, in the hospitals where they work as consultants. Similar to the trend in the United States, more births in England are taking place under the supervision of obstetricians than of general practitioners. In 1969, the rate for births handled by obstetricians in England was 69.3 percent; in 1980, the rate was 93.4 percent, with a corresponding decrease in births supervised by general practitioners (MacFarlane and Mugford, 1984:157).

On the subject of treating critically ill newborns, the British public and physicians have defended the rights of parents. For example, public controversy over the treatment of defective newborns (akin to the Infant Doe controversy in the United States) broke earlier in Great Britain than in the United States and there was more support for physicians' and parents' discretion than for governmental intervention. At the instigation of an antiabortion pressure group, Life, pediatrician Leonard Arthur was prosecuted for nontreatment of a severely compromised infant with Down's syndrome. The case was eventually thrown out of court, but not before mobilizing public opinion. In a series of polls, the British proved strongly in favor of letting physicians and parents decide the infant's fate. As a BBC-commissioned poll showed:

> By a margin of 12 to 1 the public believes that the doctor who sees to it that a severely handicapped baby dies, with the agreement of the parents, should not be found guilty of murder. (Simms, 1983:2)

The public and physicians also supported the discontinuation of care for severely handicapped newborns. Dr. John Lorber, whose clinical criteria for treating spina bifida infants were sharply rejected in the United States (Weir, 1984:67–70), and his colleague Dr. S. A. W. Salfield stated:

> There will always be some who object to selection on the grounds that life should be saved at all costs, even if the result is a life of suffering and severe handicaps for the patient and his family. We strongly disagree with this view, as does the predominant opinion of our society and the medical profession. (1981:830)

Similarly, interviews with the parents of handicapped children have shown a great deal of ambivalence about the burden of care, especially from the mothers of older children (Shepperdson, 1983). The findings of parent interviews done by the National Children's Bureau revealed a similar problem:

> The main burden of care falls on the mother. Otherwise the father is the chief source of help, but most are necessarily unavailable when some help is needed and few provide a high level of assistance in child care tasks or with housework. A few siblings help substantially but relatives, friends and neighbors give much less help, and this is mainly confined to baby-sitting or shopping. Practical help with child-care or domestic tasks from social service departments is virtually non-existent. (Simms, 1983:4)

There is tension generated by the continuing efforts of Life and other antiabortion groups. These groups drafted the Disabled Children Bill in 1981 to make withholding treatment from any newborn a legal offense, and they have persisted in their efforts to have the bill introduced in Parliament. As Aaron and Schwartz (1984) commented in their analysis of National Health Service policies, some causes evoke a tremendous emotional response from the public and thereby gain extra support. The treatment of seriously ill newborns offers a powerful incentive for private donations, which hospitals have received, and such sentiment could pave the way for increased government and area council support for increased public investment in SCBUs.

THE NETHERLANDS: DECENTRALIZATION AND PREVENTION IN HEALTH CARE

The Netherlands is an anomaly among industrialized nations because of the proportion of home births maintained in post-World War II years. Between 1961 and 1974, for example, in the United Kingdom, the percentage of home births moved from 33 percent to less than 5 percent. Home births in the Netherlands have declined at a much slower rate, from 70 percent in 1961 to 35 percent in 1988. Often idealized by home birth advocates, the Dutch boast one of the lowest infant mortality rates in the world (6.4 per 1,000) and an equally impressive perinatal mortality rate (10 per 1,000), in comparison with the United States, England, and other nations.

The social and economic conditions as well as health care policies underlying these Dutch health statistics are not easily duplicated elsewhere. Poverty, which is strongly associated with prematurity and infant death, has been virtually eliminated. Guest worker populations from less developed parts of Europe and the Third World countries account for only 6 percent of the nation's births, less than one-half the estimated percentage in the United Kingdom. A relatively healthy though not completely untroubled economy supports social welfare programs to protect economically disadvantaged individuals and families by means of income guarantees. Reports of the malnutrition and poor housing typical of England (Townsend, 1979) appear to be nonexistent in the Netherlands.

The Netherlands' health service system is highly decentralized, relying on sickness funds that are compulsory for 70 percent of the population. The remaining, most affluent 30 percent use voluntary private health insurance. Acting as a planning office, the Ministry of Health advocates primary care, and not just in maternal and infant health care. The strategy is to identify and treat health problems early using a range of workers: dentists, physical therapists, dieticians, home nurses, social workers, and clergy. Baby clinics directed by family practitioners number 2,700. Infant clinics for parent education and child guidance number 2,000. This is for a population of 13.5 million. In contrast, only seven newborn intensive care units are supported and these are in university hospitals.

Prenatal care is available and taken advantage of; the Ministry of Health claims 100 percent participation by mothers by their third month of pregnancy (Phaff, 1979). Abortion and contraception are also freely available.

Two-thirds of the Dutch people belong to Cross organizations funded by the membership and subsidized by the government. These organizations offer parenting and prenatal classes as well as the services of maternity nurses, full- or part-time, to help with household chores and the new infant. More than 60 percent of Dutch mothers combine brief hospital stays with home maternity care as a way of managing childbirth.

Expectant mothers have the choice of three childbirth professionals: the midwife, the family physician, or the obstetrician. The Ministry of Health favors selection of the midwife, who is an independent practitioner licensed to supervise prenatal care and delivery without physician supervision. Home birth is the established province of midwives and reimbursement for home birth is total. General practitioners have been retreating from the area of childbirth, presumably because the declining birth rate reduces their opportunities to keep up their skills or because the irregular hours disrupt their practices. Nevertheless, family physicians still offer mothers a childbirth option subject to full reimbursement.

If the reimbursement plan favors the choice of home birth, how is it that so many Dutch women have their babies in hospitals? Referrals of women at high risk for obstetric problems account for about one-half of the in-hospital births. Midwives and family physicians follow a list of more than 100 risk factors to designate women as needing hospital supervision, at times needing early admission for surveillance. The remaining women who have their infants in hospitals choose to do so, paying the equivalent of $50 to $100 for the service.

The choice is not between high-technology childbirth in the hospital and a total withdrawal from hospital resources in home birth. Clinics annexed to hospitals offer low-technology childbirth, with prime emergency access to hospital care. Even major hospitals, by United States standards, are conservative in medical intervention. The cesarean delivery rate in the Netherlands is between 3 percent and 4 percent. Five hundred births per year is the maximum for many hospitals. Also, many women who choose hospital birth leave in a day, suggesting that the option has a risk-hedging appeal unrelated to actual clinical need.

Nor is home birth in the Netherlands a complete withdrawal from hospital care. Government investment in transportation, good roads, and the densely populated and urban character of the country enable fast referrals and the transport during labor and immediately after delivery. Maternity homes are another non-hospital option for expectant mothers. These twenty-bed local facilities are run by three or four midwives and, while an 1865 law restricts midwives to natural childbirth methods, maternity homes are well-connected to hospitals.

Professional Competition

Despite the variety of low-technology options, childbirth in the Netherlands is becoming increasingly medicalized, that is, defined more as a pathology than a natural event. In his book on the competition between midwives and physicians, Klinkert (1980) showed that midwives are losing the contest over control of the definition of childbirth to the increasing numbers of obstetricians. Physicians' collegial ties also make a difference in the determination of where women will give birth. Family practitioners have the best access to pregnant women, yet midwives have little contact with these primary care physicians. The family practitioner can also refer a patient directly to a hospital specialist, bypassing the midwife to build up a colleague referral network. Obstetricians and gynecologists are vocal about the improved outcome in hospital births despite the selection for worst cases. Still, home birth statistics have also demonstrated improved survival rates (Fig. 10.2).

Health policy analysts have argued that the Dutch system is characterized by strong incentives for hospitalization (Maynard and Ludbrook, 1981), though until recently obstetric care has been the exception. Now that more women choose hospital birth, the chances for the integration of infants into a referral system for special care also increase. What kind of infant patient, then, is likely to receive hospital care and what professional attitudes direct treatment?

Neonatal Care. The infant likely to be treated in a Dutch special care nursery is the full-term rather than a premature infant (Table 10.1). At the university hospital unit we visited, few of the infants treated weighed less than 2,500 grams. For example, in 1977, only 212 newborns were in that category, of a total of 1,490. In 1978, the figures

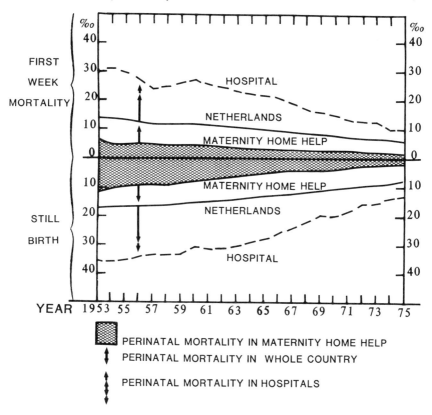

Figure 10.2. Perinatal mortality (per 1,000 live births) by type of maternity care, the Netherlands, 1953 to 1975.

were much the same: 218 of 1,510. The mortality rate for the unit in 1978 was 2.1 percent, in 1977, 2.4 percent.

These figures could indicate either that extremely small newborns are rare or that, when born, they are not brought to the unit. The former seems to be the case. Statistically, the Netherlands has for some time had proportionately fewer premature newborns than either the United States or England, around 4 percent as opposed to the 7 percent to 8 percent prematurity rate common in the United States and England and Wales (MacFarlane and Mugford, 1984:232–46).

In the context of a relatively healthy population, definitions of newborn viability and the clinical frontier obviously change. In 1977, for example, the unit admitted three infants weighing less than 500 grams, following the policy that the nursery is an appropriate place for infants perceived as born dying. As one senior physician later explained:

Table 10.1. The Netherlands—Admissions and deaths in the special care nursery, 1977, 1978, and 1984

Birth weight (grams)	Admissions			Deaths in the neonatal period		
	1977	1978	1984	1977	1978	1984
Less than 500	3			3		
500–990	11	21	47	6	16	19
1,000–1,490	38	43	95	12	7	24
1,500–1,990	53	62	71	6	3	8
2,000–2,490	107	92	86	3	2	6
2,500–2,990	265	293	68	3	2	
3,000–3,490	540	538	74	2	1	
3,500–3,990	351	355	53	1	—	
More than 4,000	122	106	29	—	1	
Total	1490	1510	523	36	32	57

> The delivery room is not a quiet place, so if the baby takes too long to die, we bring it in here. We can put it in a simple isolette and let him die quietly here. Even if the baby is 500 grams and will die within one hour, then we take him here and put him in a quiet place to die.

Twelve beds in this nursery were designated for high-risk cases needing oxygen support and other basic therapies. Twelve to fifteen other beds were also available, but the expectation of the staff was that referred infants would have problems that could be solved quickly and without much technology. When the researcher noted that few infants were on respirators, the physician in charge replied, "One week ago three babies out of eleven were on respirators and that seemed like a lot to us." Along the same lines, surgery, for instance, was not offered; patients with hernias, remediable heart problems, and less grave spina bifida lesions were referred to pediatric surgery. The dilemma of when to treat and how much is not necessarily avoided, even when technological solutions are minimized. One physician told us of two cases that illustrate how difficult making the right decision is:

> Our policy in the delivery room is to try to resuscitate a baby as well as possible, and if he makes no attempt to breathe after forty-five minutes or one hour and his heart rate is not improving, then we think we have the right to stop the resuscitation because the baby will not survive.

> But there was one baby who made no attempt to breathe—the heart rate went down, a borderline case. But he was still living. And the baby survived on his own, only with oxygen [from manual bagging]. By then it was too late to use the respirator. And the question is, would it have

been better if we had used the respirator? The baby is living, is one year old now and can't do anything.

The second infant had an equally grim outcome but for different reasons:

On the the other hand, there was a baby unexpectedly asphyxiated. Seven pounds. He was resuscitated. The color improved so well and the heart improved very well and he tried to breathe. We thought he had a good chance so we put him on the ventilator. The baby seemed to be doing well but he could not wean off the ventilator. At the end of the day, he got convulsions, developed bleeding tendencies. At 8:30, he died.

There is some indication that, as in the United States and England, central hospital pediatricians in the Netherlands are treating more very low birth weight infants (Table 10.1) as special care nurseries select more precisely for critically ill newborns. Yet practitioners in the Netherlands can avoid many of the difficult decisions faced by their colleagues in the United States and in England because the infant population there is healthier.

Relations with Families

The presence of parents, especially mothers, was more strongly felt in this nursery than in those in either the United States or England. This was due partially to the continuity between obstetric and newborn care that brought high-risk women under hospital supervision early and kept them close to their infants after birth. The special care nursery was adjacent to a room with six beds for mothers still hospitalized and was just down the corridor from rooms and a lounge for pregnant women. Mothers with infants in the nursery are generally kept separate from those rooming in with their newborns. The physicians and nurses in this nursery had also initiated an organization for parents that sponsored meetings where "They can tell their frustrations, anxieties, and tell us our limitations and faults."

The expectation was that parents could and should respond to the experience of sickness in their newborn and to the professional care provided. Another assumption was that the sequence of heroic intervention followed by evaluation includes parents, at least informally. Ultimately, the physicians manage the decision to withdraw care. Asked about the withdrawal of ventilator support in difficult cases, one physician recounted:

If even in the fourth week the child is in failure, in that case, we expect the child will not recover, to die. But we do not put that question to the parents. But later on they come to the insight that the child is not recovering at all and they ask us, "Is he getting worse?" Then we say yes. And then they ask, parents may ask, "Will you continue?" Then we say maybe we will have to [stop treatment] because there's no progress. And then they ask about the brain. And then we say we suspect [the prognosis is not good]. From both sides, the parents and staff agree the ventilator will be stopped, especially if the heart rate is slowing down. In the first [acute] period we will not ask if the parents agree. In a later period when there is no hope, we try to let parents reach that point so it doesn't seem [that we are being] cruel, but that it is their own insight.

Again, the infrequency of this kind of decision in the Netherlands is in contrast to trends in the United States and England.

BRAZIL: THIRD WORLD IN TRANSITION

Industrial Transformation

Limited versions of newborn intensive care are found in many less developed countries, despite its high cost and relative inaccessibility to the general population. Brazil offers a special example of a Third World nation that has experienced recent economic expansion simultaneous with an increased availability of medical insurance and hospitals, with resultant expansion of technology in childbirth.

Since the late 1960s, the Brazilian economy has changed from one heavily reliant on exporting a single crop (coffee) to one of state-promoted industrialization. Having successfully attracted foreign capital, the nation has been able to manufacture automobiles and other mechanical and luxury goods for the world market and for a domestic market of industrial workers and the elite.

Although the industrial sector achieved an annual growth rate of 12.2 percent between 1968 and 1974, critics of the "Brazilian Miracle" have pointed to an increasing disparity between rich and poor. Early assessments of Brazil's industrialization reported greater inequalities in income distribution (Fishlow, 1973). Women from the lower classes have been especially marginal to the economic growth, with many rural migrants becoming domestic servants to the newly affluent bourgeoisie.

The negative repercussions of this economic change on health were argued by Wood (1982), who traced an early connection between

rising infant mortality rates and a decline in real wages for industrial workers in São Paulo, the area most affected by industrial
growth. Both economic marginality and the precarious nutritional
status of substantial sectors of the urban population still contribute
to infant mortality, and even worse conditions hold in rural areas.
Widespread malnutrition has been reported in Brazil and linked to
high rates of mortality for children under the age of five. In 1970,
infant mortality rates ranged from 140 per 1,000 in the rural northeast region to 65 per 1,000 in the south (Horn, 1985).

Income Disparity and Unequal Access to Aggressive Care

Income differences in Brazil have a direct influence on who receives
hospital care and of what kind (Elling, 1980). The expansion of social insurance and social assistance plans for workers between 1954
and 1970 fostered the building and upgrading of hospitals for new
patients; a side effect of this change was a turn to hospital births
supervised by obstetricians instead of home births supervised by
midwives (Bastos, 1971). Further expansion in government insurance and in the employer/employee insurance contract called the
convenio allows 80 percent of the population in large urban centers
to have access to hospital care (Enders, 1981). Government coverage
for childbirth is 30 percent less than what the convenio pays and,
with high inflation, the slowness of the government to cover claims
is a hazard for providers. Of course, wealthy private patients suffer
no restraints at all in purchasing services. On the other hand, considerable numbers of Brazilians are classified as indigents and depend on the charity of public clinics and hospitals.

Differential access to acute care technology in reproductive medicine is reflected in the hierarchy of insurance coverage. For example, Janowitz et al. investigated the unusually high rates of cesarean
births in Brazil and observed rates of 25 percent or less for indigent
women, 40 percent for insured patients, and 75 percent for private
patients.

> Since medical conditions do not vary by payment status, they cannot
> dictate differing scheduling practices. It may, therefore, be inferred that
> financial considerations play an important role in encouraging doctors to
> plan more [cesarean sections] among private and convenio patients than
> among other women. (1982a:25)

The Janowitz study, conducted in Rio de Janeiro and Campinas,
suggests that wealthy Brazilians can and do purchase acute care

medicine, presumably with the belief that it represents progress. This differential access to acute care also is observable in services for newborns. The individual woman's coverage (or lack of it) determines the care her infant will receive. Since little transport service is funded, the rural poor are denied access to high-level infant hospital care unless they can overcome barriers of geographic distance. One 1,000-gram newborn in a unit we observed in Brasilia had been carried in by his mother on a public bus from a village 400 kilometers away. Other families used cabs or, if they had a car, drove their infant from one institution to another. Well-to-do families, if at a distance, paid for air transport.

A great diversity exists among hospitals in Brazil, even within the same city. For example, two very different sites visited for this study were within São Paulo, an industrializing city of great socioeconomic diversity. One was a governmentally and religiously funded facility for poor unwed mothers. The other was an elite private hospital. In the first, a living place was often provided for women who were between six and nine months pregnant and who, no longer considered employable as domestic servants, had nowhere to live. The cesarean birth rate at this hospital was about 7 percent, and a physician explained that cesareans were done "only if it is absolutely medically necessary." There were no respirators for newborns, no x-ray machines, and the newborns were put close to each other in small boxes instead of cribs. When we visited, nineteen infants wrapped in receiving blankets had been removed from their boxes and placed in a row on a narrow counter—their blankets touching and their heads almost touching—awaiting examination. Another room had "warm beds," but the cleaning women had opened the window, thus cooling the air. In still another room, several isolettes were available, at times for two unrelated infants to share. Infection and diarrhea were common problems. The support staff was generally unskilled but essential in supervising maternal and infant care. Physicians explained that many women who got pregnant then worked at the hospital. For example, a woman working in a separate room for babies with diarrhea had been at the hospital 15 years; she had had her baby there and then stayed on, learning by doing the work rather than by formal education.

In the private hospital, a large, modern building complete with a gift shop, there were seventy-five cribs available for newborns and the unit followed strict rules about spacing between the cribs. There were about ten isolettes. A pediatrician typically was present at deliveries, sixty-four percent of which were by cesarean section. Sophisticated monitoring equipment along with radiological and surgical resources were available. One baby we observed was scheduled for a cardiac catheterization. Nineteen physicians and forty-five skilled nurses, including one nurse with a university education, served this unit.

Care for sick infants in the government-funded hospital was clearly less than that in the private hospital. Referrals from this hospital to another did occur, but infrequently and only if research goals were satisfied. As a physician in the hospital for the poor described:

> This hospital does not have any respirators. . . . Another hospital has respirators and sometimes we can send a baby there, but not all. At that hospital, the first priority for respirators goes to their own babies. Second priority goes to babies that are interesting research cases.

Regarding surgical referrals, this physician continued, "I have developed informal relationships with a doctor at another hospital and I can send certain surgical cases there."

At another private hospital, in Rio de Janeiro, a small n.i.c.u. virtually replicated Level III criteria in the United States and was well equipped with respirators and incubators manufactured in various countries (United States, Denmark, and Brazil). Two ambulances were available for physicians to transport critically ill infants from other hospitals, provided they were private patients. Trained in the United States, the unit director also lectured in other regions of Brazil and other Latin American countries about implementing this intensive care service.

Despite the differences in resources from one Brazilian hospital to another, the attitude of the physicians in charge was uniformly in favor of doing as much as possible with the available technology. As the director of the unit for private patients in São Paulo stated:

> We resuscitate all—because of ethics—because we don't know the future outcome. We have seen babies survive well.

Present when he made this remark was a pediatrician from the government-funded maternity hospital. She added:

> At my hospital too, we do all we can, even though it is less [because of fewer resources].

When asked if there were some cases that she would not treat, she replied, "No, we are not ready for that."

Various practitioners in Brazil reported a willingness to set limits on treatment, but, as in the United States, these applied only to extreme cases. A physician at a local hospital in the interior of Brazil said:

> About a week ago at my hospital, a baby was born with no eyes, a "nose" up high, and a hole for a mouth. We did not do anything—the baby would not have a good life.

At a central hospital in Brasilia that accepted convenio patients, a baby born with external intestines was being fed but was not expected to survive.

> *Physician:* "We are just feeding it. No antibiotics—[we]will not give antibiotics. The baby will probably die of infection."
> *Researcher:* "Why have you decided not to treat?"
> *Physician:* "There are two problems. The main problem, there is no solution; [we] cannot do the surgery. Also the cost, [it is] too expensive for the family and for the state."
> *Researcher:* "Who made the decision?"
> *Physician:* "The surgeon decided, the doctors decided."

At a unit in Rio de Janeiro, physicians indicated that withdrawal of care was a delicate subject and discussion of such atypical cases was kept within a small, closed medical circle:

> *Researcher:* "Are there some cases you do not treat?"
> *First physician:* "Yes. Maybe we give antibiotics, but we do not resuscitate."
> (The second physician agreed. Both physicians looked over their shoulders as they discussed this.)
> *Researcher:* "I noticed you looked over your shoulders."
> *Second physician:* "When we do it, we do it in a way so no one suspects—so that the nurses do not suspect."

At this point in the transfer of newborn intensive care technology to Brazil, physicians espouse much of the same aggressive intervention goals as their United States counterparts. There is also an elite clientele able to pay for the service directly even when it includes private airplane flights and (as occasionally happens) paying for North American neonatologists to fly to Brazil for consultation. The main external restraint on the expansion of the service is the government health ministry. As a physician in Brasilia explained, newborn care is not a high priority of the government. However, private patients continue to have full access to newborn intensive care, no matter what restrictions apply to patients under other circumstances.

The present unplanned introduction of n.i.c.u. technology into Brazil presents peculiar contrasts. The children of the well-to-do who have access to intensive care are probably least in need of the concentration of resources surrounding them at birth. The prematurity and birth defects of the children of the poor might be better addressed by economic improvements or at least improvements in nutrition, housing, and sanitation. Even when they do survive, the environment works against their living through their first year. The pediatrician at the government maternity hospital commented on this problem as she stood at the bedside of an infant being given special care:

> When he reaches 2,000 grams he will go home and he will die. (She said this matter-of-factly and with an air of finality.) He will die because the infant mortality rate is so high in Brazil.

The physicians interviewed, however, avoided direct reference to social problems and social solutions. In this omission they confirmed Escudero's comments about the diagnosis of diseases rooted in social ills.

> When treating a malnourished patient with diarrhea, a physician is likely to record the latter term and not the former one, usually going to painstaking lengths—which are often irrelevant as far as alternative therapeutic decisions are concerned—of detailing the precise microbial etiology of the diarrhea. . . . An emphasis on the microbial causes of diseases immediately brings forth "technical" solutions for them: health care, sanitation, drugs, hospitals. An emphasis on the malnutrition of patients implies a much more general and structural criticism of societies which allow this to happen while exporting food to industrialized nations. (1980:425)

There is also a hidden agenda in the elite's selection for childbirth technologies. In a country that forbids abortion and tubal ligation and in general discourages contraception, postpartum sterilization nevertheless is a major family planning method (Janowitz et al., 1982). The cesarean delivery can be a means to the end of obtaining the otherwise forbidden surgical sterilization. Women who pay privately or who are privately insured have more postpartum sterilizations than do women insured by the convenio or indigent women.

> As a consequence of the Brazilian policy of allowing easy access to sterilization only for women with a history of cesarean deliveries, most poor, high parity women find it difficult to obtain postpartum sterilizations. (Janowitz et al., 1982b:1982)

A physician at a neonatal unit we visited in Rio de Janeiro noted an unfortunate outcome related to elective cesareans, including those for which the main goal was tubal ligation. He said physicians often did cesareans without properly testing for gestational age, the result being babies with problems such as respiratory distress. In his words, the exceptionally high cesarean rate for private patients was "tragic."

Thus, the three-tiered (indigent, convenio, and private) system of access to high technology in childbirth offers questionable solutions. Major surgery is the most dangerous method of sterilization. The mother's and the infant's clinical childbirth needs may have nothing to do with access to cesareans, and the newborn's clinical needs may have nothing to do with access to intensive care. Finally, public health and prevention would probably be a more cost-effective, practical solution to the problem of infant mortality than technology transferred from industrialized countries.

MAJOR COMPARATIVE ISSUES

As diverse as our three comparative cases are in social context and health policy, newborn intensive care in each setting raises similar problems. In these countries and the others we visited (France, West and East Germany), the dilemma of appropriate intervention on behalf of the critically ill newborn is unavoidable. This is true in the Netherlands, which has generally shunned an experimental approach, and it is true also in England and Brazil. No matter what the level of technology, physicians exercising discretion in emergency childbirth situations will be in a quandary.

The principle of the technologic imperative also seems to apply. Physicians use available resources and, especially in emergency or acute cases, will employ the limits of those resources. Technological buildup, however, does not take place in a vacuum, apart from perceived need. The relative good health of Dutch newborns is consonant with the more modest investment in childbirth technologies there. England and the United States have among the highest prematurity rates among industrialized countries, and their medical specialists have responded with increased armaments. In countries like Brazil, the relationship between medical need and use of medical resources appears reversed. However, if newborn intensive care, like cosmetic surgery and cesarean deliveries, is defined as a luxury item, then the actual need for it becomes moot. In any event, we know that professional perceptions of need can go hand-in-glove with consumer wants, and that both can foster the technologic imperative in newborn intensive care.

The organization of hospital services is another major issue for comparison. Where a woman gives birth determines her infant's patient career. In the United States, with a highly developed referral system, access to maximum sustained newborn intensive care is probably imperfect but it is the best in the world. It carries with it the jeopardy of overtreatment. In England, access is more erratic, though childbirth in a major medical center can ensure a service duplicating a Level III nursery in the United States. The special care nursery in other, smaller, and more rural English hospitals offers much less. In the Netherlands, hospitalization for childbirth and referral to newborn intensive care has a different meaning because the investment in hospital technology and specialist services is much less than in the United States or England; yet it appears to meet infant patients' needs.

Finally, public opinion and its translation into law make a tremendous difference in the license granted practitioners and institutions. Active public debate in England about childbirth technologies—as a feminist issue (Oakley, 1979), as a family support problem, and as a pro-life standard—reflects a state of dissension familiar to Americans. British physicians and nurses feel fewer legal pressures than do their United States counterparts, but the value conflicts— professional autonomy versus public interests, government responsibilities versus family privacy, physicians' authority versus women's rights—remain the same. Underlying the dissension are persisting inequities between the health of the poor and of the upper classes, inequities that neither socialized medicine nor federal programs have successfully overcome.

In contrast, the Netherlands and Brazil appear relatively free from the childbirth technology debate, though for entirely different reasons. Public opinion in Holland is focused less on the moral issues surrounding reproduction and more on the economic problems that a declining birth rate and the aging of the population produce. In addition, the multiple options for birth control and childbirth have allowed women in the Netherlands to exert selective control over when, how, and with whose professional assistance they will give birth. The situation of Brazilian women is markedly different, allowing them little latitude in planning or controlling reproduction. In addition, despite a growing working class, many women having children remain voiceless because they are economically and educationally disadvantaged. Therefore the tension between the interests of medicine, the family, and the state is not publicized.

The main lesson we learn from looking at these three national cases is that newborn intensive care can be integrated into a larger plan for maternal and child health or can exist at considerable remove from long-range programs. In either event, the service at its most developed stands in potential conflict with other health care solutions for newborn pathologies, especially prenatal care. The optimal place for newborn intensive care in the United States health care system is the subject of the next chapter.

11
Policy Recommendations

THE NEED FOR COORDINATED POLICIES

The rapid development of newborn intensive care in the United States attests to strong professional and public confidence in the service. Because the referral of more newborns to intensive care exposes the infants to sophisticated medical technologies, the same policy questions troubling adult medicine now affect neonatology. How is the appropriate and equitable selection of patients best guaranteed? How can treatment be withheld? Who should control the decisions that affect life and death?

The expansion of intensive care for neonates has taken place in the absence of a comprehensive national plan for maternal and infant health. Instead, physicians' belief in the efficacy of emergency intervention has provided the basic initiative for hospitals to support high-technology care for newborns. The base of support has been broadened by government, for example, in the financing of emergency transportation, which enabled the expansion of regional referral systems. Newborn intensive care is now entrenched in dense professional and institutional networks not easily open to change. At the center of each is the Level III nursery. Without specific and uniform policies that take the needs of newborns into account, neonatal intensive care runs the risk of subverting their interests to professional and institutional goals. Infant patients can be inappropriately referred and inappropriately treated, with no malice intended by any individual decision maker but with tremendous negative repercussions for infants, families, and society.

271

No single policy or rule can fully address this complex service. Instead, there are three main realms where decisions are made and within which change can take place. The first is the newborn intensive care unit itself. The second is the administrative province of the hospital. The third is government, which plans and oversees multiple types of health services. In this chapter we present specific recommendations for change in each arena.

Described briefly, these recommendations demand an integrated effort on the part of medical professionals, hospital administrators, and government officials. Where physician authority is paramount, in the n.i.c.u., two changes in clinical practice are recommended. The first is the formal reevaluation of a patient's status soon after admission to the Level III nursery, to avoid routine but unnecessary acute care. Second is the requirement that newborns weighing less than 1,000 or 900 grams at birth be designated as experimental cases and due special protection. In addition, n.i.c.u. physicians, in cooperation with the nursing staff and other trained personnel, should both educate parents about newborn intensive care and better integrate them into the process of deciding the course of medical treatment.

At the hospital level, mainly the major medical center, we recommend hospital review committees for their potential role in educating personnel and improving standards of care in the n.i.c.u. Training programs that give medical students and residents an opportunity to take the long view on maternal and child health are even more important. Obstetric care, neonatal care, and follow-up of infant patients should be integrated service and educational programs. Also, the administrators of major medical centers should encourage research that decreases the uncertainty now surrounding the treatment of high-risk newborns.

As for government policy, any regulation pertaining to the medical treatment of newborns should acknowledge their vulnerability to overtreatment as well as neglect. Regulations to prevent harm to human subjects from the unknown risks of experiments should apply to newborns no less than to other patients. The understanding of this fact at the federal level will make it possible for physicians to make humane decisions in the delivery room and in the intensive care nursery. In addition, government initiative is needed to improve three areas of child health. First is the improvement of prenatal care, both clinical services and education. The second is provision of adequate support for infants who survive with disabilities. Third is the upgrading of research on treatment outcome, so that solid facts support clinical decisions to the greatest extent possible.

If the best interest of the newborn were a program goal of the first order, then a coordinated effort to improve services would be possible. Unfortunately, the obstacles to comprehensive protection of the infant, both those now born and those who will be born, are considerable. After discussing each of these recommendations, we review the disincentives and incentives for constructive change.

THE N.I.C.U.

There are two basic areas of activity within the Level III nursery. One is the clinical evaluation and treatment of infant patients and the other is staff–parent relations.

Clinical Evaluation of Patients

Case Reevaluation. A major problem in the high-level nursery is the automatic, even routine nature of aggressive intervention. Even when an infant is dying, there is little or no provision for evaluating the benefits versus the detriments of continued therapy. An alternative to unremitting heroic intervention is to make reevaluation standard procedure. This can mean resuscitating all critically ill yet viable infants at birth, but allowing a reassessment of the newborn's status after twenty-four to forty-eight hours in the n.i.c.u. This approach was advocated in an early conference on newborn patients, with the understanding that it might lead to cessation of treatment in some cases:

> Thus, it is more ethical, although perhaps more agonizing, to terminate care after a period of time than to withhold resuscitative measures at the moment of birth. This should be an accepted and publicly acknowledged policy in pediatric and obstetric practice. (Jonsen et al., 1975:764)

This innovation would require the staff to reflect about continuing treatment rather than simply having the staff's perception of crises determine discussions about ultimate decisions. Formal reevaluation would also clarify the issue of commitment. If the staff decides to proceed with maximum care for a very low birth weight or defective newborn, then the staff should be consciously committed to the effort. It should also be possible, in instances when a long and difficult patient career is predictable, to fix multiple points of reevaluation of the benefits versus the harm of treatment.

Experimental versus Routine Cases.   In most Level III units, the majority of admitted patients benefit from heroic intervention and are quickly discharged. There are some newborns, however, who, though they are treated in the routine heroic manner that benefits other n.i.c.u. patients, are doubtful candidates for this therapy. A difficult kind of clinical evaluation involves drawing the distinction between routine and experimental cases. This line can never be rigidly fixed as long as we invest in progressive medicine. In addition, there are gradations in clinical status—in birth weight, estimated gestational age, and severity of disease or anomalies—that only the practitioner at bedside can judge. Nonetheless, newborn intensive care is a sufficiently mature service to yield consistent data about the survival and development prospects of certain infants. Infants born weighing less than 900 grams, for example, have uncertain chances for survival or good outcome, no matter how much intensive care they are given. They may even be particularly susceptible to iatrogenic harm. If such infant patients are going to be referred and treated, they should be clearly designated as experimental patients. The same designation should be applied to newborns with syndromes and anomalies also associated with poor chances of clinical success.

The purpose of such a designation is not necessarily to limit referral or treatment but to foster an overt acknowledgment that latent experiments are indeed taking place, sometimes as erratic forays in clinical problem solving. The best protection for newborns in this category is to have their treatment guided by a scientific protocol and to have their parents well advised of the risks of treatment and the chances of death or permanent injury associated with their infant's condition. The storming of the 500-gram barrier to neonatal survival may be an agenda that society and parents accept. However, the option for parents and the public to choose is present only when the experimental nature of the quest is openly communicated. The same is true for the treatment of infants with serious anomalies.

The issue of who chooses medical treatment for the infant or child has long troubled pediatric care. When experimentation is involved, the issue is even more troubled by the problem of who should make crucial life-and-death decisions for another (Curran and Beecher, 1969). Even if it affects relatively few infants, the informal pursuit of medical progress in neonatal intensive care only muddies these waters further, making it difficult, in some instances, to pinpoint who, in the complex bureaucratic organization, is ultimately responsible for harm done.

Staff–Parent Relations

The improvement of staff–parent relations is another way of making the intensive care unit a more protective environment for newborns. We refer here to the extra safeguard afforded when an informed, deeply concerned parent joins the circle of professionals around an infant's isolette. Not all, but the majority of parents are capable of playing this important advocacy role and thereby decreasing the odds that more impersonal forces will determine the course of treatment.

Standard Information. Much more could be done to demystify Level III activities so that parents have a better understanding of clinical and organizational processes. Verbal explanations can be clarified so that families understand their infant's likely career as a patient. To reinforce verbal explanations, parents need visual aids to understand neonatal physiology and pathologies. They also need printed information, in lay language, to take home and read. The use of respirators, monitors, and intravenous feeding is such a predictable part of n.i.c.u. procedures that, again, families could easily be advised by charts and pamphlets. In addition, parents should know about the frequent and routine use of such diagnostic procedures as x-ray films, ultrasound, and blood gas tests.

Just as important as this clinical information is material on the organization of the n.i.c.u. This could be as broad as a description of the general referral system or perinatal program. At the least, parents should be informed about the scope of service the unit offers, the available personnel, and the schedule of shifts and rotations that affect who is in charge of their infant. General information on newborn intensive care is now available in book form for the lay audience (Henig and Fletcher, 1984; Avery and Litwack, 1983), but it could easily be assembled by an individual unit or program.

Mutual Education. How much can patients teach a hospital staff? This question was raised by Strauss et al. (1982) in a study of hospitalized adult patients being taught self-care. The staff's focus on the patients' needs and on techniques ruled out the patient's being able to tell nurses and physicians about the human experience of medical technology. The assumption was that the staff had nothing to learn from patients. In the same way, dialogue with parents can be cancelled out because parents are seen only as a second order of patient. Actually, parents of n.i.c.u. patients have a great deal to teach staff members about the personal experience of infant illness and death. It is precisely this spontaneous response to the condition of n.i.c.u. patients that the Level III staff is at risk of losing. Sharing rather than denying the experience they have in common allows staff members and families (including other offspring) to resolve their inevitably strong reactions to the critical illness and suffering of infants.

Cooperation in staff–patient relations (the "mutuality" described by Strauss et al. [1982]) is enhanced by whatever kind of primary care organization can be effectively instituted for physicians and nurses. Increasing the staff members' sense of personal responsibility toward the individual patient and linking that commitment to the parents' commitment gives the newborn in the intensive care nursery the optimal set of caretakers. The integration of social workers and psychologists into the n.i.c.u. staff–family relationship is difficult to institutionalize, but worth encouraging. The experience and training of those professionals who know the family and community is invaluable, provided the staff is already committed to a broader perspective on patient care.

HOSPITAL ADMINISTRATION

The contemporary hospital combines internal bureaucratic order with the capacity to intersect with other institutions and with the community. Decisions made at the hospital level can add to the protection of the newborn in ways not available to neonatologists in the n.i.c.u. These options include review committees, the management of service programs, and the establishment of research directives, each of which can broaden the perspective on infant health.

The Hospital Review Committee

The hospital review committee has been widely approved as a guarantee that difficult infant cases will receive an equitable hearing. The report of the President's Commission for the Study of Ethical Problems in Medicine and Biomedical and Behavioral Research recommended the committee forum as a better solution than taking cases to court (1983:165). Weir (1984:268–71) recommended a committee specifically for the n.i.c.u. as a source of appeal for parents or attending physicians unable to reach agreement about treatment for the newborn. The idea that the committee can act effectively as a proxy on behalf of a hospitalized infant also appealed to the professional groups and lobbies opposed to the Baby Doe regulations. The compromise position of the federal government has been to advocate governmental intervention in clinical decisions less stridently and to encourage the formation of Infant Care Review Committees. At the request of Congress, the Department of Health and Human Services described the model committee in detail in the December 15, 1984, regulations. This committee would have the authority to override parents' or physicians' decisions and make its own judgment on behalf of the infant patient.

This decision-making role may not be the most effective part that a hospital or n.i.c.u. committee could play. According to a study presented in the Commission's report (Youngner et al., 1983) and to a survey done by the American Academy of Pediatrics (1984), few hospitals currently maintain committees with formal prognostic functions. More than half of the hospitals with special care pediatric units surveyed by the Academy reported having review committees, but these had multiple functions and varying degrees of activity.

Actual committee intervention in clinical case decisions was rare, indicating some respect accorded the current processes for resolving conflict. For instance, the easy access of the unit staff to custody orders can make committee review unnecessary. Nor is there any suggestion that committee intervention actually improved protection of any infant's interests. As the Youngner study describes review committees, they serve best as a means for physicians, nurses, social workers, and other hospital employees to clarify ethical issues, gain legal protection, shape hospital policies, and air professional disagreements. The committee chairpersons themselves saw their groups as less than effective in increasing patients' and families' abilities to influence decisions, yet very effective in educating professionals about issues relevant to life support decisions (1983:447–48). Even if Infant Care Review Committees should become widespread, there is no particular assurance that such groups would do more than represent the interests of the hospital at large, rather than act as impartial advocates for the child.

Given this bias, hospital review committees could be an effective means to the end of standardizing policy concerning the treatment of newborns and relations with families. Defining the goals of such policy should depend, however, more on hospital leadership than on committee deliberations, a process not necessarily productive of wise conclusions.

Service Programs

Major teaching hospitals in the United States have the capacity to modify existing services. The creation of Level III nurseries is a case in point. Central hospitals can also create new programs, even across institutional boundaries and in conjunction with communities. It has been possible, for example, for pediatric and general hospitals to sponsor perinatal programs that combine the resources of both institutions. By the same token, hospital administrators could address several problems noted in our study.

Continuity of Care.   The lack of continous care for newborns in the Level III nursery is, for most patients and parents, a minor problem. But there are instances, such as in the case of Darlene Bourne or of Andrew Stinson (Stinson and Stinson, 1979, 1983), when individuals suffer because of a turnover in personnel. The solutions to this problem depend primarily on how residents are integrated into the n.i.c.u. team. The overuse of pediatric residents in newborn intensive care has been a source of professional concern (American Academy of Pediatrics, 1980). The unit's need for physicians also necessitates that it accept pediatric training responsibilities potentially at odds with the well-being of patients. This is an old dilemma in the teaching hospital, but the special size and fragility of premature and other infant patients sharpens the conflict.

One solution is to structure an apprenticeship for first-year residents to familiarize them with the pace and tasks of the n.i.c.u. without demanding that they take solo responsibility for patients. This is already done while educating nurses in Level III nurseries. The effort would entail a separate effort on the part of neonatology fellows or attending physicians. A compatible approach is the extension of house officer service rotations, which are limited to second- and third-year residents. Still another partial solution is the upgrading of nurses' status so that staff members who serve continuously and take a holistic approach to patient care can assume more clinical responsibilities. Another solution would be the early designation of an attending physician to assume primary responsibility for difficult borderline cases. A comprehensive solution to the problem of discontinuous care will require hospital administrators' assessing teaching versus clinical responsibilities as they are expressed in both residency and nurse training programs in the n.i.c.u.

Interhospital and Community Programs.   The growth of the referral system on which newborn intensive care relies demonstrates the important capacity of the central hospital to organize cooperative behavior among professionals. Even without interhospital programs, perinatal programs requiring close cooperation of pediatricians and obstetricians have developed in large general hospitals. The centralization of obstetric services along with neonatal intensive care (McCormick, Shapiro, and Starfield, 1985) has facilitated this kind of cross-specialty effort. Much needs to be done, however, to create less ambivalent professional relations between neonatologists and obstetricians. Competition between the two specialties is probably inevitable, especially as neonatology increasingly concerns itself with fetal development. Still, hospital administrators can foster active communication and cooperation in high-risk cases that would improve accountability in treatment. Obstetricians should know firsthand how infant patients fare. In the same way, neonatologists should envision the newborn in the context of the mother's health, not only to better understand the causes of specific clinical problems but to humanize their perspective on the infant patient.

Beyond the major hospital, in the regionalized referral network, the central hospital can play an important role in outreach programs. Many major hospitals already sponsor continuing education courses. A more effective approach is the targeting of hospitals in the referral network so that physicians and nurses in more local communities become familiar with proper delivery room procedures for high-risk newborns. The communication of clinical standards for referral is another important task for which not only the Level III nursery physicians but hospital administrators should take responsibility.

Perhaps the greatest breadth the major hospitals can give to newborn intensive care is in residency programs that combine pediatric and obstetric experience. Two hospitals we visited sent residents to local clinics where both prenatal care and pediatric follow-up were given. This put the activity of the Level III nursery in the broader context of which it is a part. Perinatal programs in major hospitals do not necessarily emphasize prenatal care, but address only the time spent in the hospital.

Finally, when hospitals are forced to come to terms with the untreatable nature of some newborn pathologies, the infant and pediatric hospice may prove a humane and practical solution. As Silverman (1982) has argued, the hospice, as a place where natural death can take place, has served adult patients and can serve infant patients and their families as well. This service can be independent of a hospital or linked to intensive care. In either event, the best palliative care should be given the dying infant out of the context of the n.i.c.u. where the emergency rescue mandate preoccupies the staff.

Follow-up Clinics.   Follow-up care and evaluation for infants who have been n.i.c.u. patients varies from nonexistent to exemplary. Based on their experience at the Meyer Center for Pediatric Development at Baylor College in Houston, Desmond, Vorderman, and Salinas (1980) emphasize that the early course of the postintensive care infant is rarely smooth. Parents who were relieved that their infants survived often face months of adjusting to the special needs, including recurring eating and lung problems, of their infants. For the minority of parents with permanently disabled infants, special medical problems evolve into long-term and usually stressful responsibilities.

The narrow time perspective of the Level III nursery precludes consideration of these consequences, yet decisions made in the unit can create long-term needs. An important role the hospital can play is in the provision of clinical follow-up services. As we noted, at Northeast Pediatric, the follow-up clinic was on a volunteer basis, which is not a recommended arrangement if the service is to be professionally valued. In addition, there is the understandable tendency for neonatologists to perceive former patients selectively, that is, to emphasize clinical victories over partial successes. The model follow-up clinic should be independent of the n.i.c.u. but a vigorous educator (via written reports, seminars, and rounds) of n.i.c.u. physicians about the repercussions of aggressive intervention.

Research Directions.   Massive research investments have already been made in reproductive medicine, perinatology, and neonatology. The most prudent at present would be in the follow-up evaluation of former n.i.c.u. patients. Progress in newborn intensive care must be based on more than just survival statistics. As Murphy, Nichter, and Liden (1982) pointed out, there are many problems inherent in this kind of research: finding subjects, selecting samples from the population, accurately assessing infant and child development, and sorting out the antecedents of specific medical problems. Even so, the measurement of major problems—cerebral palsy, hydrocephalus, mental disability, blindness, and deafness—has been possible in the past. The need now is to keep follow-up evaluation at a pace commensurate with clinical innovation or to limit experimentation.

The growing use of computers, especially in regionalized programs, suggests new ways of researching treatment outcome and the efficiency of services. The accurate collection and interpretation of hospital data will depend, however, on collaboration among investigators to standardize scientific protocols in line with sophisticated epidemiologic techniques.

THE GOVERNMENT OVERVIEW

There are several specific points at which government policy influences newborn intensive care. Regulatory control is one, funding research is another, and third is the support of health and medical services.

Regulations

Despite extensive legal and congressional action, the Baby Doe rule may prove to have no effect on newborn patient care other than its symbolic value for the physicians, hospital administrators, antiabortion groups, and advocates for the disabled who influenced its phrasing (Murray, 1985). On the other hand, the exclusive emphasis of the regulation on medical neglect, while ignoring the dangers of overtreatment in the n.i.c.u., is an important legal interpretation of physicians' and parents' responsibilities toward the newborn patient. The withholding of care is permissible only when an infant is unambiguously beyond medical care. Neonatologists who want to reflect on permanent, serious neurological compromise in the newborn who is not dying should not, according to this rule, let such considerations affect treatment decisions. The closed world of the Level III nursery may permit greater discretion than the rule allows. But we should remember that neonatologists are more a part of the corporate institutional structure than are private practitioners. That structure will protect n.i.c.u. physicians from liability up to a certain point. Yet it demands bureaucratic accountability, including adherence to a regulation that potentially affects governmental support of hospital services. A balanced approach to regulatory control would appreciate that appropriate care of the newborn patient avoids the dangers of overtreatment as well as of undertreatment.

The general applicability of government regulations gives them importance. When they fail to address the ordinary activities that threaten, in this instance, individual patients' rights, then regulations tend to lose their protective power. With the Baby Doe controversy, the medical neglect of some infants, especially those with

Down's syndrome or spina bifida, has been designated as a problem. This is in part because of the great change in public attitudes toward the mentally and physically disabled. It is also partly due to special and perhaps increased sentimental investment in infants. Nonetheless, balanced regulatory control would take into account the dangers of overtreating newborns and caution practitioners and hospital administrators against this more common jeopardy.

Going beyond simply recognizing the vulnerability of the newborn patient to overtreatment would entail acknowledgment that certain infant patients are protected by human subjects research regulations. Infant patients and their parents are entitled to an initiative on the part of the federal government to prevent undue risks in medical treatment and to promote physicians' fully advising parents of the benefits and deficits of treatment. Most physicians are probably generally aware of the ethical issues in human subjects research (Barber et al., 1973), but many physicians involved in newborn intensive care rely on informal clinical problem solving, an approach that masks the experimental nature of some case decisions. If the federal government has the power to raise professional and public consciousness of potential medical neglect of newborns, it also has the power to promote informed consent and caution in experimentation.

Costs and Program Choices

Prenatal Care.   The government has a unique responsibility in planning how health care dollars are spent. A major choice is between implicit and explicit rationing, that is, the limiting of resources, or the reallocation of resources (Mechanic, 1979). With limited resources, physicians have to define priorities in treating and to distinguish between services that might appear necessary for a given patient. The newborn intensive care unit may be the most difficult environment in which to make those decisions. For a better guarantee of equity, governmental decisions regarding the allocation of support among different levels of medical care are in order, especially when there are preventive as well as emergency solutions for the same health problem.

Concern about the cost of newborn intensive care is largely limited to immediate and long-term expenses for very premature infants in the birth weight range (less than 900 grams) that we call experimental. There are other, full-term infants whose long-term prognosis is predictably grim and costly, often due to asphyxia, infection, or accidents at birth. In any effort to reduce the costs of care, the prevention of neonatal problems appears to be the most reasonable strategy. In terms of the emotional experience of pregnancy and childbirth, it is hard to imagine a more difficult course than a complete lack of prenatal counseling, ending in a difficult delivery, premature birth, and the infant's death or serious disabilities. This is the worst-case scenario we should plan to prevent.

The top priority should be universal access to good prenatal care, a goal which other industrialized nations have been much more successful in achieving than the United States. Lack of effort is not the reason; the lack of coordination between federal and state programs is. The Institute of Medicine Report *Preventing Low Birthweight* (1985:30) cites "the nation's patchwork, nonsystematic approach to making prenatal services available to those who need them." The report recommends a consolidation of governmental effort and goes on to describe the importance of early pregnancy care and risk assessment to increase the likelihood of full-term births. The importance of a public information campaign targeted at high-risk mothers (teenagers, smokers, and the economically disadvantaged) is also crucial in improving participation in programs and generally informing women about self-care in pregnancy. Even among full-term newborns, prenatal management can also reduce the incidence of death and serious injury (Philips et al., 1984).

This kind of allocation choice requires a societal understanding of the value of prevention in health programs. As Victor Fuchs commented:

> If society believes that some of the resources going to intensive newborn care could be more fruitfully used, say, to prevent high-risk births or to vaccinate preschool children, society must make the difficult choice. If it is left to the individual physician or parent at the time of crisis, further escalation of costs is inevitable. (1983:49)

A greater investment of funds in the prevention of premature birth should be complemented by the leadership of concerned physicians who have the status and expertise to influence public opinion and instruct other professionals.

Services for the Disabled

As long as society is willing to support newborn intensive care and there is the probability that some infant survivors will be disabled mentally or physically, then society also incurs the obligation that these children receive the necessary services to make their lives as rewarding as they can be. Parents and families should not bear this burden alone, especially when government regulation encourages aggressive intervention even in experimental newborn cases and increases the likelihood that compromised infants will survive. Since prematurity and other newborn problems are more common in very low-income populations, the economic burden of the disabled child is potentially greater for families in these groups. Further, in all classes, the caring responsibilities for sick and handicapped infants are generally assumed by women, whether as single parents or as the partner expected to manage home care.

Research Directions

Governments, state and federal, are in an advantageous position to research the efficacy of both clinical and organizational aspects of newborn intensive care. Neither specific nurseries nor hospitals can claim a disinterested overview of how the last twenty years have affected the general population or how the next twenty might be planned to greater advantage.

At least two national centers, the National Perinatal Epidemiology Center in England and the French National Institute of Health and Medical Research (INSERM) offer models for the central assessment of national and regional programs in maternal and child health, as well as clinical practice. The evaluation of its eight sizable regional perinatal projects by the Robert Wood Johnson Foundation (McCormick, Shapiro, and Starfield, 1985) offers a privately funded model on a national scale, one that has methodological lessons to offer public agencies. Coordinating research among hospitals is complicated by differences ranging from record forms to ethnic variety in the local population. Still, the reliability possible in large-scale, scientific studies is indispensable to the development of treatment standards. It is also indispensable to the modification, if necessary, of hospital services.

DISINCENTIVES TO CHANGE

After reviewing the close association between poverty and illness, Kosa, Zola, and Antonovsky wrote:

> It would be unwise to abandon the dream of ending poverty and wiping out class differences in health, but it would be even more foolish to for-

get about the smaller goals which lie within politically feasible boundaries. (1969:335)

The major problem dealt with in the Level III nursery is prematurity and this is indeed related to poverty. Medicine is a poor solution to social ills, but this has never protected its practitioners from having to deal with the results of social problems. In some instances, as in the organization of physicians against nuclear weapons, members of the profession have used their authority to shape public opinion. Advocacy of prenatal care to lessen rates of premature birth offers obstetricians and pediatricians a unique chance to promote health care policies, which, if they do not change the world, at least could reduce the tragedies of newborn death and disability. As an exclusive approach, acute emergency intervention conservatively sidesteps the causes of prematurity by focusing on medical crises at birth. However, only part of the impetus behind newborn intensive care is this misapplication of medical care. In each of the three policy realms where change is possible, there are serious disincentives to modifying newborn intensive care.

The clinical reevaluation of cases and the categorical distinction between experimental and routine admissions are proposals that n.i.c.u. physicians might understandably resist. Both modifications could improve the appropriate selection and treatment of newborns, but they also could reduce the volume of work and weaken the association of neonatology with progressive medicine. By admitting that there are limits to medical intervention, whether in a bedside reevaluation or in the definition of extremely premature infants as experimental patients, n.i.c.u. physicians would increase the options to withhold care. This action translates easily to fewer admissions and shorter hospital stays. As one neonatologist succinctly remarked in discussing these proposals with us, "It means empty beds."

In addition, the central claim of neonatology to medical advance is the pursuit of the low birth weight frontier as an integral part of n.i.c.u. activities. To require a more scientific approach, including clinical trials and follow-up studies, also requires unit physicians to become rigorous scientific investigators or to admit to their company the researchers whose plans they would have to follow. Whether many Level III nurseries can support this extension of physicians' responsibility or incorporate researchers are open questions. If a Level III nursery admits very low birth weight newborns, its progressive reputation is assured. In contrast, if the unit staff treats only routine cases, say, mildly premature newborns, it verges on an emergency service with no particular advances to contribute to medicine and no special status for its practitioners in major medical centers.

As for the informed participation of parents in the n.i.c.u., no referral service that relies on professional and institutional networks will necessarily founder because family members are not integrated into clinical decision making. Parents have special guardianship responsibilities toward their infants, yet these are and essentially must be held in abeyance while a hospitalized newborn is in mortal danger. Most parents consent to the authority of physicians and the n.i.c.u. team because they want their infants to survive. In these ultimate terms, the work of the unit staff can be exclusively clinical management.

For physicians to take the parents' experience of newborn intensive care more seriously also means their accepting work that is generally undervalued in the hospital context, namely social work. Highly specialized, acute care medicine, like neonatology, is particularly prone to separation from family and social issues in patient care.

These obstacles to constructive change at the unit level are compounded by the interests of major hospitals in competitively maintaining themselves as high-technology, acute care centers. Once the investment is made in a Level III nursery, institutional finances virtually dictate its maximum use. Patients who have short hospital stays and require many diagnostic and therapeutic procedures may ideally suit the hospital budget by paying back on the investment. Many n.i.c.u. patients are in this category. The current integration of obstetric and neonatal services within and between hospitals bespeaks a strategic appreciation of how not only to recruit pregnant women as patients but also to increase the options for newborn referral to intensive care.

Formally categorizing certain newborns as experimental cases, which physicians might well resist, could also have negative repercussions for hospitals. It could, for example, threaten the private and public insurance reimbursements that underwrite hospital services. The justification for coverage relies on a normative sense of what medicine should attempt. In the United States, the boundaries of clinical experiments seldom retract. Some experimental procedures, such as organ transplantation, are judged important even at a time of enormous increases in hospital care costs. But the redefinition of an entire category of patients as experimental implies that their treatment costs should come from a research budget or that they should perhaps not be awarded the priority given to patients with predictably better outcomes. Either way, the stipulation that certain very low birth weight infants are at maximum risk could be used as an effective way to curtail service use and limit insurance coverage, to the possible disadvantage of hospitals and patients.

The fostering of prenatal and newborn follow-up services could produce mixed budgetary results for major medical centers. Just as elite physicians' services can be defined as those most distant from the poor, hospitals, too, have reason to disdain front-line work. Mothers who are socially and economically disadvantaged are most in need of prenatal care. Their reliance on Medicaid and charity make them less desirable as clients than privately insured women, at least in times of reduced public support for health care. Sponsorship of follow-up clinics could be equally undesirable if there were a pronounced selection for publicly funded patients whose coverage might not meet the costs engendered by providing the service.

In the long run, effective prenatal care and education could diminish the need for Level III nurseries, depriving some hospitals of returns on their investments in neonatal technology. In the same way, follow-up research might diminish use of the Level III nursery if clinical outcome failed to justify treatment for certain case types on a general scale. More ambitious research programs could also reveal the duplication of intensive care services by offering a precise answer to the question, how many n.i.c.u.'s does a city or state need? Any retraction of present regionalized systems would decentralize intensive care, so that local hospitals with Level I and II nurseries would keep the infant patients now referred to major medical centers.

At the governmental level, newborn intensive care is essentially the product of deep societal ambivalence concerning human reproduction, death, and poverty. With the highest rate of teenage pregnancies among industrialized nations (Jones et al., 1985), we have left education about pregnancy and childbirth largely to individual initiative, as if there were only private consequences to newborn death and illness. Instead of programs for more healthy pregnancies and sensitivity to the risks of chronic disease and handicaps among children, we have invested instead in the incorporation of the newborn into the framework of adult, disease-oriented hospital services. The present imbalance between the prevention of newborns' problems and the rapid development of childbirth technologies accurately reflects the high value we Americans place on "magic bullet" solutions in medical care, especially for high-risk patients. Neither what happens before emergency acute medical intervention nor what happens after is of compelling interest; in our culture, that is the individual's problem, not the public's.

INCENTIVES TO CHANGE

The incentives for making newborn intensive care a more humane service may be more pragmatic than altruistic. From a professional point of view there is no market advantage in promoting newborn intensive care as miracle medicine. While individual parents may be marginal to the clinical work of the n.i.c.u. staff, the number of families with n.i.c.u. experience is growing annually. Their experiences are multiplied many times over and communicated with increasing frequency in the mass media. This collective testimony, not always positive, forms the basis for public support of newborn intensive care. Distrust of n.i.c.u. physicians is already reflected in the Baby Doe rule and could lead to more stringent controls on the service, to the possible detriment of the many newborns who benefit from it. It is therefore essential for practitioners to be concerned about clinical outcome and the education of parents regarding the limits of medical intervention. As David Mechanic has advised concerning adult medicine:

> Although the medical profession may have contributed to such excessive expectations by exaggerating the effects of medical advances, it is in the interests of both patients and physicians to have the public better informed about the limitations of medical care as well as its benefits. The challenge is to educate the patient without encouraging further distrust of physicians and their work.(1979:13)

In the same way, hospitals must operate as service institutions with clients to satisfy and budgets to balance. Many hospitals currently have to confront new consumer attitudes towards medical care. Prospective parents can pick and choose from among different childbirth alternatives, as the developers of perinatal programs well know. Further, hospital administrators must contend with the strain that even a few long-term borderline cases impose on the institutional allocation of resources. Entire charity funds can be depleted or other services undercut by experimental n.i.c.u. ventures. Those research experiments that potentially benefit infant patients are justifiable. Others have neither moral nor practical merit.

For society at large, newborn intensive care is a practical investment insofar as it effectively saves newborns from both death and serious physical injury. In instances when newborn intensive care systemically prolongs the life of dying infants or fails to prevent increases in the number of seriously impaired children and adults, an assessment of the clinical standards and organization of the service is due.

At the core of these practical incentives should be the well-being of the newborn. Defining what is a good life for another person presumes a weighty authority. With regard to newborns, this authority is exercised daily by society, professionals, and parents. It is in the power of these caregivers to better protect all infants from death, disability, and suffering. That the newborns most in medical need come from the most economically disadvantaged families should warn us that even an efficient hospital service is no cure for social problems. Instead, newborn intensive care should be part of a more general program that promotes better health for women and protects citizens from extreme poverty.

Bibliography

Aaron, Henry J., and William B. Schwartz. 1984. *The painful prescription: Rationing hospital care.* Washington, D.C.: Brookings Institution.

Abbott, Andrew. 1981. Status and status strain in the professions. *American Journal of Sociology* 86:819–835.

Aiken, Linda H. 1983. Nurses. In *Handbook of health, health care, and the health professions.* ed. David Mechanic, 407–431. New York: Free Press.

American Academy of Pediatrics. 1980. Estimates of need and recommendation for personnel in neonatal pediatrics. *Pediatrics* 65:850–853.

———. 1984. Survey on infant care review committees. Presented at the American Academy of Pediatrics Annual Meeting, 18 Sept., Chicago, Illinois. Mimeo.

American Medical Association, Judicial Council. 1982. Opinions of the Judicial Council of the American Medical Association. Chicago: American Medical Association. Mimeo.

Annas, George J. 1983. Baby Doe redux: Doctors as child abusers. *The Hastings Center Report* 13:26–27.

Ariès, Philippe. 1962. *Centuries of childhood: A social history of family life.* Translated from the French by Robert Baldick. New York: Knopf.

Avery, Mary Ellen, and Georgia Litwack. 1983. *Born early.* Boston: Little, Brown.

Barber, Bernard, et al. 1973. *Research on human subjects.* New York: Russell Sage.

Bastos, M.V. 1971. Brazil's multiple social insurance programs and their influence on medical care. *International Journal of Health Services* 1:378–389.

Becker, Howard S., Blanche Geer, Everett C. Hughes, and Anselm L. Strauss. 1961. *Boys in white. Student culture in medical school.* Chicago: University of Chicago Press.

Belknap, Ivan. 1956. *Human problems of a state mental hospital.* New York: McGraw-Hill.

Benfield, D. Gary, Susan A. Leib, and Jeanette Reuter. 1976. Grief response of parents after referral of the critically ill newborn to a regional center. *New England Journal of Medicine* 294:975–978.

Bernstein, Paul. 1980. *Workplace democracy: Its internal dynamics.* New Brunswick, N.J.: Transaction.

Bloom, Samuel W., and Robert N. Wilson 1979. Patient-practitioner relationships. In *Handbook of medical sociology*, ed. Howard E. Freeman, Sol Levine, and Leo G. Reeder, 275–294. Englewood Cliffs, N.J.: Prentice-Hall.

Bogdan, Robert, Mary Alice Brown, and Susan Bannerman Foster. 1982. Be honest but not cruel: Staff/parent communication on a neonatal unit. *Human Organization* 64:10–16.

Bok, Sissela. 1982. *Secrets: On the ethics of concealment and revelation.* New York: Pantheon.

Bosk, Charles. 1979. *Forgive and remember: Managing medical failure.* Chicago: University of Chicago Press.

Boyle, Michael H., et al. 1983. Economic evaluation of neonatal intensive care of very-low-birthweight infants. *New England Journal of Medicine* 308:1330–1337.

Britton, S, P. S. Fitzhardinge, and S. Ashley. 1981. Is intensive care justified for infants weighing less than 801 grams at birth? *Journal of Pediatrics* 99:937–943.

Bucher, Rue, and Joan Stelling. 1977. Becoming professional. Beverly Hills, Ca.: Sage.

Bucher, Rue, and Anselm Strauss. 1961. Professions in process. *American Journal of Sociology* 66:325–334.

Budetti, Peter, et al. 1981. *The implications of cost-effectiveness analysis of medical technology: Case study # 10: The costs and effectiveness of neonatal intensive care.* Washington, D.C.: Office of Technology Assessment, Congress of the United States.

Butler, J. C. 1978. *Regionalized perinatal services.* The Robert Wood Johnson Foundation Special Report No. 2. Princeton, N.J.

Campbell, D.M. 1984. Why do physicians in neonatal care units differ in their admission thresholds? *Social Science and Medicine* 18:365–374.

Cassell, Eric J. 1972. Being and becoming dead. *Social Research* 39:528–542.

———. 1975. Preliminary explorations of thinking in medicine. *Ethics in Science and Medicine* 2:1–12.

Cassem, N.H., and T.P. Hackett. 1972. Sources of tension for the CCU nurse. *American Journal of Nursing* 72:1426–1430.

Chalmers, Iain. 1983. Randomized controlled trials in perinatal medicine. *European Journal of Obstetrics, Gynecology, and Reproductive Biology* 15:300–303.

Cherniss, Cary. 1980. *Professional burnout in human service organizations.* New York: Praeger.

Children's Defense Fund. 1984. *American children in poverty.* Washington, D.C.: Children's Defense Fund.

Childress, James F. 1984. Ensuring care, respect, and fairness for the elderly. *Hastings Center Report* 14:27–31.

Clarke, Thomas A., et al. 1984. Job satisfaction and stress among neonatologists. *Pediatrics* 74:52–57.

Clyman, Ronald I., et al. 1979. What pediatricians say to mothers of sick newborns: An indirect evaluation of the counseling process. *Pediatrics* 63:719–723.

Coser, Rose Laub. 1962. *Life in the ward.* East Lansing, Mich.: Michigan State University.

———. 1979. *Training in ambiguity.* New York: Free Press.

Crane, Diana. 1977. *The sanctity of social life: Physicians' treatment of critically ill patients.* New Brunswick, N.J.: Transaction. First published in 1975, New York: Russell Sage.

Curran, William J., and Henry K. Beecher. 1969. Experimentation in children: A reexamination of legal ethical principles. *Journal of the American Medical Association* 10:77–83.

Daniels, Arlene Kaplan. 1969. The captive professional: Bureaucratic limitations in the practice of military psychiatry. *Journal of Health and Social Behavior* 10:255–265.

Dann, M., et al. 1964. A long-term follow-up study of small premature infants. *Pediatrics* 33:945–955.

Davis, Fred. 1966. Preface. In *The nursing profession: Five sociological essays,* ed. F. Davis, vii–xii. New York: Wiley.

Davitz, L., and J. Davitz. 1975. How do nurses feel when patients suffer? *American Journal of Nursing* 75:1505–1510.

Department of Health and Social Security. 1971. Report of the expert group on special care for babies. DHSS Reports on Public Health and Medical Subjects No. 127 London: Her Majesty's Stationery Office.

Desmond, Murdina, Abbie Vorderman, and Martha Salinas. 1980. The family and premature infant after neonatal intensive care. *Texas Medicine* 76:60–63.

Duff, Raymond S., and Campbell, A.G.M. 1973. Moral and ethical dilemmas in the special-care nursery. *New England Journal of Medicine* 289:890–894.

———. 1976. On deciding the care of severely handicapped or dying persons: With particular reference to infants. *Pediatrics* 57:487–493.

Duxbury, Mitzi, et al. 1984. Head nurse leadership style with staff burnout and job satisfaction in neonatal intensive care units. *Nursing Research* 33:97–101.

Elling, Ray H. 1980. *Cross-national study of health systems: Political economies and health care.* New Brunswick, N.J.: Transaction.

Enders, Wayne T. 1981. Subjective evaluation and utilization of hospitals by low-income urban residents in Porto Allegre, Brazil. *Social Science and Medicine* 15:525–536.

Escudero, José Carlos. 1980. On lies and health statistics: Some Latin American examples. *International Journal of Health Services* 10:421–434.

Fagerhaugh, S., and A. Strauss. 1977. *The politics of pain management: Staff-patient interaction.* Menlo Park, Calif.: Addison-Wesley.

Field, Mark G. 1953. Structured strain in the role of the Soviet physician. *American Journal of Sociology* 58:493–502.

Fishlow, Albert. 1973. Some reflections on post-1964 Brazilian economy. In *Authoritarian Brazil,* ed. A. Stephan, 69–118. New Haven: Yale University Press.

Fitzpatrick, M. Louise. 1977. Nursing. *Signs* 2:818–834.

Fletcher, Joseph. 1972. Indicators of humanhood: A tentative profile of Man. *Hastings Center Report* 2:1–4.

———. 1974. Four indicators of humanhood—The enquiry matures. *Hastings Center Report* 4:4–7.

Fox, Renée C. 1957. Training for uncertainty. In *The student-physician: Introductory studies in the sociology of medical education,* ed. Robert K. Merton, George G. Reader, and Patricia L. Kendall, 207–241. Cambridge: Harvard University Press.

———. 1959. *Experiment perilous.* Glencoe: Free Press.

Fox, Renée C., and Judith P. Swazey. 1974. *The courage to fail: A social view of organ transplants and dialysis.* Chicago: University of Chicago Press.

Frader, Joel E. 1979. Difficulties in providing intensive care. *Pediatrics* 64:10–16.

Freidson, Eliot. 1960. Client control and medical practice. *American Journal of Sociology* 65:374–382.

———. 1970. *Profession of medicine: A study of the sociology of applied knowledge.* New York: Dodd, Mead and Co.

———. 1976. *Doctoring together.* New York: Elsevier North Holland.

Fuchs, Victor R. 1968. The growing demand for medical care. *New England Journal of Medicine* 279:190–195.

———. 1983. *How we live. An economic perspective on Americans from birth to death.* Cambridge: Harvard University Press.

Gamsu, H. R. 1983. Neonatal intensive care in the four Thames regions: Some problems and solutions. In *Neonatal intensive care. A dilemma of resources and needs,* 13–20. London: The Spastics Society.

Glaser, William A. 1966. Nursing leadership and policy: Some cross-national comparisons. In *The nursing profession: Five sociological essays,* ed. F. Davis, 1–59. New York: Wiley.

Glaser, Barney G., and Anselm L. Strauss. 1968. *Time for dying.* Chicago: Aldine.

Ginzberg, Eli, ed. 1977. *Regionalization and health policy.* Washington, D.C.: U.S. Dept. of Health, Education, and Welfare, Public Health Service, Health Resources Administration. DHEW Publication No. [HRA] 77-623.

Goffman, Erving. 1959. *The presentation of self in everyday life.* Garden City, N.Y.: Doubleday.

———. 1961. *Asylums: Essays on the social situation of mental patients and other inmates.* Garden City, N.Y.: Doubleday.

Gribbins, Ronald E., and Richard E. Marshall. 1982. Stress and coping in the NICU staff nurse: Practical implications for change. *Critical Care Medicine* 10:865–867.

———. 1984. Stress and coping strategies of nurse managers in the NICU. *American Journal of Perinatology* 1:268–271.

Guillemin, Jeanne. 1981. Babies by cesarean: Who chooses, who controls? *Hastings Center Report* 11:15–18.

Guillemin, Jeanne Harley, and Lynda Lytle Holmstrom. 1983. Legal cases, government regulations, and clinical realities in newborn intensive care. *American Journal of Perinatology* 1:89–97.

Gustafson, James M. 1973. Mongolism, parental desires, and the right to life. *Perspectives in Biology and Medicine* 16:529–557.

Hack, Maureen, et al. 1980. Changing trends of neonatal and postneonatal deaths in very low-birth-weight infants. *American Journal of Obstetrics and Gynecology* 137:797–800.

Hack, M., A. A. Fanaroff, and I. R. Merkatz. 1979. The low birthweight infant—Evolution of a changing outlook. *New England Journal of Medicine* 301:1162–1165.

Hackel, Alvin. 1978. Regionalization and the Northern California Infant Medical Dispatch Center. Newborn Air Transport. Conference sponsored by Mead Johnson Nutritional Division, 9–10 February, Denver, Colorado. Mimeo.

Hancock, Emily. 1976. Crisis intervention in a newborn nursery intensive care unit. *Social Work in Health Care* 1:421–433.

Henig, Robin N., and Anne B. Fletcher. 1984. *Your premature baby: The complete guide to the premie during that crucial first year.* New York: Ballentine.

Hollender, Marc H. 1958. *The psychology of medical practice.* Philadelphia: W. B. Saunders.

Holmstrom, Lynda Lytle, and Ann Wolbert Burgess. 1983. *The victim of rape: Institutional reactions.* New Brunswick, N.J.: Transaction. First published in 1978, New York: Wiley.

Horn, James J. 1985. Brazil: The health care model of the military modernizers and technocrats. *International Journal of Health Services* 15:47–68.

Hughes, Everett C. 1942. The study of institutions. *Social Forces* 20:14–20.

———. 1951. Mistakes at work. *Canadian Journal of Economics and Political Science* 17:320–327.

———. 1956. The making of a physician: General statement of ideas and problems. *Human Organization* 14:21–25.

———. 1958. Licence and mandate. In *Men and their work.* Glencoe, Ill.: Free Press. 78–89.

———. 1984. Social role and the division of labor. In *The sociological eye: Selected papers.* New Brunswick, N.J.: Transaction. 304–310. First published in 1955, *Bulletin of the Committee on Human Development,* Chicago: University of Chicago Press. 32–38.

Hunter, Rosemary S., et al. 1978. Antecedents of child abuse and neglect in premature infants: A prospective study in a newborn intensive care unit. *Pediatrics* 61:629–635.

Institute of Medicine. 1985. *Preventing low birthweight.* Washington, D.C.: National Academy Press.

Janowitz, Barbara, et al. 1982a. Cesarean section in Brazil. *Social Science and Medicine* 16:19–25.

———. 1982b. Interval sterilizations. *Social Science and Medicine* 16:1979–1983.

Janowitz, Morris. 1960. *The professional soldier.* New York: Free Press.

Jones, E. F., et al., 1985. Teenage pregnancy in developed countries: Determinants and policy implications. *Family Planning Perspectives* 17:53–63.

Jonsen, Albert R., et al. 1975. Critical issues in newborn intensive care: A conference report and policy proposal. *Pediatrics* 55:756–768.

Kanter, Rosabeth Moss. 1977. *Men and women of the corporation.* New York: Basic Books, 1977.

Kitchen, William H., and Laurence J. Murton. 1985. Survival rates of infants with birth weights between 501 and 1,000 g. *American Journal of Diseases of Children* 139:470–471.

Klaus, Marshall H., and Avroy A. Fanaroff. 1979. *Care of the high-risk neonate.* 2d ed. Philadelphia: W. B. Saunders.

Klaus, Marshall, and John H. Kennell. 1976. *Maternal-infant bonding: The impact of early separation or loss on family development.* St. Louis, Mo.: C. V. Mosby.

Klinkert, J.J. 1980. *Midwives and doctors: Past and present of some professions in health care.* Brussels: Alphen.

Kosa, John, Irving Kenneth Zola, and Aaron Antonovsky. 1969. Health and poverty reconsidered. In *Poverty and health. A sociological analysis,* ed. J. Kosa, A. Antonovsky, and I. K. Zola, 319–339. Cambridge: Harvard University Press.

Kramer, Marcia J. 1976. Ethical issues in neonatal intensive care: An economic perspective. In *Ethics of newborn intensive care*, ed. A. R. Jonsen and M. J. Garland, 75–93. San Francisco: Health Policy Program, University of California, San Francisco.

Kumar, S. P., et al. 1980. Follow-up studies of very low birth weight infants (1,250 grams or less) born and treated within a perinatal center. *Pediatrics* 66:438–444.

Leifer, Myra. 1980. *Psychological effects of motherhood. A study of first pregnancy.* New York: Praeger.

Levin, Betty Wolder. 1985. Consensus and controversy in the treatment of catastrophically ill newborns. In *Which Baby Shall Live?* ed. Thomas H. Murray and Arthur L. Caplan, 169–205. Clifton, New Jersey: Humana Press.

Lifton, Robert Jay. 1979. Advocacy and corruption in the healing professions. In *Nourishing the humanistic in medicine*, ed. W.R. Rogers and D. Bernard, 53–72. Pittsburgh: University of Pittsburgh Press.

Light, Donald, Jr. 1975. The sociological calendar: An analytic tool for fieldwork applied to medical and psychiatric training. *American Journal of Sociology* 80:1145–1163.

Lorber, John. 1971. Results of treatment of myelomeningocele. *Developmental Medicine and Child Neurology* 13:279–303.

Lorber, John, and S. A. W. Salfield. 1981. Results of selective treatment of spina bifida cystica. *Archives of Diseases in Childhood* 57:822–830.

Lortie, Dan C. 1958. Anesthesia: From nurse's work to medical specialty. In *Patients, physicians, and illness: Sourcebook in behavioral science and medicine*, ed. E. Gartly Jaco, 405–412. New York: Free Press.

Lubove, Roy. 1965. *The professional altruist: The emergence of social work as a career 1880–1930.* Cambridge: Harvard University Press.

McCormick, Marie C. 1985. The contribution of low birthweight to infant mortality and childhood morbidity. *New England Journal of Medicine* 312:82–90.

McCormick, Marie, Sam Shapiro, and Barbara Starfield. 1985. The regionalization of perinatal services. *Journal of the American Medical Association* 252:799–804.

McCormick, Richard A. 1974. To save or let die: The dilemma of modern medicine. *Journal of the American Medical Association* 229:172–176.

MacFarlane, Alison, and Miranda Mugford. 1984. *Birth counts: Statististics of pregnancy and childbirth.* London: Her Majesty's Stationery Office.

McKinlay, John B. 1982. Towards the proletarianization of physicians. In *Professionals as workers: Mental labor in advanced capitalism*, ed. C. Derber, 37–62. Boston: G. K. Hall.

Marcuse, Herbert. 1982. Some social implications of modern technology. In *The Essential Frankfort School Reader*, ed. A. Arato and E. Gebhardt, 138–182. First published in 1941, *Studies in Philosophy and Social Science* 9:414–439.

Marram, Gwen, et al. 1976. Cost-effectiveness of primary and team nursing. Wakefield, Mass.: Contemporary Publishing.

Marshall, Richard E., and Christine Kasman. 1980. Burnout in the neonatal intensive care unit. *Pediatrics* 65:1161–1165.

Martin, William. 1957. Preferences for types of patients. In *The student physician. Introductory studies in the sociology of medical education*, ed. R. K. Merton, G. Reader, and P. L. Kendall, 189–205. Cambridge: Harvard University Press.

Maynard, Alan, and Anne Ludbrook. 1981. Thirty years of fruitless endeavor? An analysis of government intervention in the health care market. In *Health, Economics, and Health Economics,* ed. J. van der Gaag and M. Perlman, 45–65. New York: North-Holland Publishing.

Mechanic, David. 1979. *Future issues in health care: Social policy and the rationing of medical services.* New York: Free Press.

Melbin, Murray. 1978. Night as frontier. *American Sociological Review* 43:3–22.

Merton, Robert K., and Elinor Barber. 1963. Sociological ambivalence. In *Sociological theory, values, and sociocultural change: Essays in honor of Pitirim A. Sorokin.* ed. E. A. Tiryakian, 91–120. New York: The Free Press.

Merton, Vanessa, Robert K. Merton, and Elinor Barber. 1983. Client ambivalence in professional relationships: The problem of seeking help from strangers. In *New directions in helping.* ed. B. M. DePaulo, A. Nadler, and J.D. Fisher, 13–44. New York: Academic Press.

Millman, Marcia. 1977. *The unkindest cut: Life in the backrooms of medicine.* New York: Morrow Quill.

Mills, C. Wright. 1951. *White Collar.* New York: Oxford University Press.

Moore, Wilbert E., and Melvin M. Tumin. 1949. Some social functions of ignorance. *American Sociological Review* 14:787–795.

Murphy, Catherine P. 1983. Models of the nurse-patient relationship. In *Ethical problems in the nurse-patient relationship.* ed. C. P. Murphy and H. Hunter, 9–24. Boston: Allyn and Bacon.

Murphy, Timothy, Charles A. Nichter, and Craig B. Liden. 1982. Developmental outcome of the high-risk infant: A review of methodological issues. *Seminars in Perinatology* 6:353–364.

Murray, Thomas H. 1985. The final, anticlimatic rule on Baby Doe. *Hastings Center Report* 15:5–9.

Newman, Lucille F. 1980. Parents' perceptions of their low birth weight infants. *Paediatrician* 9:182–190.

Oakley, Ann. 1979. A case of maternity: Paradigms of women as maternity cases. *Signs* 4:44–61.

Parsons, Talcott. 1951. The social system. New York: The Free Press.

Parsons, Talcott, and Robert F. Bales. 1955. *Family, socialization and interaction process.* New York: Free Press.

Parsons, Talcott, and Renée Fox. 1952. Illness, therapy, and the modern urban American family. *Journal of Social Issues* 8:31–44.

Pedroso, Odair P., et al. 1978. São Paulo. In *Health care in big cities,* ed. Leslie H. W. Paine, 194–218. New York: Saint Martin's Press.

Phaff, J. M. L. 1979. The organization of obstetrics in the Netherlands. Geneva: World Health Organization Perinatal Study Group. Mimeo.

Phibbs, C. S., R. L. Williams, and R. H. Phibbs. 1981. Newborn risk factors and cost of newborn intensive care. *Pediatrics* 68:313–321.

Philips, Joseph B. III, et al. 1984. Characteristics, mortality and outcome of higher birthweight infants who require intensive care. *American Journal of Obstetrics and Gynecology* 149:875–879.

Playa, Antonio O., Lucy M. Cohen, and Julian Samora. 1968. Communication between physicians and patients in outpatient clinics: Social and cultural factors. *Milbank Memorial Fund Quarterly* 46:161–213.

President's Commission for the Study of Ethical Problems in Medicine and Biomedical and Behavioral Research. 1983. Seriously ill newborns. In *Decisions to forego life-sustaining treatment: Ethical, medical, and legal issues in treatment decisions.* Washington, D.C.: U.S. Government Printing Office.

Quint, Jeanne C. 1965. Institutionalized practices of informational control. *Psychiatry* 28:119–132.

———. 1966. Awareness of death and the nurse's composure. *Nursing Research* 15:49–55.

Ramsey, Paul. 1970. The patient as person. New Haven: Yale University Press.

———. 1978. *Ethics at the edges of life: Medical and legal intersections.* New Haven: Yale University Press.

Rapoport, Robert N., Rhona Rapoport, and Irving Rosow. 1959. *Community as doctor.* London: Tavistock Publications.

Rhoden, Nancy K., and John D. Arras. 1985. Withholding treatment from Baby Doe: From discrimination to child abuse. *Milbank Memorial Fund Quarterly/Health and Society* 63:18–51.

Robertson, John A., and Norman Fost. 1976. Passive euthanasia of defective newborn infants legal considerations. *Journal of Pediatrics* 88:883–889.

Roemer, Milton I. 1977. *Comparative national policies on health care.* New York: Marcel Dekker.

Rosini, Lawrence A., et al. 1974. Group meetings in a pediatric intensive care unit. *Pediatrics* 53:371–374.

Roth, Julius A. 1963. *Timetables: Structuring the passage of time in hospital treatment and other careers.* Indianapolis, Ind.: The Bobbs-Merrill Co.

Rothschild-Whitt, Joyce. 1979. The collectivist organization. *American Sociological Review* 44:509–527.

Russell, Louise B. 1979. *Technology in hospitals: Medical advances and their diffusion.* Washington, D.C.: The Brookings Institution.

Ryan, George M., Jr. 1975. Towards improving the outcome of pregnancy: Recommendations for the regional development of perinatal health services. *Obstetrics and Gynecology* 46:375–384.

Scheff, Thomas J. 1963. Decision rules, types of error, and their consequences in medical diagnosis. *Behavioral Science* 8:97–107.

Sells, Clifford J., et al. 1983. Mortality in infants discharged from a neonatal intensive care unit. *American Journal of Diseases of Children* 137:44–47.

Shapiro, Sam, et al. 1980. Relevance of correlates of infant deaths for significant morbidity at 1 year of age. *American Journal of Obstetrics and Gynecology* 136:363–373.

———. 1983. Changes in infant morbidity associated with decreases in neonatal mortality. *Pediatrics* 72:408–415.

Shaw, Anthony, Judson G. Randolph, and Barbara Manard. 1977. Ethical issues in pediatric surgery: A national survey of pediatricians and pediatric surgeons. *Pediatrics* 60 (Supplement):588–599.

Shaw, Nancy Stoller. 1974. *Forced labor: Maternity care in the United States.* New York: Pergamon.

Shepperdson, Billie. 1983. Abortion and euthanasia of Down's syndrome children—The parent's view. *Journal of Medical Ethics* 9:152–157.

Sherman, Miriam. 1980. Psychiatry in the neonatal intensive care unit. *Clinics in Perinatology* 7:33–46.

Silverman, William A. 1979. Incubator-baby side shows. *Pediatrics* 64:127–141.

———. 1980. *Retrolental fibroplasia: A modern parable.* New York: Grune and Stratton.

———. 1982. A hospice setting for humane neonatal death. *Pediatrics* 69:239–240.

———. 1985. *Human experimentation: A guided step into the unknown.* New York: Oxford University Press.

Simms, Madeleine. 1983. Severely handicapped infants: A discussion document. *The New Humanist* 98:15–22.

Singleton, Edward B. 1981. Radiologic considerations of intensive care in the premature infant. *Radiology* 140:291–300.

Slater, Philip. 1961. Parental role differentiation. *American Journal of Sociology* 67:296–311.

Smith, David H. 1974. On letting some babies die. *The Hastings Center Report* 4:129–138.

Solnit, Albert, and Mary H. Stark. 1961. Mourning and the birth of a defective child. *Psychoanalytic Study of the Child* 16:523–537.

Sosnowitz, Barbara G. 1984. Managing parents on neonatal intensive care units. *Social Problems.* 31:390–402.

Stahlman, Mildred T. 1984. Newborn intensive care: Success or failure? *Journal of Pediatrics* 105:162–167.

Starr, Paul. 1982. *The social transformation of American medicine.* New York: Basic Books.

Stinson, Robert, and Peggy Stinson. 1979. On the death of a baby. *The Atlantic* 244:64–72.

———. 1983. *The long dying of Baby Andrew.* Boston: Little, Brown.

Strauss, Anselm L. 1966. The structure and ideology of American nursing. In *The nursing profession*, ed. F. Davis, 60–108, New York: Wiley.

———. 1968. The intensive care unit: Its characteristics and social relationships. *Nursing Clinics of North America* 3:7–15.

Strauss, Anselm L, et al. 1982. The work of hospitalized patients. *Social Science and Medicine* 16:977–986.

Sugarman, Muriel. 1979. Toward really improving the outcome of pregnancy: What you can do. *Birth and the Family Journal* 6:109–118.

———. 1981. The psychological aspects of neonatal intensive care: Theoretical and practical considerations. Mimeo.

Szasz, Thomas S., and Marc H. Hollender. 1956. A contribution to the philosophy of medicine: The basic models of the doctor-patient relationship. *A.M.A. Archives of Internal Medicine* 97:585–592.

Thomas, Lewis. 1977. On science and the technology of medicine. In *Doing better and feeling worse*, ed. J. Knowles, *Daedalus* 106:35–42.

Todres, I. David, et al. 1977. Pediatricians' attitudes affecting decision-making in defective newborns. *Pediatrics* 60:197–201.

———. 1986. Physicians' changing attitudes towards newborn patients. *Pediatrics* (in press).

Townsend, Peter. 1979. *Poverty in the United Kingdom: A survey of household resources and standards of living.* London: Penguin.

Tyson, Jon, et al. 1984. Effect of nursing-staff support groups on the quality of newborn intensive care. *Critical Care Medicine* 12:901–906.

Ver Steeg, Donna F., and Croog, Sydney H. 1979. Hospitals and related health care delivery settings. In *Handbook of medical sociology.* ed. Howard E.

Freeman, Sol Levine, and Leo G. Reeder, 308–334. Englewood Cliffs, N.J.: Prentice-Hall.

Walker, Donna-Jean B., et al. 1984. Cost-benefit analysis of neonatal intensive care for infants weighing less than 1,000 grams at birth. *Pediatrics* 74:20–25.

Warner, Kenneth E. 1975. A "desperation-reaction" model of medical diffusion. *Health Services Research* 10:369–383.

Weir, Robert F. 1984. *Selective nontreatment of handicapped newborns: Moral dilemmas in neonatal medicine.* New York: Oxford University Press.

Wertz, Richard W., and Wertz, Dorothy C. 1977. Lying-in: A history of childbirth in America. New York: The Free Press.

Wilson, Ann L. 1978. Neonatal air transport: Its stress on families. Newborn Air Transport. Conference sponsored by Mead Johnson Nutritional Division, 1978 February 9–10, Denver, Colorado. Mimeo.

Wood, Charles H. 1982. The political economy of infant mortality in São Paulo, Brazil. *International Journal of Health Services* 12:215–229.

World Health Organization. 1976. *Health aspects of human rights.* Geneva: World Health Organization.

Wynn, Margaret and Arthur Wynn. 1976. Prevention of handicap of perinatal origin. An introduction to French policy and legislation. London: Foundation for Education and Research in Childbearing.

Youngner, Stuart J., et al. 1983. A national survey of hospital ethics committees. In *Deciding to forego life-sustaining treatment,* 443–457. Washington, D.C.: The President's Commission for the Study of Ethical Problems in Medicine and Biomedical and Behavioral Research.

Zelitzer, Viviana A. 1985. *Pricing the priceless child: The changing value of children.* New York: Basic Books.

Zerubavel, Eviatar. 1979. *Patterns of time in hospital life.* Chicago: University of Chicago Press.

Glossary

ambiguous genitalia   Coexistence of both male and female sexual organs.

amniocentesis   Passage of a needle through the abdominal wall into the uterus to obtain and analyze amniotic fluid.

amniotic fluid   The fluid in which the fetus develops, the physiologic roles of which are protective, nutritive, and excretory.

anencephaly   The congenital absence or severe reduction in size of both cerebral hemispheres of the brain.

anomaly   A congenital or hereditary defect.

anoxia   The reduction or lack of oxygen in body tissue impairing physiologic function; severe degrees of anoxia are associated with neurologic compromise.

Apgar score (Apgars)   A scoring system developed by anesthesiologist Virginia Apgar to assess the newborn's condition (heart rate, respiratory effort, muscle tone, reflex irritability, and color) at one and five minutes after birth. A score of 10 is perfect; 3 or less indicates a severely depressed infant.

apnea   Cessation of breathing.

apneic spell   Period of apnea longer than 20 seconds and/or one accompanied by bradycardia (slow heart beat) and cyanosis (bluish skin color).

arrhythmia   Any departure from the normal heart beat rhythm.

asphyxia   Condition caused by lack of oxygen; if severe, it can result in brain damage.

bag   To assist an infant's breathing by manually pumping a hand-held bag attached to a face mask on the infant.

bilirubin level   A test for the product of the chemical breakdown of old red blood cells; an elevated level indicates infant jaundice.

blood gas test   The measurement of the levels of oxygen and carbon dioxide in an infant's blood. Measurement of the acidity (pH) of the blood is usually included in "blood gases."

blood-urea nitrogen test (BUN)   Test that measures urea levels in serum or plasma; increases in BUN values suggest renal failure or dehydration.

bradycardia   Slowing of the heart beat.

brain bleed   Common expression for intraventricular hemorrhage (IVH), bleeding into the ventricles of the brain.

brain shunt   The surgical implantation of a valve-regulated device to treat hydrocephalus. See *hydrocephalus.*

bronchopulmonary dysplasia (BPD)   Chronic lung disorder occurring in low birth weight infants with severe hyaline membrane disease who required respiratory therapy.

cannula   Tube, e.g., nasal cannula.

cannulate   To insert a cannula.

cardiac massage   Rhythmic manual compression of the heart to restore and maintain circulation.

catheter   Flexible tubular instrument used to withdraw or infuse fluids.

catheterization   Insertion of a catheter, e.g., cardiac catheterization for diagnostic tests.

cesarean delivery   Delivery of an infant by surgical incision through the mother's abdominal and uterine wall.

chest tube   A tube inserted in the chest to remove air or fluid that is between the lung and chest wall and causes compression of the lung. See *pneumothorax.*

chromosomal defect   A defect in the part of the cell nucleus that contains genetic information, i.e., the chromosome, which contains genes.

code   A plan of action for specific medical emergency situations, e.g., a code indicating how long to continue resuscitation efforts or whether to attempt resuscitation. A "no code" means "do not resuscitate."

complete blood count (CBC)   A count of the different types of blood cells and their proportions; used to determine the presence of infection.

computerized axial tomography (CT or CAT scan)   A procedure in which x-ray films taken across several planes of the body are integrated by computer.

continuous positive airway pressure (CPAP)   Respirator pressure applied continuously to an infant's airway while the infant breathes spontaneously.

cortex, cerebral   Surface layer of gray matter on the cerebral hemispheres associated with higher mental, motor, and visceral functions.

cretinism   A condition caused by a lack of thyroid secretion and characterized by stunted mental and physical development.

C-section   See *cesarean delivery.*

deceleration   Decrease in the fetal heart rate in relation to the associated uterine contraction; early, late, and variable decelerations indicate obstetrical complications.

diethylstilbestrol (DES)   Drug given to prevent miscarriages and associated with birth defects in the second generation. A "DES daughter" is the daughter of a mother to whom DES was given during pregnancy.

digoxin ("dig") A preparation of digitalis used to treat heart failure.

"do not resuscitate" order (DNR) See *code*.

Down's syndrome A set of congenital anomalies associated with a chromosomal abnormality, typically trisomy 21.

echo See *ultrasound*.

electroencephalogram (EEG) A measure of the brain's electrical activity.

electrolysis test A measure of the molecules in the blood that carry an electrical charge, such as sodium, potassium, and chloride.

endotracheal tube (ETT) A tube inserted into the trachea and at specific times connected to a respirator.

epinephrine ("epi") Medication consisting of a hormone that, among other effects, raises blood pressure and stimulates the heart.

evoked potentials A neurological test that measures basic brain functioning.

exchange transfusion A transfusion that replaces the blood of an infant, used to treat high bilirubin levels.

extubate To remove the endotracheal tube.

failure to thrive A pronounced lag in infant weight gain and physical development.

fetal alcohol syndrome Syndrome caused by excessive alcholic intake during pregnancy; the infant is undersized and may have various anomalies.

gastrostomy A surgically created opening through the abdominal wall into the stomach that is used for feeding.

gavage Feeding by means of a tube inserted through the nose or mouth and into the stomach of an infant.

gestational age The estimated period of time from fertilization to birth; gestational age is one of the main ways the development of infants is categorized. About 80% of the population is born between 38 and 42 weeks of gestational age.

gram The metric equivalent of 0.035 ounces. Regarding birth weight, the equivalents of some important dividing lines are as follows: 2,500 g = 5.47 lb; 1,500 g = 3.28 lb; 1,000 g = 2.19 lb; 500 g = 1.09 lb.

hemodialysis Cleansing of the blood by means of an artificial kidney machine.

hood, oxygen Plastic shield placed over a baby's head to direct the flow of oxygen.

hyaline membrane disease (HMD) A disease of the immature lung of the premature infant. When the infant exhales, the lungs collapse and are unable to remain aerated. Also known as *respiratory distress syndrome* (RDS).

hydrocephalus Cranial enlargement due to obstruction in the circulation of cerebrospinal fluid.

hyperbilirubinemia Excessively high levels of bilirubin in the blood that cause infant jaundice and can be treated by phototherapy or exchange transfusion. See *bilirubin level*.

hypernatremia, hypernatremic Excessively high level of sodium in the blood.

hypoplasia Incomplete growth of an organ, e.g., hypoplastic lung.

hypothyroidism A severe thyroid condition in infants that can result in cretinism.

hypotonia A condition of diminished muscle tone and resistance.

iatrogenic effect Adverse condition caused by medical intervention either as a side effect of treatment or through an error in judgment.

indomethacin A drug that causes a patent ductus arteriosus to close. See *patent ductus arteriosus.*

induction Medical precipitation of labor. See *pitocin.*

Intralipid A nutritious soybean oil–egg lecithin emulsion that provides necessary fats and calories to the growing infant.

intravenous (IV) Within the vein, e.g., intravenous line, intravenous feeding, intravenous drug administration.

intraventricular hemorrhage (IVH) Bleeding into the ventricle of the brain.

intubation The insertion of a tube into a patient; in the n.i.c.u., it usually refers to the endotracheal tube.

in vitro fertilization Fertilization of the human egg occurring in a test tube or other artificial environment.

Isuprel Trade name for the drug isoproterenol, used to stimulate heart rate and contractions.

kilogram One thousand grams. See *gram.*

LA/Ao, left atrium/aorta ratio A measure used in echocardiography to determine the degree of shunt through a patent ductus arteriosus.

ligation The application of a ligature or tie, e.g., to close a patent ductus arteriosus.

lumbar puncture (LP) See *spinal tap.*

meconium A dark green mucilaginous substance in the intestine of the newborn infant, resulting from a mixture of amniotic fluid and intestinal secretions; its presence in the amniotic fluid at birth may indicate fetal or neonatal complications, e.g., asphyxia or pneumonia. See *persistent fetal circulation.*

meningomyelocele A form of spina bifida characterized by a cystic lesion of the spinal column with a resulting neurological dysfunction. See *spina bifida.*

metabolic acidosis A shift in the normal acid–base status of the body that can affect breathing and circulation.

morbidity Illness in a population, often expressed as a rate.

mortality Death in a population, often expressed as a rate. Specific mortality categories are as follows: (1) perinatal, death rate during the first week of life; (2) neonatal, death rate during the first four weeks of life; (3) infant, death rate during the initial 12 to 14 months of life.

murmur, heart Additional sound generated by the heart that often reflects a heart defect. At times, a murmur may be associated with a normal heart.

necrotizing enterocolitis An inflammation of the gastrointestinal tract that may progress to gangrene of the intestines.

neonate The infant during the first four weeks of life.

parenteral nutrition The intravenous feeding of selected concentrations of nutrients for long-term sustenance.

patent ductus arteriosus (PDA) Aperture in the heart of the premature infant, causing blood to flow from the aorta to the pulmonary artery and resulting in the recirculation of arterial blood through the lungs.

Pavulon Trade name for the muscle relaxant pancuronium; sometimes given to infants who resist mechanical ventilation.

perinatal Refers to the physiologic condition of the mother and fetus in late pregnancy and just after birth.

persistent fetal circulation (PFC) The constriction of pulmonary blood vessels associated with a number of conditions, including the aspiration of meconium by the infant, or occurring spontaneously.

phenylketonuria A genetic defect of metabolism that, when severe, results in mental retardation and neurologic problems.

platelet A disk-shaped blood cell known primarily for its function in blood coagulation.

pneumothorax A spontaneous or traumatic rupture of the lung, with air escaping into the pleural cavity between the lung and chest wall.

preeclampsia A toxic condition of late pregnancy that can result in premature birth.

prematurity The status of the neonate prior to full-term development.

Priscoline Trade name for the drug tolazoline, which relaxes the vascular spasm associated with persistent fetal circulation.

respirator An apparatus used to artificially ventilate an infant's lungs.

respiratory distress syndrome (RDS) See *hyaline membrane disease.*

retrolental fibroplasia (RLF) Damage to the retina of the eye associated with the administration of high levels of oxygen. Low birth weight newborns are especially vulnerable to this condition.

sepsis The presence of pathogenic microorganisms, or their toxins, in the blood or tissue.

spina bifida A major anomaly of the spinal column in which a cystic lesion forms on the infant's back causing paralysis below that point. The condition is due to defective closure of the developing neural tube.

spinal tap The insertion of a needle between the lumbar vertebrae into the spinal canal for the withdrawal of spinal fluid.

toxemia A toxic condition resulting from the body's absorption of bacteria at the site of infection.

trisomy The presence of extra chromosomes; each additional chromosome causes a specific anomalous syndrome, e.g., trisomy 18, trisomy 13, trisomy 21. See also *Down's syndrome.*

trisomy 18   The condition caused by the presence of an extra chromosome 18; characteristics include severe mental retardation and gastrointestinal and renal deformities.

ultrasound   The diagnostic use of extremely high auditory frequencies to visually display sound echos from internal organs.

ventricle   A chamber or cavity in the heart or brain.

Subject Index

Name Index

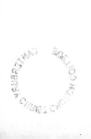